Symbols Summary

gf = gluten-free

GF lines or facility; or
No chance of cross-contamination

Gluten Testing is performed

Gluten-Free based on review of ingredient label
(as no GF list was provided)

Procedures to Mitigate Cross-Contamination are in place,
although there are shared facilities or equipment

Cross-Contamination is possible; or, Made with "gluten-free ingredients" (with no mention of overall status by the company)

For the full key, see page 21 >>

D1449660

Quick Reference Table of Contents

DAIRY & EGGS

BEVERAGES

BAKING AISLE

CONDIMENTS cont'd

**SNACKS &
CONVENIENCE
FOODS**

**BABY FOOD &
FORMULA**

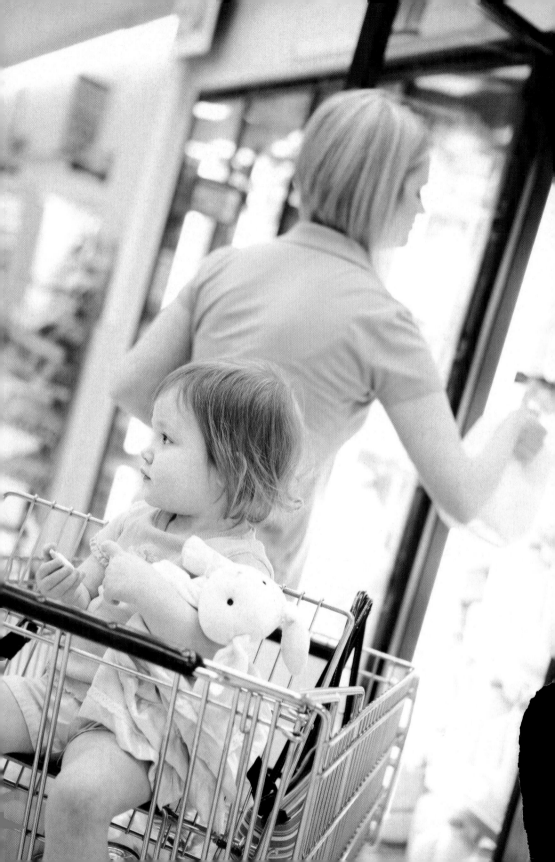

INTRODUCTION

Do me (and yourself) a favor—before you take this guide shopping, sit on your couch and just skim through the listings for a minute.

You will notice something amazing.

There are prepared meals that have gravy on them. Yes, honest-to-goodness rich, creamy gravy that's thickened with cornstarch, not wheat flour. And I know what you're thinking, "great, but it's probably hard to find and expensive." I have good news for you: it's a mainstream brand that I found at my friend's local supermarket in Illinois and here at home in Virginia.

You'll also find cereal—more cereal than ever before. Remember the days when there was just one, lonely cereal box in your pantry? Well, we've finally got the attention of not one, but several cereal companies who've reformulated their products and production lines especially to be gluten-free. Yup, they did it just for us!

Just a couple years ago, the savvy gluten-free shopper wouldn't even take a second look at anything with gravy or teriyaki sauce (which often has wheat). But with all the attention gluten-free has been getting, now, you just never know...

That said, caution is still in order. In our research, we were elated to come across a gluten-free teriyaki sauce from a famous condiments brand. But, we also found out that the marinade version was not gluten-free. They both had similar packaging, and if I were in a rush, I could see myself confusing the two. I mean, I wouldn't expect the sauce version to be safe, but the marinade version not to be.

FREE NEWSLETTER

For product updates, coupons and the latest in gluten-free news, sign up for the free online Triumph Dining newsletter. Just visit this URL to subscribe:

www.triumphdining.com

You can unsubscribe at anytime, and your information will NEVER be sold or shared.

And, for up-to-date info on gluten-free living, check out Triumph's blog here:

www.triumphdining.com/blog

And that's the funny thing about having expectations. Sometimes, they keep us from having an open mind and make us miss the awesome new possibilities out there (hello, gluten-free teriyaki chicken for dinner, yum!). But, they can also help us stay out of trouble (like that nagging thought that prompts me to read labels extra closely when dealing with something that's not normally gluten-free, like teriyaki sauce).

So, while a lot has changed for the gluten-free shopper in the past few years, gluten-free grocery shopping still remains a challenge. Despite advances in the gluten-free marketplace, relatively few products are clearly labeled "gluten-free." Because there's no uniform definition of gluten-free, many companies don't broadcast that they're gluten-free. They'll only tell you if you ask.

But, a typical grocery store carries over 40,000 products. That's a lot of companies to ask! As individual consumers searching for gluten-free products, we're often left guessing in grocery store aisles, or calling dozens of manufacturers on a regular basis. This guide gives us a better way. It's designed to help you save valuable time and money anywhere you shop.

To that end, I hope you'll continue to share any comments, suggestions, or questions you have with me. If there's something we could be doing better, or some help we can provide you, please tell me. Your feedback is very important to us, and I read every e-mail personally. In fact, you'll notice that we added more brands and an index this year. These are improvements we made based on feedback from customers like you. We're listening.

Wishing you a happy, healthy, and gluten-free year,

Ross Cohen

President
Triumph Dining
ross@triumphdining.com

GENERAL TIPS FOR GROCERY SHOPPING

Everyone knows how to grocery shop—we've all been doing it most of our adult lives. The interesting thing is that each person approaches shopping slightly differently. Some people spend hours methodically comparing prices in search of the best deal, and others race through the store as quickly as possible so they can move on to other things. There's no right or wrong way to shop, but what follows are a few basic tips and ideas to help make your gluten-free shopping trips a little more successful—no matter what your personal shopping style is.

Choosing a Grocery Store

Some grocery stores are simply better for the gluten-free shopper than others. Generally, I prefer to do my shopping in stores that cater to gluten-free clientele in some way—it makes my shopping easier, and I prefer to support the businesses that focus on my needs.

A store's focus on gluten-free customers can manifest itself in several ways:

1. Grouping gluten-free goods in one section, like Kroger does;

2. Stocking an extensive selection of gluten-free products—many smaller, specialty stores like Martindale's in Springfield, PA, Against the Grain in Salt Lake City, UT, and Gluten-Free Trading Company in Milwaukee, WI pride themselves on carrying hundreds or thousands of specialty, gluten-free items;

3. Labeling gluten-free foods—either in the grocery aisle like Whole Foods, or on packaging itself; Wegman's in New York marks their gluten-free, private label foods with a little "G";

4. Publishing a list of gluten-free items that can be found in their stores, like the Trader Joe's chains (which is why it's not printed here).

Stores that fit into these categories will tend to have more options for gluten-free customers, resulting in a better shopping experience. Try to frequent these types of stores when you can.

But, we understand that not everyone lives near a Trader Joe's, or can afford to buy all their groceries from premium and specialty stores. That's why this guide is designed to help you find gluten-free options in any grocery store—whether or not it specifically caters to gluten-free customers.

Common Pitfalls to Avoid

One ongoing concern for people on the gluten-free diet is cross-contamination. It can happen anywhere, there's no way to know whether it's happened to a product, and it's rarely ever flagged for us. Also, the Food Allergen Labeling and Consumer Protection Act does not set specific standards for using cross-contamination advisory statements or require manufacturers to identify the possibility of inadvertent cross-contamination. (See the next chapter for a more in-depth discussion of the FALCPA.)

And, concerns about cross-contamination extend beyond grocery store shelves, to bulk bins, deli/meat counters, and the prepared foods sections.

Bulk Bins

Bulk bins are largely left unattended by grocery store personnel. There's often no way to tell that other customers haven't inadvertently shared serving scoops across products, potentially contaminating anything that otherwise would have been gluten-free. And, there's no indication whether products rotate through the bins or, if they do, whether the bins are thoroughly cleaned before transitions. In other words, the bin that holds a seemingly gluten-free product today could have been full of wheat flour last week. For these reasons, we recommend avoiding bulk bins and buying packaged items, instead.

The Deli Counter

Deli counters and prepared food sections present a different challenge. Here, store personnel directly handle food products meant for your consumption. The easiest way to navigate these challenges is to think of the deli counter and prepared food section like "mini restaurants." (For more information about issues to consider in gluten-free restaurant dining, please refer to *The Essential Gluten-Free Restaurant Guide*, also available from Triumph Dining.)

Before you make a purchase, you need to understand both the ingredients in the food and the preparation methods used to create it. There are many issues to consider in making a decision about these foods. Some examples include: Do gluten-containing meats go in the deli slicer?

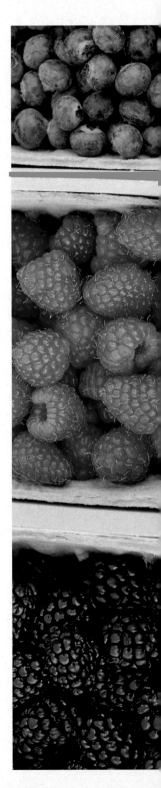

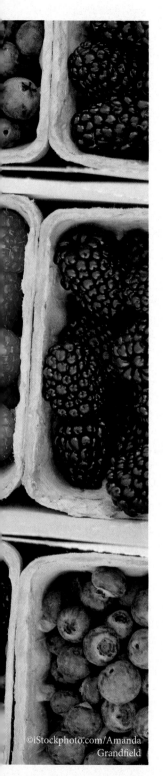

What, if any, precautions are taken in the prep area to avoid cross-contamination? Are there ingredient labels on the prepared foods? How accurate are those labels?

Often times, however, it's challenging to interface with the employees who prepared these foods. At some grocery stores we've seen, the prepared foods are made off-site or by an early morning crew that's long since cleared out by the time the typical person shops, making it hard to get questions answered about dish contents and preparation methods. For these reasons, we recommend frequenting deli counters and prepared food sections only when you've done sufficient due diligence to confirm the products you're purchasing truly are gluten-free.

Selecting Your Groceries

Despite a restricted diet, there are still many wonderful foods for gluten-free shoppers to choose from. When given a choice, I prefer to support the companies that cater to the needs of gluten-free customers. Some of these companies produce specialty products for the gluten-free market. Others have dedicated manufacturing lines and/or carefully test their products for gluten. Please consider buying their products and calling or writing in to let them know you appreciate their efforts. The more we support these businesses, the more products we'll have to choose from in the future.

Consider Your Information Source

When thinking about which products to purchase and evaluating information available to you, please keep in mind that primary source information, like ingredient statements on packages and manufacturer statements, is always better and more reliable than secondary source information, like postings on message boards and compilation lists (this guide included). Think of it like a game of telephone—the more people who handle information before you receive it, or the older that information gets, the greater chance there is of it having inaccuracies or other problems.

Always Read Labels

The goal of this guide is to drastically cut your label-reading time, but the reality is that no product obviates the need for label-reading entirely. Product formulations can change without notice, companies can make mistakes on their gluten-free list, and people compiling information can make mistakes, as well. That's why you need to read labels every time you make a purchase, and regularly contact the company to confirm the gluten-free status of the products you consume.

Never Make Assumptions

When contacting companies, please keep in mind that the FDA has yet to issue a rule defining the term "gluten-free." Meanwhile, there's a lot of conflicting information on the gluten-free diet, even among dieticians, support groups and the many other experts in the field. Some believe that blue cheese is gluten-free, others do not. And, the emerging question about the suitability of oats in the gluten-free diet adds even more confusion. So, don't expect a company to guess what your definition of gluten-free is. Always ask questions to make sure you understand what their particular definition of gluten-free is.

Where to Find More Information

This guide pre-supposes that you are already familiar with the gluten-free diet. But for those just starting out, there are some excellent resources available to help you understand the gluten-free diet and to make informed choices. For example, there are a host of helpful resources available from local and national support groups, widely available books and online materials. Doctors and nutritionists are also an excellent source of information. In short, please be proactive about educating yourself. When it comes to the gluten-free diet, an educated shopper really is a healthy shopper!

GLUTEN FREE OATS?

Ask your doctor to see if "gluten-free" oats may be right for you. Recent research suggests that moderate consumption of oats can be safe for most Celiacs. However, there's a catch . . . it's only pure, uncontaminated oats.

In contrast, normal oats and oat products, like the ones found at your local grocer, are usually cross-contaminated with wheat during harvest, transport, or processing. Consequently, they are unsafe for the gluten-free diet.

However, pure, uncontaminated oats are available. They have to be specially grown and processed to avoid cross-contamination, so they are harder to find and more expensive than traditional oats. But if you're hankering for oatmeal-raisin cookies or a crunchy bowl of granola, you may finally have a safe option!

BOB'S RED MILL
(800) 553-2258

CREAM HILL ESTATES
(866) 727-3628

GLUTEN FREE OATS
(307) 754-2058

Effective January 1, 2006, the Food Allergen Labeling and Consumer Protection Act of 2004 (FALCPA), set requirements for the labeling of eight major allergens on packaged foods. This is a quick overview of the elements of the FALCPA that are likely to be relevant to consumers on a gluten-free diet.[1]

Allergens Covered

The FALCPA covers eight major allergens that are credited with causing 90% of all food allergies. Those allergens include: milk, eggs, fish, crustacean shellfish, tree nuts, peanuts, soybeans and, most importantly, wheat. The FDA notes that, for the purposes of the FALCPA, wheat includes common wheat, durum wheat, club wheat, spelt, semolina, Einkorn, emmer, kamut and triticale.

Allergens Not Covered

It's important to note that the FALCPA does **not** cover barley or rye. Nor does it cover oats, which are likely to be cross-contaminated with wheat.

Labeling: What's Required

The FALCPA requires food manufacturers to identify allergens in ingredient lists in one of two ways:

1. In the ingredient listing, the common or usual name of the major food allergen must be followed in parentheses by the name of the food source from which the major allergen is derived. For example: "Enriched flour (wheat flour…)," or

2. Immediately following the ingredient listing, a "Contains" statement must indicate the name of the food source from which the major food allergen is derived. For example: "Contains: milk, wheat and eggs."

Allergens present in flavorings, coloring and additives must also be identified in one of the two ways listed above.

Labeling: What's Not Required

It is important to note that the FALCPA does not apply to major food allergens that are unintentionally added to food as a result of cross-contamination. Cross-contamination can result during the growing and harvesting of crops, or from the use of shared storage, transportation or production equipment.

---

[1]Please note this brief overview is not meant to be comprehensive, nor is it intended as medical or legal advice. If you have questions about food labeling laws or their impact on your dietary choices and decision making, please consult a legal professional, dietician or doctor, as appropriate.

The FALCPA also does not address the use of advisory labeling, including statements designed to identify the possibility of cross-contamination. The FALCPA does not require the use of such statements, nor does it specifically articulate standards of use for advisory statements.

Application

The FALCPA applies to all packaged foods sold in the U.S. that are regulated by the FDA and that are required to have ingredient statements.

It's important to note that the FALCPA does not apply to meat products, poultry products and egg products that fall under the authority of the USDA.

The Big Picture

What does this all mean for people following the gluten-free diet? There are three important limitations of the FALCPA to keep in mind:

- As far as gluten is concerned, the FALCPA does not cover it. The FALCPA covers wheat, but not rye, barley or other potentially troublesome grains.
- The FALCPA covers only products regulated by the FDA that require ingredient lists. For any product that does not require an ingredient list (such as raw fruits), or that falls outside the FDA's jurisdiction (such as meat, poultry and egg products that fall under the authority of the USDA), the FALCPA does not require manufacturers to identify major allergens.
- The FALCPA does not require manufacturers to identify the possibility of inadvertent cross-contamination, nor does it set specific standards for using advisory statements warning of potential cross-contamination.

The important thing to remember is that, despite improved labeling laws, hidden gluten in grocery items is still a very real possibility. Gluten can come from non-wheat sources, result from cross-contamination, or can occur in products not covered by the FALCPA. For those reasons, it's important to remain vigilant and carefully scrutinize the products you buy. It's not enough to just read labels; contacting manufacturers directly is often necessary.

What is Gluten-Free Anyway?

One final note on the FALCPA: The FALCPA required the FDA to issue a rule to define and permit the use of the term "gluten-free" on food labels by August 2008 (clearly, this ruling has been delayed by quite some time). We expect that ruling in the future, but when it comes, it will not require food companies to label gluten-free products as such. Rather, the the FDA will establish a uniform standard definition of the term "gluten-free" to be used voluntarily by food manufacturers, likely after some period of notice to allow companies time to comply. For more information, please visit the FDA at www.fda.gov.

Our goal is for this guide to make your shopping trips easier, safer, and full of choices. There are a few things you need to know about this guide's content and organization to help us fulfill on that goal.

PRODUCTS FEATURED

Our guide covers over 30,000 products from hundreds of different brands. The products listed are groceries likely to be found in typical American grocery stores like Safeway, Kroger, Hy-Vee, etc. They include brand names, as well as private label brands from some of the larger grocery chains. In cases where the grocery chain's name is different from their private label brand, we've also put the chain's name in parentheses next to the private label brand name.

When "All" are Gluten-Free

Some brands publish a list enumerating each gluten-free item, while others chose to simply say all foods in a particular category are gluten-free. In the latter case, we list the brand name in the appropriate category and sub-category, followed by a description of the products covered and the word "All," where applicable. For

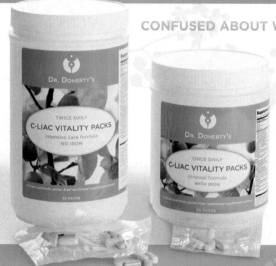

example, if a company, let's call it "Brand X," tells us that all its cheeses are gluten-free, it will be listed under "Brand X," followed by "Cheeses (All)." Alternatively, sometimes the brand communicated that all of their products were gluten-free, in which case, they will be noted in the guide as "Brand X (All)."

"All BUT"

Sometimes, the brand communicated that all but a few of its products were gluten-free. In those cases, they're listed as "Brand X (All BUT . . .)." That qualifier will always appear with Brand X across all categories to cut down on the need to cross-reference multiple sub-categories as you shop.

PRODUCTS NOT FEATURED

You will not find "boutique" gluten-free brands in this guide, unless they are likely to be found in typical grocery stores. This list is also far from comprehensive; there are smaller brands and new items popping up all the time. Just because a product isn't listed in these pages, doesn't mean it's not gluten-free. If there's something you're interested in that's not listed in this guide, call the company directly or let us know, and we'll look into adding it for the next edition.

There are some brands missing from the product listings because they simply do not provide or maintain lists of their gluten-free products. Unfortunately, companies are not required to maintain or share their gluten-free lists, so not every company can be listed in this guide.

We haven't listed some items that are generally accepted and widely known to be gluten-free. For example, plain dairy milk is not listed. However, we have listed flavored milk, sour cream and other items that contain ingredients (e.g., thickeners or other additives) that may be a concern to some shoppers. Of course, what is "generally accepted" and "widely known" to be gluten-free is subjective. So while one person may find

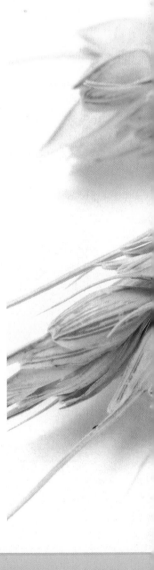

NAVIGATION TIP

The Easy Reference Table of Contents on the inside front cover is a quick visual reference for the different categories and sub-categories. Or, use the index in the back, if you prefer.

an entire sub-category of items we cover in the guide to be obviously gluten-free, some will not. We try to be as inclusive as possible for the sake of the latter audience.

Finally, for the sake of simplicity, this guide only lists items on a company's gluten-free list. We have excluded items that were reported to contain gluten.

GENERAL OVERVIEW OF ORGANIZATION

The product list is organized into a three tier system: first by category, then by subcategory, then by product name.

Organization by Category

The products listed in this guide are arranged like a typical grocery store. The list is organized first by master categories that align with aisles in a grocery store, like those for Dairy and Eggs, Snacks and Frozen Foods. Our belief is that organizing the guide by grocery aisle will make your trip through the store quicker—you can follow along in the guide as you shop through the store.

There are a few exceptions to the link between master category and grocery aisle: in some cases our consumer research found it more helpful to organize items by general category as opposed to aisle. For example, while refrigerated orange juice is often found in the Dairy and Eggs aisle, you'll find it listed here in the Beverages category.

Organization by Sub-Category

Each master category is further sub-divided by sub-categories that align with the particular types of food products found in the master category aisle. For example, sub-categories within the Snacks master category include: Chips, Cookies, Crackers, etc. Sub-categories are organized alphabetically within the master category.

Organization by Brand & Product

Within these subcategories, you'll find individual products listed alphabetically by brand name (in bold), then product name (not in bold). While we've done our best to organize the products into the "correct" category and sub-category, we hope you'll understand it was a subjective process and there will be some variance.

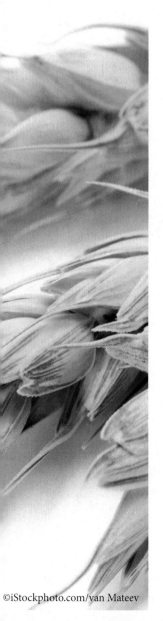

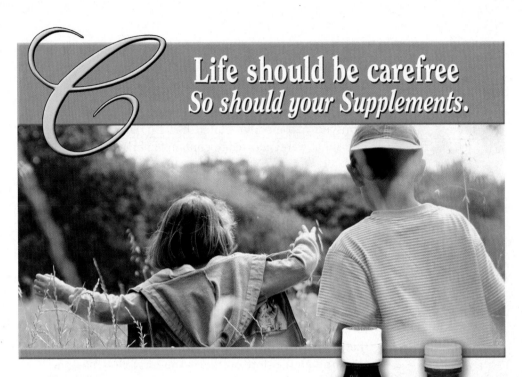
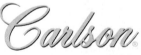

Information on all items listed, except the items in gray (more about these later) is obtained directly from the brand, manufacturer or brand representative (we refer to these as the "company" for short). Occasionally, they also send along additional information, ranging from legal disclaimers to in-depth notes on manufacturing procedures.

In order to make this guide portable and convenient, it's not practical to reprint all these notes provided by a company. But, there are a few exceptions. We know that you want to know which items may pose cross-contamination concerns and conversely, when companies go the extra mile by having dedicated production lines or gluten testing, for example. Therefore, those and other relevant situations are marked with special symbols.

We'll discuss each symbol in-depth here, but don't worry, there's a cheatsheet on page 1 to jog your memory when you're actually at the store.

Placement of Symbols

If a symbol applies to all of a brand's listed products, we placed the symbol next to the brand name. If it only applies to a particular product, the symbol will only appear next to that specific product. For example, if Brand X's entire line comes with a cross-contamination warning, the disclaimer icon will appear next to the Brand X name. If the warning only applies to its Chocolate Chip flavor, we place the symbol next to the Chocolate Chip flavor listing only.

Limitation of Symbols

Another thing to keep in mind is that any information, including disclaimers like cross-contamination warnings, are provided by companies at their discretion. Unfortunately, companies are not required by law to warn shoppers of cross-contamination, so just because a company does not have a cross-contamination warning does not mean it's not an issue! We sincerely hope that the FDA will resolve this issue in the near future.

SYMBOLS IN-DEPTH

Glasses Symbol

Some prominent brands do not maintain or share gluten-free lists. When you're gluten-free, your choices are, by definition, limited. The goal of this book is to open up more choices, not limit them.

Therefore, in cases where brands do not have a gluten-free list, but DO have a policy of accurately labeling for gluten, no matter how small the amount, Triumph independently reviewed each product's ingredients (based solely on reviewing the product labeling) to determine which are gluten-free.

The information for these particular product listings did not come directly from the brand or manufacturer, as with the other products in this guide, so we have distinguished them with a special reading-glass symbol and gray text color.

This feature was introduced in the 2nd edition, and it proved popular, so here it is again!

Gluten Testing Symbol

This symbol indicates that a company has tested its ingredients, finished products, machinery and/or equipment, etc. for gluten.

Gluten-Free Processing Symbol

Here's another happy symbol: this symbol indicates that the company reports any of the following:

- They use gluten-free lines, equipment or facilities; or,
- Items are produced in a gluten-free environment; or,
- Cross-contamintion is not an issue for whatever reason (be it because they have a dedicated facility, rigorous testing policies, etc.).

Cross Contamination/Shared Equipment Symbol **RED**

A company may get this symbol if it reports any of the following:

- Cross-contamination may be an issue; or,
- Their products are made on equipment, lines or in a plant that also process gluten-containing items; or,
- Their products are made with gluten-free ingredients, but they would not provide information on whether the manufacturing process is gluten-free.

So, does this symbol mean that you need to avoid these products entirely? The answer is complicated, I'm afraid. I don't like the answer any more than you're going to, but this is the world we live in and the hand the FDA has dealt us.

Some companies—too many, in my opinion—use language like the above bullet points in the hopes that it will cut down on litigation. In other words, they don't want to get sued. In these cases, it's not their Quality Control teams that are writing these disclaimers, but their legal teams.

So it's very possible that these products may be safe with little to no chance of cross-contamination, but the companies want to cover their legal bases by noting the chance, no matter how remote.

Unfortunately, there are also many cases where there may be a legitimate chance of cross-contamination. There's no surefire way to distinguish these "real" cross-contamination risks from an overzealous legal department. Trust me, we've tried!

Cross Contamination
Symbol **ORANGE**

This is a new symbol for the 3rd edition. We are usually loathe to add more symbols. In fact, the 1st edition had six, and we cut that down to four in our 2nd edition.

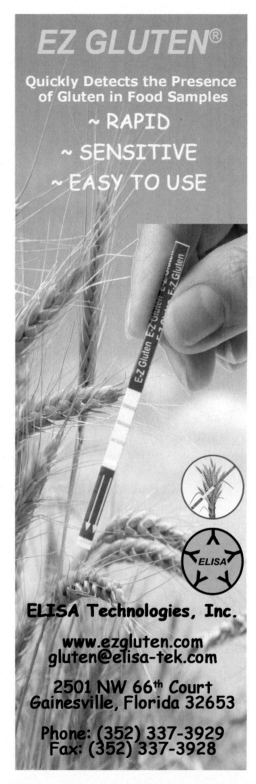

But, something felt wrong about lumping together companies that write "cross-contamination is a possibility" and those that state "cross contamination is a possibility but all our personnel are trained in handling allergenic materials, which are stored separately, and we sanitize and swab test shared machinery between each product run."

That's why we introduced this new symbol. It covers companies that noted cross-contamination or shared equipment, like the RED cross-contamination scenario, but also informed us about counter measures they have in place. Such measures may include the following:

- Special handling and/or segregation of gluten-containing ingredients or products; or,
- Scheduling of equipment and machinery so that gluten-containing items are processed at different times than gluten-free items; along with,
- Thorough cleaning/sanitization procedures of machinery and equipment between gluten-containing and gluten-free product batches.

Of course, this is not an exhaustive list of the many different methods companies take to minimize cross-contamination. But, I think you get the picture!

Strange Bedfellow

So you probably have this symbols thing down by now. But, then you may see ⓘ and ⚥ together. And you may rightly wonder, how can something be made on a dedicated gluten-free line or facility and the company still wants to have the cross-contamination symbol. Well, an example scenario may be that they have four lines in a plant, and three are dedicated gluten-free, but the fourth is used for gluten-containing items. So, in this case, there is both a gluten-free line (⚥) and non-gluten-free facility (ⓘ).

Final Thoughts

This guide was created in response to a loose-leaf binder our founder used to carry. The binder was a collection of hundreds of gluten-free lists from hundreds of companies. It was a monster to carry and even worse to update. We're talking entire days spent calling companies and listening to bad hold music.

We've come a long way from loose-leaf binders and frantic calls to food companies right before dinner. And we hope that all this research we've done helps to make your life easier. We are the only guide that takes the time to give you these symbols because we think they're relevant to good decision-making and that you deserve the extra information. Please use it, and use it wisely.

LIMITATIONS OF THE GUIDE

While we hope that this guide makes gluten-free shopping easier, we do recognize that it has some limitations, which we would like to call out so that you can make informed shopping decisions.

Gluten-Free Lists

As mentioned in previous chapters, there is currently no FDA rule defining gluten-free and generally no consensus in the community as to an exact definition. (Consider the controversies surrounding blue cheese and oats, just to name a few.) So when a company reports that its products are gluten-free, there is the possibility that their definition of gluten-free may differ from yours.

In addition, the information published in this guide for each food item has been obtained directly from that item's manufacturer, the entity that licensed the manufacturing, or an affiliate, unless otherwise noted. It's impossible for us to verify the accuracy of the information companies report to us.

Always Read Labels

It's important to keep in mind that product formulations and ingredient sourcing can and do change without notice, companies can make mistakes on their gluten-free list, and people compiling and categorizing large volumes of information (like the content for this guide) can make mistakes, as well. For these reasons, Triumph Dining cannot assume any liability for the correctness or accuracy of any information presented in this guide. You should read labels every time you make a purchase and regularly contact companies to confirm the gluten-free status of the products you consume.

Contact the Company with Questions

Please contact companies directly with any questions or for updates. Any information provided in this guide was obtained from the company (unless otherwise noted), and they will always be your best source of information on their products.

A Question of Semantics

Since there is still no FDA regulation defining the term "gluten-free" and no requirement that companies report the possibility of cross-contamination, as consumers, we're still very much on our own. A company may claim its products are "gluten-free" and free of "cross-contamination," but since there's no universally accepted definition of either term, you may still not be getting the whole story. Therefore, a product's appearance in this guide does not mean that the product is entirely free of gluten (besides, that would likely be an impossible standard, as the most sensitive, sophisticated commercially-available tests for gluten do not measure to 0 ppm). However, you may find our symbols useful in deciding whether a product is suitable for you. Please see page 21 for more details.

This guide is largely a compilation of the information over 1,000 companies provide when consumers reach out to them asking about the gluten-free status of their products.

Common Sense is Your Best Guide

A guide like this should never be a replacement for your own knowledge, common sense and diligence. This guide is intended as a starting point only, and not a final determination that a listed product is gluten-free, suitable for the gluten-free diet, or safe for you personally to consume. It is not a substitute for reading labels and contacting companies. Rather, this guide is designed to help you hone in on the products most likely to be suitable for the gluten-free diet, so that you can focus your label-reading and company-contacting efforts on the most promising products, without wasting dozens and dozens of hours chasing dead ends. Always exercise caution when using any lists, even this one or ones directly from a brand. People make mistakes, so if something doesn't feel right, it probably isn't.

Some Final Notes

The information published in this guide is intended for use in the United States and with products manufactured with the intent to be sold in the United States only. Products sold or intended to be sold outside the United States may have completely different ingredients than their U.S. counterparts, and may not be gluten-free.

This guide is for limited educational purposes only and is not medical advice. If you have questions about the gluten-free diet, what ingredients are appropriate to consume, whether or not particular items are appropriate for your consumption, etc., please consult with your physician.

For the foregoing reasons, Triumph Dining cannot assume any liability for any losses or damages resulting from your use of this product listing. It's up to you to determine whether a product is appropriate based on your individual dietary needs. For more information about a particular company's testing practices, standards and thresholds, please contact that company directly.

Use of this guide indicates your acknowledgement of and agreement to these terms.

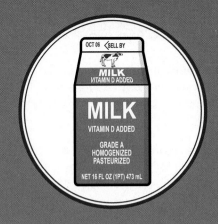

DAIRY & EGGS

BUTTER

Cabot
Cabot's Products (All)

Challenge 🍽
Butter (All)

Crystal Farms
60/40 Butter Blend
Salted Butter
Unsalted Butter

Darigold
Darigold (All)

Giant
Salted Butter Quarters
Unsalted Butter Quarters

Great Value (Wal-Mart)
Salted Butter Quarters
Unsalted Butter Quarters

Hy-Vee
Sweet Cream Butter Quarters
Sweet Cream Butter Solid
Sweet Cream Whipped Butter
Unsalted Sweet Butter Quarters

Keller's Creamery 🍽
Butter

Kerrygold
Butters (All)

Kroger ⓘ
Butter

Lucerne (Safeway)
Butter

Meijer
Butter AA Quarters

Nature's Promise (Giant)
Organic Butter

Nature's Promise (Stop & Shop)
Organic Butter

Plugrá 🍽
Plugrá

Publix ()
Butter - Salted
Butter - Unsalted
Butter - Whipped, Salted
Butter - Whipped, Unsalted
Sweet Cream Butter

Purity Dairies
Milk and Cultured Products (All)

Stop & Shop
Salted Butter Quarters
Unsalted Butter Quarters

Straus Family Creamery 🍽
Butter (All)

Tillamook
Butter (All)

Winn-Dixie ⓘ
Unsalted Butter

BUTTERMILK

Darigold
Darigold (All)

Giant
1% Buttermilk

Hood
Buttermilk

Lucerne (Safeway)
Buttermilk - Fat Free
Buttermilk - Low Fat
Buttermilk - Regular

Shamrock Farms
Buttermilk

CHEESE & CHEESE SPREADS

A & E Cheese
Pre-Sliced American Cheese
Pre-Sliced Colby Jack Cheese
Pre-Sliced Havarti Cheese
Pre-Sliced Mild Cheddar Cheese
Pre-Sliced Mozzarella Cheese
Pre-Sliced Muenster Cheese
Pre-Sliced Pepper Jack Cheese
Pre-Sliced Provolone Cheese
Pre-Sliced Swiss Cheese
Shredded Colby Jack Cheese
Shredded Mexican Mix Cheese
Shredded Mild Cheddar Cheese
Shredded Mozzarella Cheese
Shredded Sharp Cheddar

Alouette
Baby Brie - Herb
Baby Brie - Plain
Chive and Spring Onion Spreadable Cheese
Cilantro Lime Spreadable Cheese
Creamy Onion & Shallots Spreadable Cheese
Crème de Brie - Herb
Crème de Brie - Original
Créme Fraîche
Elegante Roasted Garlic/Pesto
Elegante Roasted Pepper/Olive
Elegante Sundried Tomato & Garlic
Garlic & Herbs Spreadable Cheese
Garlic Supreme Spreadable Cheese
Light Cucumber Dill Spreadable Cheese
Light Garlic & Herbs Spreadable Cheese
Peppercorn Parmesan Spreadable Cheese
Savory Vegetable Spreadable Cheese
Spinach Artichoke Spreadable Cheese
Sundried Tomato Spreadable Cheese

Alpine Lace ()
Cheese Products

Applegate Farms ⓘ
Applegate Farms (All BUT Chicken Nuggets, Chicken Pot Pie, & Chicken Strips)

Athenos ⌒
Blue Cheese Crumbled Natural
Chunk Mild
Chunk with Basil & Tomato
Chunk with Black Peppercorn
Chunk with Garlic & Herb
Crumbled Mild
Crumbled Reduced Fat
Crumbled Traditional
Crumbled Traditional (Value Size)
Crumbled with Basil & Tomato
Crumbled with Basil & Tomato Reduced Fat
Crumbled with Black Peppercorn
Crumbled with Garlic & Herb
Crumbled with Lemon Garlic & Oregano
Crumbled with Roasted Bell Peppers & Garlic
Feta Crumbled Reduced Fat
Feta Crumbled with Basil & Tomato Natural
Feta Crumbled with Garlic & Herb Natural
Feta Traditional Chunk Packed In Brine Natural
Gorgonzola Crumbled Natural
Traditional Feta Crumbled Natural

BelGioioso Cheese
BelGioioso Cheese (All)

Betts ⌁
Cheese Spreads (All)

Boar's Head
Cheeses (All)

Borden
Borden Cheese Products (All)

Boursin
Boursin Cheese (All Flavors)

Cabot
Cabot's Products (All)

Cantaré Foods
Burrata
Mascarpone

Mozzarella
Ricotta

Chavrie
Chavrie
Chavrie with Basil/Roasted Garlic

Cracker Barrel &
Cheese Sticks - Extra Sharp Cheddar 2% Milk Reduced Fat
Cheese Sticks - Natural Extra Sharp Cheddar White
Cheese Sticks - Natural Sharp Cheddar
Cracker Cuts - Extra Sharp
Cracker Cuts - Extra Sharp Cheddar
Cracker Cuts - Extra Sharp Cheddar 2% Milk Reduced Fat
Cracker Cuts - Extra Sharp Cheddar Cheese Cuts
Cracker Cuts - Vermont Sharp White
Emmentaler Swiss
Extra Sharp
Extra Sharp Cheddar 2% Milk Reduced Fat Shredded
Extra Sharp White
Extra Sharp White Cheddar
Fontina
Havarti
Natural Baby Swiss
Natural Cheddar Vermont Sharp White
Natural Extra Sharp Cheddar
Natural Extra Sharp Cheddar 2% Milk Reduced Fat
Natural Extra Sharp White Cheddar Reduced Fat
Natural Sharp Cheddar
Natural Sharp Cheddar 2% Milk Reduced Fat
Natural Sharp Cheddar Slices
Natural Sharp White Cheddar Reduced Fat
Natural Vermont's Sharp White Cheddar 2% Milk Reduced Fat
Sharp White Cheddar
White Colby

Crystal Farms
2% and Fat Free IWS
Aerosol Cheese (All Flavors)
American Deluxe Sliced

American IWS
Blue Cheese & Gorgonzola
Cheese Spread Loaf
Jar Cheese (All Flavors)
Natural Cheeses - Chunks & Shreds (All Varieties and Flavors)
Parmesan and Romano - Shaker & Shredded
Ricotta (All Varieties)
Sliced American Cheese
Stick Cheeses
String Cheese
Swiss, Sharp, Pepper Jack IWS

Dofino
Dofino (All)

Finlandia Cheese
Finlandia Cheese (All)

Friendship Dairies 8
Friendship Products (All)

Giant
Colby and Monterey Blend (All Varieties) ()
Colby Half Moon Single Slices ()
Fat Free White Cheese Singles ()
Feta (All Varieties) ()
Havarti (All Varieties) ()
Horseradish Cheddar Cheese ()
Mexican Cheese Blend ()
Mild Cheddar (All Varieties) ()
Mild Longhorn Style Cheddar (All Varieties) ()
Monterey Jack (All Varieties) ()
Mozzarella (All Varieties) ()
Muenster (All Varieties) ()
Neufchatel Cheese ()
NY Extra Sharp Cheddar (All Varieties) ()
NY Sharp Cheddar (All Varieties) ()
Parmesan Cheese (All Varieties) ()
Port Wine Cheddar Cheese ()
Provolone (All Varieties) ()
Ricotta (All Varieties) ()
Sharp Cheddar (All Varieties) ()
Sharp Cheddar Cold Pack Cheese Food ()
String Cheese ()
Swiss Cheese (All Varieties) ()
Taco Cheese Blend ()
Vermont Sharp Cheddar (All Varieties) ()

Wisconsin Sharp (All Varieties)

Great Value (Wal-Mart)

100% Parmesan Grated Cheese
2% Milk American Deluxe Reduced Fat Pasteurized Process Cheese with Added Calcium
2% Milk Reduced Fat Mild Cheddar Cheese Chunk
2% Milk Reduced Fat Sharp Cheddar Cheese Chunk
American Pasteurized Prepared Cheese Product Singles
American Reduced Fat Pasteurized Process Cheese Food Singles
Cheese Wow American Cheese
Cheese Wow Cheddar Cheese
Cheese Wow Pepper Jack Cheese
Colby And Monterey Jack Cheese Chunk
Colby And Monterey Jack Cheese Cubes
Deluxe American Pasteurized Process Cheese Singles
Deluxe White American Pasteurized Process Cheese Singles
Extra Sharp Cheddar Cheese Chunk
Fancy Shredded Colby & Monterey Jack Cheese
Fancy Shredded Colby And Monterey Jack Cheese
Fancy Shredded Fiesta Blend Cheese
Fancy Shredded Italian Blend Cheese
Fancy Shredded Low-Moisture Part-Skim Mozzarella Cheese
Fancy Shredded Mild Cheddar Cheese
Fancy Shredded Mozzarella Cheese
Fancy Shredded Parmesan Blend
Fancy Shredded Parmesan Cheese
Fancy Shredded Pizza Blend Cheese
Fancy Shredded Sharp Cheddar Cheese
Fancy Shredded Swiss Cheese
Fancy Shredded Taco Blend Cheese
Fat Free Pasteurized Process Cheese Product Singles
Feather Shredded Colby & Monterey Jack Cheese
Feather Shredded Mild Cheddar Cheese
Feather Shredded Mozzarella Cheese
Longhorn Style Colby Cheese Chunk
Longhorn Style Mild Cheddar Cheese Chunk
Medium Cheddar Cheese Chunk
Medium Cheddar Chunk
Melt 'n Dip Pasteurized Processed Cheese Spread
Mild Cheddar Cheese Chunk
Mild Cheddar Cheese Cubes
Monterey Jack Cheese Chunk
Mozzarella Cheese Chunk
Muenster Cheese Chunk
Natural Colby Cheese Chunk
Neufchatel Cheese
Pepper Jack Cheese Chunk
Pepper Jack Cheese Cubes
Sharp Cheddar Cheese Chunk
Sharp Cheddar Chunk
Shredded Mild Cheddar Cheese
Shredded Mozzarella Cheese
Shredded White Sharp Cheddar Cheese
Sliced Mild Cheddar Cheese
Sliced Mozzarella Cheese
Sliced Pepper Jack Cheese
Sliced Provolone Cheese
Sliced Swiss Cheese
Swiss Cheese Chunk
White American Pasteurized Prepared Cheese Product Singles
White Mild Cheddar Cheese Chunk
White Sharp Cheddar Cheese Chunk

Heluva Good

Solid Block Style Cheese (All)

Hy-Vee

American Singles
Cheeze-Eze
Colby 1/2 Moon Longhorn Cheese
Colby Cheese
Colby Hunk Cheese
Colby Jack 1/2 Moon Longhorn Cheese
Colby Jack Cheese
Colby Jack Cheese Cubes
Colby Jack Hunk Cheese
Colby Jack Slices
Colby Longhorn Cheese
Colby Slice Singles
Extra Sharp Cheddar Cheese

Fancy Shredded 4 Italian Cheese
Fancy Shredded Cheddar Jack Cheese
Fancy Shredded Colby Jack Cheese
Fancy Shredded Mild Cheddar 2%
  Cheese
Fancy Shredded Mild Cheddar Cheese
Fancy Shredded Mozzarella 2% Milk
Fancy Shredded Mozzarella Cheese
Fat Free Singles
Fat Free Swiss Cheese Slices
Finely Shredded Colby Jack Cheese
Finely Shredded Mild Cheddar Cheese
Grated Parmesan Cheese
Hot Pepper Cheese
Lil' Hunk Colby Jack Cheese
Lil' Hunk Mild Cheddar Cheese
Medium Cheddar Cheese
Medium Cheddar Longhorn Cheese
Mild Cheddar Cheese
Mild Cheddar Cheese Cubes
Mild Cheddar Hunk Cheese
Mild Cheddar Slices
Monterey Jack Cheese
Monterey Jack Hunk Cheese
Mozzarella Cheese
Mozzarella Hunk Cheese
Muenster Cheese
Muenster Cheese Slices
Pepper Jack Cheese
Pepper Jack Cheese Cubes
Pepper Jack Hunk Cheese
Pepper Jack Singles
Pepper Jack Slices
Provolone Cheese
Provolone Cheese Slices
Sharp Cheddar Cheese
Sharp Cheddar Hunk Cheese
Sharp Cheddar Longhorn Cheese
Shredded Colby Jack Cheese
Shredded Mexican Blend Cheese
Shredded Mild Cheddar Cheese
Shredded Mozzarella Cheese
Shredded Parmesan Cheese
Shredded Pizza Cheese
Shredded Sharp Cheddar Cheese
Shredded Taco Cheese
Sliced Low-Moisture Part-Skim
  Mozzarella

Swiss Cheese
Swiss Singles
Swiss Slices

Isaly's ()
Cheese Items (All)

Jarlsberg
Jarlsberg (All)

Kerrygold
Cheeses (All)

Kraft Cracker Cuts
Cheese Cuts - Colby & Monterey Jack
  Natural Marbled
Cheese Cuts - Natural Mild Cheddar
Cheese Cuts - Sharp Cheddar

Kraft Deli Deluxe
American 2% Milk Slices
American Slices
American White Slices
Sharp Cheddar Slices
Swiss Slices

Kraft Deli Fresh
Colby Jack Slices
Mild Cheddar Slices
Natural Swiss Slices
Pepper Jack Spicy Slices
Provolone Slices
Sharp Cheddar Slices
Swiss 2% Milk Reduced Fat Slices
Swiss Slices

Kraft Easy Cheese
American
Cheddar
Sharp Cheddar

Kraft Grated Cheese
Parmesan & Romano Medium 100%
Parmesan 100%
Parmesan Original
Parmesan Reduced Fat
Parmesan Shredded
Parmesan, Romano & Asiago Shredded
Romano 100% Grated

Kraft Natural Cheese
Cheddar & Monterey Jack 2% Cubes
Cheddar & Monterey Jack Marbled
Cheddar Bacon
Cheddar Extra Sharp
Cheddar Mild

Cheddar Mild 2% Cubes
Cheddar Mild 2% Milk Reduced Fat
Cheddar Sharp
Cheddar Sharp 2% Cubes
Colby
Colby & Monterey Jack
Colby & Monterey Jack 2% Cubes
Colby & Monterey Jack Marbled
Colby 2% Milk Reduced Fat
Colby Longhorn Style
Extra Sharp Cheddar
Medium Cheddar
Mild Cheddar
Mild Cheddar Longhorn Style 2% Milk
Monterey Jack
Monterey Jack 2% Milk Reduced Fat
Mozzarella Low-Moisture Part-Skim
Organic Cheddar
Pepper Jack
Roasted Garlic Cheddar
Sharp Cheddar
Sharp Cheddar 2% Milk Reduced Fat
Smoky Swiss & Cheddar

Kraft Natural Cheese Sticks ᨃ
Extra Sharp Cheddar
Mild Cheddar
Sharp Cheddar 2% Milk Reduced Fat

Kraft Natural Crumbles ᨃ
Blue Cheese
Feta Cheese
Italian Style
Mediterranean Style
Mexican Style 2% Milk Reduced Fat
Mozzarella
Reduced Fat Colby & Monterey Jack
Sharp Cheddar
Three Cheese Monterey Jack/Colby &
   Cheddar

Kraft Natural Shredded Cheese ᨃ
Cheddar Fat Free
Cheddar Mild 2% Milk Finely Shredded
   Reduced Fat
Cheddar Mild 2% Milk Reduced Fat
Cheddar Sharp
Colby & Monterey Jack
Colby & Monterey Jack 2% Milk
   Shredded

Colby & Monterey Jack Finely Shredded
Colby & Monterey Jack Shredded
Italian Style Five Cheese
Mexican Cheddar Jack
Mexican Cheddar Jack with Jalapeno
   Peppers
Mexican Four Cheese
Mexican Four Cheese 2% Milk
Mexican Style Four Cheese
Mild Cheddar
Mild Cheddar Finely Shredded
Monterey Jack
Mozzarella
Mozzarella & Parmesan Finely Shredded
Mozzarella 2% Milk Reduced Fat
Mozzarella Fat Free
Mozzarella Low Moisture
Mozzarella Low Moisture Finely
   Shredded
Mozzarella Low Moisture Part Skim
Organic Cheddar
Organic Mozzarella
Pizza Mozzarella & Cheddar
Sharp Cheddar 2% Milk Reduced Fat
Sharp Cheddar Finely Shredded
Sharp Cheddar Finely Shredded 2%
   Milk
Swiss

Kraft Singles ᨃ
Aged Swiss
American
American 2% Milk Slices
American Fat Free Slices
American Slices
Organic American Slices
Pepperjack 2% Milk Slices
Select American Slices
Sharp Cheddar
Sharp Cheddar 2% Milk Slices
Sharp Cheddar Fat Free Slices
Swiss 2% Milk Slices
Swiss Fat Free Slices
Swiss Slices
White American
White American 2% Milk
White American Fat Free Slices

Kraft String-Ums ✎
  Mozzarella String Cheese
Kraft Twist-Ums & String-Ums ✎
  Mozzarella & Cheddar
  Mozzarella & Cheddar Super Long
Kroger ⓘ
  Bar Cheeses
  Cubed Cheeses
  Shredded Cheeses
  Sliced Cheeses
Laughing Cow ⛉
  Laughing Cow Cheese (All)
Lifeway ⛉
  Lifeway Products (All BUT Probiotic
    Wellness Bars)
Lucerne (Safeway)
  Cheese (All Varieties)
  Ricotta Cheese
  String Cheese
Maggio ⛉
  Mozzarella (Solid Block Style)
  Ricotta
Meijer
  2% Individual Wrap American
  2% Individual Wrap Sharp
  American Cheese Spray (Aerosol)
  Cheddar - Fancy Shred
  Cheddar - Medium Bar
  Cheddar - Midget Horn
  Cheddar - Mild Bar
  Cheddar - Mild Chunk
  Cheddar - Sharp Bar
  Cheddar - Sharp Chunk
  Cheddar - Sharp Fancy Shred
  Cheddar - Sharp Shredded
  Cheddar - Shred
  Cheddar - Shred (Zip Pouch)
  Cheddar - Shred Sharp (Zip Pouch)
  Cheddar - Sliced Longhorn Half Moon
  Cheddar - X-tra-Sharp Bar
  Cheddar Jack Fancy Shred (Zip Pouch)
  Cheddar/Monterey Jack Bar
  Cheese (Individually Wrapped)
  Cheese Cheddar (Aerosol)
  Cheese Sharp Cheddar (Aerosol)
  Cheese Swiss (Individually Wrapped)
  Cheezy Does It Jalapeno

Cheezy Does It Processes Spread Loaf
Cheezy Does It Spread Loaf
Colby Bar
Colby Chunk
Colby Jack Bar
Colby Jack Fancy Shred
Colby Jack Longhorn Half Moon
Colby Jack Sliced Single
Colby Longhorn Full Moon
Colby Longhorn Half Moon (Sliced)
Colby Midget Horn
Colby Shred Fancy
Fancy Italian Blend Shred
Fancy Mexican Blend Shred
Fancy Mexican Blend Shred
Fancy Shred Colby Jack
Fancy Shred Mild Cheddar
Fancy Shred Mozzarella
Fancy Shred Nacho/Taco
Hot Pepper Jack Chunk Cheese
Individual Wrap Slice Pepper
Low Moisture Part Skim Mozzarella Bar
Low Moisture Part Skim Mozzarella
  Shred
Low Moisture Part Skim Mozzarella
  Square
Low Moisture Part Skim String Cheese
Marble Cheddar (C&W Cheddar)
Mexican Shred
Monterey Jack Chunk
Mozzarella Shred
Mozzarella Single Slice
Muenster Slice Single
Parmesan and Romano Cheese (Grated)
Parmesan Cheese (Grated)
Parmesan Cheese 1/3 Less Fat
Pepper Jack Bar
Pepperjack Sliced Stack Pack
Pizza Shred Mozzarella/Cheddar
Processed American Cheese Slices
Processed Fat Free Sharp Individual
  Slices
Provolone Stacked Slice
Ricotta Cheese - Part Skim
Ricotta Cheese - Whole Milk
String Cheese
Swiss Chunk
Swiss Slice Single

Swiss Sliced Sandwich/Cut

Midwest Country Fare (Hy-Vee)
American Sandwich Slices
Shredded Cheddar Cheese
Shredded Mozzarella Cheese

Mini Babybel 🍼
Mini Babybel Cheese (All)

Montrachet
Chives
Herbs
Original Flavor

Old Chatham Sheepherding Company
Old Chatham Sheepherding Company
(All)

Polly-O Cheese ✍
Fat Free Ricotta
Lite Ricotta
Mozzarella Fat Free
Mozzarella Parmesan Finely Shredded
Mozzarella Part Skim
Mozzarella Shredded Fat Free
Mozzarella Shredded Lite
Mozzarella Shredded Part Skim
Mozzarella Shredded Whole Milk
Original Ricotta
Parmesan Grated
Part Skim Ricotta
Pizza Mozzarella - Provolone Romano
Parmesan Shredded

Primo Taglio (Safeway)
American Cheddar
Caesar Jack Cheese
Crumbled Danish Blue
Danish Havarti
Hot Pepper Jack
Imported Ages White Cheddar
Lacy Swiss Cheese
Muenster
Provolone
Regular Jack Cheese
Shredded Asiago
Smoked Fontina Cheese

Publix ()
Asiago Wedge
Blue Crumbled
Cheddar - Extra Sharp (All Forms:
Block, Chunk & Shreds)

Cheddar - Medium (All Forms: Block,
Chunk & Shreds)
Cheddar - Mild (All Forms: Block,
Chunk & Shreds)
Cheddar - Sharp (All Forms: Block,
Chunk & Shreds)
Cheese Spread (Processed Cheese)
Colby (All Forms: Block, Chunk &
Shreds)
Colby Jack (All Forms: Block, Chunk &
Shreds)
Creative Classic Queso Blanco
Creative Classic Queso de Freir
Crumbled Feta
Crumbled Goat
Crumbled Reduced Fat Feta
Deluxe American Cheese Slices
(Processed Cheese)
Feta Chunk
Garden Jack Stick
Garlic and Herb Cheese Spread
Gorgonzola Crumbled
Grated Parmesan
Horseradish Jack Stick
Hot Pepper Cheese Spread
Italian 6-Cheese Blend - Shredded
Mexican 4-Cheese Blend - Shredded
Monterey Jack & Cheddar - Shredded
Monterey Jack (All Forms: Block, Chunk
& Shreds)
Monterey Jack with Jalapeño Peppers
(All Forms: Block, Chunk & Shreds)
Mozzarella (All Forms: Block, Chunk &
Shreds)
Muenster (All Forms: Block, Chunk &
Shreds)
Parmesan Wedge
Parmesan, Grated
Provolone (All Forms: Block, Chunk &
Shreds)
Reduced Fat Feta Chunk
Reduced Fat Pepper Jack
Ricotta
Salsa Jack Stick
Shredded Parmesan
Singles - Pasteurized Process American
Cheese Food

Singles - Pasteurized Process American Cheese Food (Thick Slice)

Singles - Pasteurized Process Swiss Cheese Food

Swiss (All Forms: Block, Chunk & Shreds)

Redwood Hill Farm

Cheeses (All)

Rosenborg

Rosenborg (All)

Safeway

Grated Parmesan Cheese

Quick Cheese - Sharp Cheddar

Select - Shredded Parmesan Cheese

Saladena

Feta Crumbles Mediterranean

Feta Crumbles Plain

Goat Crumbles Plain

Goat Crumbles Provencal

Sargento

Artisan Blends Shredded Authentic Mexican Cheese

Artisan Blends Shredded Double Cheddar Cheese

Artisan Blends Shredded Mozzarella & Provolone Cheese

Artisan Blends Shredded Parmesan & Romano Cheese

Artisan Blends Shredded Parmesan Cheese

Artisan Blends Shredded Swiss Cheese

Artisan Blends Shredded Whole Milk Mozzarella Cheese

Artisan Blends Shredded Wisconsin Sharp White Cheddar Cheese

BistroBlends Shredded Chipotle Cheddar Cheese

BistroBlends Shredded Italian Pasta Cheese

BistroBlends Shredded Mozzarella & Asiago Cheese with Roasted Garlic

BistroBlends Shredded Mozzarella Cheese with Sun-Dried Tomatoes & Basil

BistroBlends Shredded Nacho & Taco Cheese

BistroBlends Shredded Sharp Wisconsin & Vermont Cheddar Cheese with Real Bacon

BistroBlends Shredded Taco Cheese

Chef Style Shredded Mild Cheddar Cheese

Chef Style Shredded Mozzarella Cheese

Chef Style Shredded Sharp Cheddar Cheese

Chipotle Cheddar Cheese Snacks

Colby-Jack Cheese Snacks

Colby-Jack Cubes Snacks

Deli Style Sliced Aged Swiss Cheese

Deli Style Sliced Baby Swiss Cheese

Deli Style Sliced Chipotle Cheddar Cheese

Deli Style Sliced Colby Cheese

Deli Style Sliced Colby-Jack Cheese

Deli Style Sliced Gouda Cheese

Deli Style Sliced Havarti Cheese

Deli Style Sliced Jarlsberg Cheese

Deli Style Sliced Medium Cheddar Cheese

Deli Style Sliced Mild Cheddar Cheese

Deli Style Sliced Monterey Jack Cheese

Deli Style Sliced Mozzarella Cheese

Deli Style Sliced Muenster Cheese

Deli Style Sliced Pepper Jack Cheese

Deli Style Sliced Provolone Cheese

Deli Style Sliced Reduced Fat Colby-Jack Cheese

Deli Style Sliced Reduced Fat Medium Cheddar Cheese

Deli Style Sliced Reduced Fat Pepper Jack Cheese

Deli Style Sliced Reduced Fat Swiss Cheese

Deli Style Sliced Sharp Cheddar Cheese

Deli Style Sliced Sharp Provolone Cheese

Deli Style Sliced Swiss Cheese

Deli Style Sliced Vermont Sharp White Cheddar Cheese

Fancy Shredded 4 Cheese Mexican Cheese

Fancy Shredded 6 Cheese Italian Cheese

Fancy Shredded Cheddar Jack Cheese

Fancy Shredded Colby-Jack Cheese

Fancy Shredded Mild Cheddar Cheese
Fancy Shredded Monterey Jack Cheese
Fancy Shredded Mozzarella Cheese
Fancy Shredded Pizza Double Cheese
Fancy Shredded Sharp Cheddar Cheese
Grated Parmesan & Romano Cheese
Grated Parmesan Cheese
Hard Grating Parmesan Cheese
Light String Cheese Snacks
Limited Edition Shredded New York
  Sharp White Cheddar Cheese
Limited Edition Sliced New York Sharp
  White Cheddar Cheese
Mild Cheddar Cheese Cubes Snacks
Mild Cheddar Cheese Snacks
Mild Cheddar Snack Bars
Pepper Jack Cheese Snacks
Reduced Fat Colby-Jack Sticks
Reduced Fat Deli Style Sliced Provolone
  Cheese
Reduced Fat Sharp Cheddar Sticks
Reduced Fat Shredded Colby-Jack
  Cheese
Sharp Cheddar Cheese Sticks
Shredded Reduced Fat 4 Cheese Italian
  Cheese
Shredded Reduced Fat 4 Cheese
  Mexican Cheese
Shredded Reduced Fat Mild Cheddar
  Cheese
Shredded Reduced Fat Mozzarella
  Cheese
Shredded Reduced Fat Sharp Cheddar
  Cheese
String Cheese Snacks
SunBursts Snacks
Twirls Snacks
Vermont Sharp White Cheddar Sticks

Smart Balance
Smart Balance (All)

Stop & Shop
Colby and Monterey Blend (All
  Varieties) ()
Colby Half Moon Single Slices ()
Fat Free White Cheese Singles ()
Feta (All Varieties) ()
Havarti (All Varieties) ()

Horseradish Cheddar Cheese ()
Mexican Cheese Blend ()
Mild Cheddar (All Varieties) ()
Mild Longhorn Style Cheddar (All
  Varieties) ()
Monterey Jack (All Varieties) ()
Mozzarella (All Varieties) ()
Muenster (All Varieties) ()
NY Extra Sharp Cheddar (All Varieties) ()
NY Sharp Cheddar (All Varieties) ()
Parmesan Cheese (All Varieties) ()
Port Wine Cheddar Cheese ()
Provolone (All Varieties) ()
Ricotta (All Varieties) ()
Sharp Cheddar (All Varieties) ()
Sharp Cheddar Cold Pack Cheese Food ()
String Cheese ()
Swiss Cheese (All Varieties) ()
Taco Cheese Blend ()
Vermont Sharp Cheddar (All Varieties) ()
Vermont White Cheddar Cheese ()
Wisconsin Sharp (All Varieties) ()

Thummann's
Cheeses (All)

Tillamook
Cheese (All)

Ukrop's
Pimento Cheese Spread (Deli)

Velveeta 🐮
2% Milk Cheese
Cheese - Slices
Cheese - Slices Extra Thick
Mexican Mild Cheese
Pepper Jack Cheese
Regular Cheese

Winn-Dixie ⓘ
2% Milk Singles
American Pasteurized Cheese Product
Naturally Aged Sharp Cheddar
Singles Swiss Pasteurized Processed
  Cheese

CHEESE ALTERNATIVES

Lisanatti
Cheese Alternatives

Publix ()
  Imitation Mozzarella Cheese - Shredded
    (Processed Cheese)
Rice
  Rice (All)
Vegan
  Vegan (All)
Vegan Gourmet ⓘ 🛡
  Cheddar
  Monterey Jack
  Mozzarella Cheese Alternative
  Nacho
Veggie
  Veggie (All)
Veggy
  Veggy (All)

COTTAGE CHEESE

Axelrod 🛡
  Cottage Cheese
Breakstone's ᔐ
  Cottage Doubles Apples & Cinnamon
    Lowfat Cottage Cheese & Topping
  Cottage Doubles Blueberry Lowfat
    Cottage Cheese & Topping
  Cottage Doubles Peach Lowfat Cottage
    Cheese & Topping
  Cottage Doubles Pineapple Lowfat
    Cottage Cheese & Topping
  Cottage Doubles Raspberry Lowfat
    Cottage Cheese & Topping
  Cottage Doubles Strawberry Lowfat
    Cottage Cheese & Topping
  Large Curd Lowfat 2% Milkfat Cottage
    Cheese
  Large Curd Smooth & Creamy 4%
    Milkfat Min Cottage Cheese
  Liveactive Lowfat with Mixed Berries
    Cottage Cheese
  Liveactive Lowfat with Pineapple
    Cottage Cheese
  Small Curd 2% Milkfat Low Fat Cottage
    Cheese
  Small Curd 4% Milkfat Min Cottage
    Cheese
  Small Curd Fat Free Cottage Cheese

  Small Curd Low Fat with Pineapple
    Cottage Cheese
  Small Curd Smooth & Creamy 4%
    Milkfat Min Cottage Cheese
Cabot
  Cabot's Products (All)
Creamland Dairies ()
  Cottage Cheese
Crowley Foods 🛡
  Cottage Cheese
Daisy Brand 🛡
  Cottage Cheese
Darigold
  Darigold (All)
Friendship Dairies 🛡
  Friendship Products (All)
Giant
  Cottage Cheese - Low Fat ()
  Cottage Cheese - No Salt Added ()
  Cottage Cheese - Nonfat ()
  Cottage Cheese - Pineapple ()
  Cottage Cheese - Regular ()
Great Value (Wal-Mart)
  1% Lowfat Small Curd Cottage Cheese
  2% Lowfat Small Curd Cottage Cheese
  2% Small Curd Cottage Cheese
  4% Large Curd Cottage Cheese
  4% Small Curd Cottage Cheese
  Fat Free Small Curd Cottage Cheese
Hood
  Cottage Cheese (All)
Hy-Vee
  4% Large Curd Cottage Cheese
  4% Small Curd Cottage Cheese
Knudsen ᔐ
  Cottage Doubles Apples & Cinnamon
    Lowfat Cottage Cheese & Topping
  Cottage Doubles Blueberry Lowfat
    Cottage Cheese & Topping
  Cottage Doubles Peach Lowfat Cottage
    Cheese & Topping
  Cottage Doubles Pineapple Lowfat
    Cottage Cheese & Topping
  Cottage Doubles Raspberry Lowfat
    Cottage Cheese & Topping

Cottage Doubles Strawberry Lowfat
   Cottage Cheese & Topping
Free Nonfat Cottage Cheese
Free Nonfat Cottage Cheese On The Go
Liveactive Lowfat with Mixed Berries
   Cottage Cheese
Liveactive Lowfat with Pineapple
   Cottage Cheese
Lowfat & Pineapple Cottage Cheese
Single Serve Lowfat Cottage Cheese On
   The Go
Small Curd 4% Milkfat Min Cottage
   Cheese
Small Curd Lowfat 2% Milkfat Cottage
   Cheese
Small Curd Lowfat Cottage Cheese

Light n' Lively ∾
Fat Free Cottage Cheese
Lowfat Cottage Cheese
Lowfat Snack Size Cottage Cheese

Lucerne (Safeway)
Cottage Cheese (All BUT Fruit Added)

Midwest Country Fare (Hy-Vee)
1% Small Curd Cottage Cheese
4% Small Curd Cottage Cheese

Nancy's ⚇
Nancy's Products (All)

Penn Maid ⚇
Cottage Cheese

Publix ()
Fat Free (All Styles and Flavors)
Large Curd, 4% Milkfat (All Styles &
   Flavors)
Low Fat (All Styles & Flavors)
Low Fat with Pineapple
Small Curd, 4% Milkfat (All Styles &
   Flavors)

Purity Dairies
Milk and Cultured Products (All)

Shamrock Farms
Cottage Cheese

Stop & Shop
Cottage Cheese - Calcium Added ()
Cottage Cheese - Lowfat ()
Cottage Cheese - Nonfat with Pineapple ()

CREAM

Creamland Dairies ()
Whipping Cream
Giant
20% Light Whipping Cream
Heavy Whipping Cream
Great Value (Wal-Mart)
Heavy Whipping Cream
Light Cream
Hood
Creams (All)
Kroger ⓘ
Whipping Cream
Lucerne (Safeway)
Whipping Cream - Heavy
Whipping Cream - Light
Whipping Cream - Regular
Meijer
Ultra Pasteurized Heavy Whipping
   Cream
Publix ()
Heavy Whipping Cream
Whipping Cream
Purity Dairies
Milk and Cultured Products (All)
Stop & Shop
Heavy Whipping Cream
Light Cream
Whipping Cream
Straus Family Creamery ⚇
Cream (All)
Winn-Dixie ⓘ
Heavy Cream

CREAM CHEESE

Breakstone's ∾
Temptee Whipped Cream Cheese
Crystal Farms
Cream Cheese (All Flavors and
   Varieties)
Giant
Cream Cheese - Fat Free ()
Cream Cheese - Garden Vegetable ()
Cream Cheese - Lite ()

Cream Cheese - Regular ()
Cream Cheese - Sour Cream & Chive ()
Cream Cheese - Strawberry ()
Cream Cheese - Whipped ()

Great Value (Wal-Mart)

Chive & Onion Cream Cheese Spread
Cream Cheese Brick
Cream Cheese Spread
Fat Free Cream Cheese Brick
Light Cream Cheese
Strawberry Cream Cheese Spread
Whipped Cream Cheese Spread

Hy-Vee

1/3 Less Fat Than Cream Cheese
Blueberry Cream Cheese
Cream Cheese
Fat Free Cream Cheese
Fat Free Soft Cream Cheese
Fat Free Strawberry Cream Cheese
Garden Vegetable Cream Cheese
Onion/Chive Cream Cheese
Soft Cream Cheese
Soft Light Cream Cheese
Strawberry Cream Cheese
Whipped Cream Cheese Spread

Kroger ⓘ

Cream Cheeses

Lucerne (Safeway)

Cream Cheese - Fat Free
Cream Cheese - Garden Vegetable
Cream Cheese - Light
Cream Cheese - Neufchatel
Cream Cheese - Onion/Chive
Cream Cheese - Soft Bars
Cream Cheese - Strawberry
Cream Cheese - Whipped Spread

Nancy's 🍷

Nancy's Products (All)

Nature's Promise (Giant)

Organic Cream Cheese ()

Nature's Promise (Stop & Shop)

Organic Cream Cheese ()

Philadelphia Cream Cheese 〰

Blueberry Cream Cheese
Cheesecake Cream Cheese Spread
Chive & Onion Cream Cheese Spread
Chive & Onion Light Cream Cheese

Fat Free Cream Cheese
Garden Vegetable Cream Cheese
Honey Nut Cream Cheese
Light Cream Cheese
Light Garden Vegetable Cream Cheese
Neufchatel 1/3 Less Fat Cream Cheese
Original Cream Cheese
Peaches 'n Cream Cream Swirls Cream
    Cheese
Pineapple Cream Cheese
Raspberry Cream Cheese Spread
Regular Cream Cheese
Regular Cream Cheese Spread Original
Regular Whipped Cream Cheese
Roasted Garlic Light Cream Cheese
Salmon Cream Cheese
Strawberry Cream Cheese
Strawberry Fat Free Cream Cheese
Strawberry Light Cream Cheese
Whipped Cinnamon 'n Brown Sugar
    Cream Cheese
Whipped Cream Cheese
Whipped Garlic 'n Herb Cream Cheese
Whipped Mixed Berry Cream Cheese
Whipped Ranch Cream Cheese
Whipped with Chives Cream Cheese

Publix ()

Fat Free (All Styles)
Light - Soft (All Flavors)
Neufchatel
Regular
Regular - Soft (All Flavors)

Simply Enjoy (Giant)

Smoked Salmon Dill Sandwich Spread

Simply Enjoy (Stop & Shop)

Smoked Salmon Dill Sandwich Spread

Stop & Shop

Cream Cheese - Chive & Onion (Lite,
    Regular & Whipped) ()
Cream Cheese - Garden Vegetable (Lite,
    Regular & Whipped) ()
Cream Cheese - Honey Walnut (Lite,
    Regular & Whipped) ()
Cream Cheese - Plain (Lite, Regular &
    Whipped) ()
Cream Cheese - Strawberry (Lite,
    Regular & Whipped) ()

Fat Free Cream Cheese ◯
Neufchatel Cheese ◯

Ukrop's
Cream Cheese and Olive Spread (Deli)

Vegan Gourmet ⓘ ☷
Cream Cheese Alternative

Winn-Dixie ⓘ
Soft Cream Cheese with Strawberries

EGG SUBSTITUTES

All Whites
All Whites (All)

Better'n Eggs
Better'n Eggs (All)

Better'n Eggs Plus
Better'n Eggs Plus (All)

Ener-G ☷
Egg Replacer

Giant
100% Egg Whites
Eggs Made Simple

Hy-Vee
Egg Substitute (Refrigerated)

Lucerne (Safeway)
Best of The Egg

Meijer
Egg Substitute (Refrigerated)

Orgran ☷
Orgran (All)

Publix ◯
Egg Stirs

ReddiEgg
ReddiEgg No Fat No Cholesterol Real
Egg Product (All)

Stop & Shop
100% Egg Whites
Eggs Made Simple

EGGNOG & OTHER NOGS

Creamland Dairies ◯
Eggnog

Eagle Brand
EggNog

Hood
Cinnamon Eggnog
Gingerbread Eggnog
Golden Eggnog
Light Eggnog
Pumpkin Eggnog
Sugar Cookie Eggnog
Vanilla Eggnog

Kroger ⓘ
Eggnog - Liquid
Eggnog - Powdered

Lucerne (Safeway)
Egg Nog (All varieties)

Publix ◯
Low Fat Egg Nog
Original Egg Nog

Purity Dairies
Milk and Cultured Products (All)

Stop & Shop
Egg Nog - Light
Egg Nog - Regular

Turkey Hill ⓘ
Drink Products (All)

HALF & HALF

Creamland Dairies ◯
Half and Half

Darigold
Darigold (All)

Giant
Half & Half - Fat Free
Half & Half - Regular

Great Value (Wal-Mart)
Half & Half

Hood
Simply Smart Fat Free Half & Half

Lucerne (Safeway)
Half & Half - Fat Free
Half & Half - Light
Half & Half - Regular

Meijer
Ultra Pasteurized Heavy Half & Half

Publix ◯
Fat Free Half & Half
Half & Half

Purity Dairies
Milk and Cultured Products (All)
Shamrock Farms
Fat Free French Vanilla Half & Half
Fat Free Half & Half
Fat Free Hazelnut Half & Half
Stop & Shop
Half & Half - Fat Free
Half & Half - Regular

HUMMUS

Athenos ⬳
Artichoke & Garlic Hummus
Black Olive Hummus
Cucumber Dill Hummus
Greek Style with Lemon Garlic &
Oregano Hummus
Neo Classic Original Hummus
Neo Classic Original with Sesame Seeds
& Parsley Hummus
Neo Classic Roasted Garlic with Garlic
& Parsley Hummus
Neo Classic Roasted Red Pepper with
Red Peppers & Parsley Hummus
Original Hummus
Pesto Hummus
Roasted Eggplant Hummus
Roasted Garlic Hummus
Roasted Red Pepper Hummus
Scallion Hummus
Spicy Three Pepper Hummus
Cedar's Mediterranean Foods
Hummus Varieties (All)
Emerald Valley Kitchen
Emerald Valley Kitchen (All)
Fantastic World Foods
Original Hummus
Garden Fresh Gourmet ⌇
Hummus (All)
Tribe Hummus
Hummus - All Natural (All)
Hummus - Organic (All)

MARGARINE & SPREADS

Benecol
Benecol Spreads (All)
Brummel & Brown
Margarine (All)
Spreads (All)
Canoleo
Canoleo
Country Crock
Spread and Spreadable Butter Products
(All)
Crystal Farms
Margarine and Spreads (All Types)
Earth Balance ()
Original Spread
Giant
48% Margarine Spread
Great Value (Wal-Mart)
48% Vegetable Oil Soft Spread
Margarine Quarters
Hy-Vee
100% Corn Oil Margarine
Best Thing Since Butter
Rich & Creamy Soft Margarine
Soft Margarine
Soft Spread
Vegetable Margarine Quarters
I Can't Believe It's Not Butter!
Margarine and Spread Products (All)
Kroger ⓘ
Margarine
Vegetable Spreads
Meijer
Margarine Corn Oil Quarters
Margarine Soft Sleeve
Margarine Soft Tub
Spread 48% Crock
Spread 70% Quarters
Spread No Ifs Ands Or Butter
Promise
Margarine and Spread Products (All)
Publix ()
Corn Oil Margarine Quarters
Homestyle Spread - 48% Vegetable Oil
Homestyle Squeeze Spread - 60%
Vegetable Oil

It Tastes Just Like Butter Spread - 70%
Vegetable Oil
Original Spread Quarters - 70%
Vegetable Oil

Safeway
Light Homestyle Spread
Margarine
Vegetable Oil Spreads - 70%, 37% Light
& 70% 1/4 Lb Sticks (Homestyle)

Smart Balance
Smart Balance (All)

MILK, CHOCOLATE & FLAVORED

Creamland Dairies ()
Chocolate Milk

Giant
1% Low Fat Chocolate Milk

Great Value (Wal-Mart)
1% Lowfat Chocolate Milk
1/2% Lowfat Chocolate Milk
2% Chocolate Milk

Hood
Calorie Countdown Dairy Beverages
(All Flavors & Fat Levels)
Chocolate Milk - Full Fat (All Sizes)
Chocolate Milk - Low Fat (All Sizes)
Simply Smart Fat Free Chocolate Milk

Lucerne (Safeway)
Chocolate Milk

Meijer
1% Chocolate Milk Lowfat
1% Chocolate Milk Lowfat No Sugar
Added
Chocolate Milk
Strawberry Milk

Nesquik
Ready-to-Drink Milk (All Flavors)

Publix ()
Chocolate Milk
Low Fat Chocolate Milk

Purity Dairies
Milk and Cultured Products (All)

Rosenberger's Dairies
Milk

Safeway
Milk Drinks - Chillin Chocolate
Milk Drinks - Marvelous
Milk Drinks - Mocha Cappuccino
Milk Drinks - Vanilla Shake
Milk Drinks - Very Berry Strawberry

Shamrock Farms
Chocolate Milk
Dulce de Leche Milkshake
Strawberry Milkshake
Vanilla Milkshake

Silk
Silk Soymilk (All)

Turkey Hill ⓘ
Drink Products (All)

MILK, LACTOSE-FREE

Giant
Lactose Free Milk - Calcium Added
Lactose Free Milk - Skim
Lactose Free Milk - Whole

Lactaid ✓
Calcium Fortified Milk
Chocolate Milk

Lucerne (Safeway)
Lactose Free Fat Free Milk

Meijer
Lactose Free Milk 2% with Calcium
Lactose Free Milk Fat Free with Calcium

Stop & Shop
Lactose Free Milk - Calcium Fortified
Fat Free
Lactose Free Milk - Whole

Winn-Dixie ⓘ
Reduce Fat Lactose Free Milk

SOUR CREAM

Axelrod ♒
Sour Cream

Breakstone's ⌒
All Natural Sour Cream
Free Fat Free Sour Cream
Grade A Pasteurized Homogenized Sour
Cream

Reduced Fat Sour Cream

Cabot
Cabot's Products (All)

Cascade Fresh
Cascade Fresh (All)

Creamland Dairies
Sour Cream

Crowley Foods
Sour Cream

Daisy Brand
Sour Cream

Darigold
Darigold (All)

Friendship Dairies
Friendship Products (All)

Giant
Sour Cream - Lite
Sour Cream - Nonfat

Great Value (Wal-Mart)
Fat Free Sour Cream
Light Sour Cream
Sour Cream

Hood
Sour Cream (All)

Hy-Vee
Light Sour Cream
Sour Cream

Knudsen
Fat Free Sour Cream
Hampshire 100% Natural Sour Cream
Hampshire Sour Cream
Light Sour Cream

Kroger ⓘ
Sour Cream

Lucerne (Safeway)
Sour Cream - Low Fat
Sour Cream - Non Fat
Sour Cream - Regular

Nancy's
Nancy's Products (All)

Penn Maid
Sour Cream

Publix
Fat Free Sour Cream (All Styles)
Light Sour Cream (All Styles)
Regular Sour Cream (All Styles)

Purity Dairies
Milk and Cultured Products (All)

Stop & Shop
Sour Cream - Light
Sour Cream - Nonfat

Tillamook
Sour Cream (All)

Vegan Gourmet ⓘ
Sour Cream Alternative

SOYMILK & MILK ALTERNATIVES

Almond Dream ✔
Original
Unsweetened Original

Blue Diamond Growers
Almond Breeze Non-Dairy Almond Milk ⓘ

Eden Foods ⓘ ✔
EdenBlend - Organic
Edensoy Unsweetened - Organic

Great Value (Wal-Mart)
Chocolate Soymilk
Original Soymilk
Vanilla Soymilk

HealthMarket (Hy-Vee)
Organic Chocolate Soy Milk
Organic Original Soy Milk
Organic Vanilla Soy Milk

Hy-Vee
Chocolate Soy Milk
Chocolate Soymilk (Refrigerated)
Enriched Original Rice Milk
Enriched Vanilla Rice Milk
Original Soy Milk
Original Soy Milk (Refrigerated)
Vanilla Soy Milk
Vanilla Soy Milk (Refrigerated)

Kroger ⓘ
Rice Drink - Plain
Rice Drink - Vanilla
Soy Drink- Plain
Soy Drink- Vanilla

Nature's Promise (Giant)
Ricemilk - Plain
Ricemilk - Vanilla

Soymilk - Chocolate
Soymilk - Plain
Soymilk - Vanilla

Nature's Promise (Stop & Shop)
Chocolate Soymilk
Organic Soymilk - Chocolate
Organic Soymilk - Plain
Organic Soymilk - Vanilla
Ricemilk - Plain
Ricemilk - Vanilla

Pacific Natural Foods ⓘ
Hazelnut - Original
Low Fat Rice - Plain
Low Fat Rice - Vanilla
Organic Almond Chocolate
Organic Low-Fat Almond - Original
Organic Low-Fat Almond - Vanilla
Organic Soy - Unsweetened
Organic Unsweetened Almond Vanilla
Select Soy - Low-Fat Plain
Select Soy - Low-Fat Vanilla
Ultra Soy - Plain
Ultra Soy - Vanilla

Publix GreenWise Market ()
Soy Milk - Chocolate
Soy Milk - Plain
Soy Milk - Vanilla

Rice Dream ✓
Classic Carob
Classic Original
Classic Vanilla
Enriched Chocolate
Enriched Original
Enriched Vanilla
Heartwise Original
Heartwise Vanilla
Horchata
Supreme - Chocolate Chai
Supreme - Vanilla Hazelnut

Safeway
Select - Organic Soy Beverage
Select - Organic Vanilla Soy Beverage
   (Low Fat)

Silk
Silk Soymilk (All)

Soy Dream ✓
Chocolate Enriched

Original
Original Enriched
Vanilla
Vanilla Enriched

Vitasoy
Fiber Fortified Unsweeteened
Fiber Fortififed Sweet
Fortified Sweet Soymilk
Fortified Unsweetened Soymilk
Sweetened Soymilk

WestSoy ✓
Lite Plain
Lite Vanilla
Non Fat Plain
Non Fat Vanilla
Organic Original
Plus Plain
Plus Vanilla
Rice Plain
Rice Vanilla
Shake Chocolate
Soy Slender Chocolate
Unsweetened Almond
Unsweetened Chocolate

ZenSoy
ZenSoy Products (All)

WHIPPED TOPPINGS

Cabot
Cabot's Products (All)

Cool Whip ⌇
Extra Creamy Whipped Topping
Lite Whipped Topping
Regular Whipped Topping

Crystal Farms
Aerosol Whip Cream

Dream Whip ⌇
Regular Whipped Topping Mix

Giant
Sweetened Whipped Light Cream

Great Value (Wal-Mart)
Aerosol Extra Creamy Sweetened
   Whipped Cream
Aerosol Sweetened Whipped Light
   Cream

Hood
Instant Whipped Cream
Sugar Free Light Whipped Cream

Hy-Vee
Real Whipped Cream
Real Whipped Lite Cream

Lucerne (Safeway)
Aerosol Whipping Cream - Light & Non Dairy

Meijer
Ultra Pasteurized Non Dairy (Aerosol)
Ultra Pasteurized Whip Cream (Aerosol)

Publix ()
Whipped Heavy Cream (Aerosol Can)
Whipped Light Cream (Aerosol Can)
Whipped Topping - Fat Free (Aerosol Can)

Soyatoo! ()
Rice Whip (All)
Soy Whip (All)

Stop & Shop
Sweetened Whipped Light Cream

YOGURT

Axelrod ⅄
Yogurt

Brown Cow ✓
Yogurts (All BUT Fruit & Whole Grains)

Cabot
Cabot's Products (All)

Cascade Fresh
Cascade Fresh (All)

Crowley Foods ⅄
Yogurt

Dannon ()
Plain Activia (24 ounce container)
Plain Lowfat
Plain Natural
Plain Nonfat

Darigold
Darigold (All)

Fage Total Yogurt ⅄
Fage Total Yogurt (All)

Friendship Dairies ⅄
Friendship Products (All)

Giant
Grab'Ums Yogurt To Go - Cotton Candy/Melon ()
Grab'Ums Yogurt To Go - Strawberry/Blueberry ()
Grab'Ums Yogurt To Go - Tropical Punch/Raspberry ()
Lowfat Blended - Blueberry ()
Lowfat Blended - Cherry ()
Lowfat Blended - Peach ()
Lowfat Blended - Raspberry ()
Lowfat Blended - Strawberry ()
Lowfat Blended - Strawberry-Banana ()
Lowfat Blended - Vanilla ()
Lowfat Fruit on the Bottom - Blueberry ()
Lowfat Fruit on the Bottom - Boysenberry ()
Lowfat Fruit on the Bottom - Cherry ()
Lowfat Fruit on the Bottom - Lemon ()
Lowfat Fruit on the Bottom - Mixed Berry ()
Lowfat Fruit on the Bottom - Pineapple ()
Lowfat Fruit on the Bottom - Raspberry ()
Lowfat Fruit on the Bottom - Strawberry ()
Lowfat Fruit on the Bottom - Strawberry/Banana ()
Lowfat Plain ()
Lowfat Vanilla ()
Nonfat Light - Banana ()
Nonfat Light - Blueberry ()
Nonfat Light - Caramel ()
Nonfat Light - Cherry ()
Nonfat Light - Cherry Vanilla ()
Nonfat Light - Coffee ()
Nonfat Light - Raspberry ()
Nonfat Light - Strawberry ()
Nonfat Light - Strawberry/Banana ()
Nonfat Light - Vanilla ()
Nonfat Plain ()

Glenoaks Yogurt
Drinkable Yogurt (All Flavors)

Great Value (Wal-Mart)
Benefit Blueberry Probiotic Light Nonfat Yogurt (4 Pack)

Benefit Peach Probiotic Light Nonfat Yogurt (4 Pack)

Benefit Raspberry Probiotic Light Nonfat Yogurt (4 Pack)

Benefit Strawberry Probiotic Light Nonfat Yogurt (4 Pack)

Benefit Vanilla Probiotic Light Nonfat Yogurt (4 Pack)

Blended Banana Yogurt

Blended Black Cherry Lowfat Yogurt

Blended Blueberry Lowfat Yogurt

Blended Cherry Vanilla Lowfat Yogurt

Blended Key Lime Lowfat Yogurt

Blended Mango Lowfat Yogurt

Blended Mixed Berry Lowfat Yogurt

Blended Peach Lowfat Yogurt

Blended Pina Colada Lowfat Yogurt

Blended Raspberry Lowfat Yogurt

Blended Strawberry Banana Lowfat Yogurt

Blended Strawberry Lowfat Yogurt

Blended Vanilla Lowfat Yogurt

Fat Free Plain Nonfat Yogurt

Light Banana Cream Nonfat Yogurt

Light Banana Cream Pie Nonfat Yogurt

Light Black Cherry Nonfat Yogurt

Light Blueberry Nonfat Yogurt

Light Lemon Chiffon Nonfat Yogurt

Light Mixed Berry Nonfat Yogurt

Light Peach Nonfat Yogurt

Light Raspberry Nonfat Yogurt

Light Strawberry Banana Nonfat Yogurt

Light Strawberry Nonfat Yogurt

Light Vanilla Nonfat Yogurt

Hy-Vee

Banana Cream Non Fat Yogurt

Black Cherry Low Fat Yogurt

Blueberry Low Fat Yogurt

Blueberry Non Fat Yogurt

Cherry Non Fat Yogurt

Cherry-Vanilla Low Fat Yogurt

Fat Free Plain Yogurt

Key Lime Pie Fat Free Yogurt

Lemon Chiffon Non Fat Yogurt

Lemon Low Fat Yogurt

Mixed Berry Low Fat Yogurt

Non Fat Vanilla Yogurt

Peach Non Fat Yogurt

Peach Yogurt

Plain Low Fat Yogurt

Raspberry Low Fat Yogurt

Raspberry Non Fat Yogurt

Strawberry Banana Low Fat Yogurt

Strawberry Banana Non Fat Yogurt

Strawberry Low Fat Yogurt

Strawberry Non Fat Yogurt

Yogurt To Go - Strawberry

Yogurt To Go - Strawberry & Blueberry

Yogurt To Go - Strawberry/Banana & Cherry

La Yogurt ()

Plain - Fat Free

Plain - Low Fat

Plain - Whole Milk

Lifeway ⚱

Lifeway Products (All BUT Probiotic Wellness Bars)

Lucerne (Safeway)

Fat Free Yogurt (All Varieties)

Pre-Stirred Low Fat Yogurt (All Varieties)

Yo-Cups (All Varieties)

Yo-On-The-Go (All Varieties)

Meijer

Blended Boysenberry

Blended Strawberry

Blended Strawberry-Banana

Blended Tropical Fruit

Fruit/Bottom Blueberry

Fruit/Bottom Peach

Fruit/Bottom Raspberry

Fruit/Bottom Strawberry

Lite Banana Crème

Lite Black Cherry

Lite Blueberry

Lite Cherry-Vanilla

Lite Coconut Cream

Lite Lemon Chiffon

Lite Mint Chocolate

Lite Peach

Lite Raspberry

Lite Strawberry

Lite Strawberry-Banana

Lite Vanilla

Lowfat Blended Blueberry
Lowfat Blended Cherry
Lowfat Blended Mixed Berry
Lowfat Blended Peach
Lowfat Blended Pina Colada
Lowfat Blended Raspberry
Lowfat Vanilla
Tube-Yo-Lar Strw/Blue
Tube-Yo-Lar Troppnch/Rasp
Tube-Yo-Lar Wtr/Strw/Ban

Nancy's
Nancy's Products (All)

Old Chatham Sheepherding Company
Old Chatham Sheepherding Company (All)

Penn Maid
Yogurt

Publix
Apple Pie Light - Fat Free Yogurt
Banana Crème Pie Light - Fat Free Yogurt
Banana Fruit On The Bottom Yogurt
Black Cherry Creamy Blend Yogurt
Black Cherry Fruit On The Bottom Yogurt
Black Cherry with Chocolate - Limited Edition
Blackberry Fruit On The Bottom Yogurt
Blueberry - No Sugar Added Yogurt
Blueberry Creamy Blend Yogurt
Blueberry Fruit On The Bottom Yogurt
Blueberry Light - Fat Free Yogurt
Cappuccino Light - Fat Free Yogurt
Caramel Crème Light - Fat Free Yogurt
Cherry Fruit On The Bottom Yogurt
Cherry Light - Fat Free Yogurt
Cherry Vanilla Light - Fat Free Yogurt
Coconut Crème Pie Light - Fat Free Yogurt
Cranberry Raspberry - No Sugar Added Yogurt
Creamy Blends Black Cherry & Mixed Berry - Multi Pack
Creamy Blends Blueberry & Strawberry Banana - Multi Pack
Creamy Blends Peach and Strawberry - Multi Pack

Egg Nog - Limited Edition
Fat Free Light "Active" Peach Yogurt
Fat Free Light "Active" Strawberry Yogurt
Fat Free Light "Active" Vanilla Yogurt
Fat Free Plain Yogurt
Guava Fruit On The Bottom Yogurt
Honey Almond Light - Fat Free Yogurt
Key Lime Pie Light - Fat Free Yogurt
Kids Blue Raspberry & Cotton Candy - Multi Pack
Kids Grape Bubblegum & Watermelon - Multi Pack
Kids Strawberry & Blueberry - Multi Pack
Kids Strawberry Banana & Cherry - Multi Pack
Lemon Chiffon Light - Fat Free Yogurt
Mandarin Orange Light - Fat Free Yogurt
Mango Fruit On The Bottom Yogurt
Mixed Berry Fruit On The Bottom Yogurt
Peach - No Sugar Added Yogurt
Peach Creamy Blend Yogurt
Peach Fruit On The Bottom Yogurt
Peach Light - Fat Free Yogurt
Piña Colada Light - Fat Free Yogurt
Pineapple Fruit On The Bottom Yogurt
Pumpkin Pie - Limited Edition
Raspberry Fruit On The Bottom Yogurt
Raspberry Light - Fat Free Yogurt
Strawberry - No Sugar Added Yogurt
Strawberry Creamy Blend Yogurt
Strawberry Fruit On The Bottom Yogurt
Strawberry Light - Fat Free Yogurt
Strawberry with Chocolate - Limited Edition
Strawberry/Banana Fruit On The Bottom Yogurt
Strawberry/Banana Light - Fat Free Yogurt
Tropical Blend Fruit On The Bottom Yogurt
Vanilla - No Sugar Added Yogurt
Vanilla Creamy Blend Yogurt
Vanilla Light - Fat Free Yogurt

Redwood Hill Farm
Yogurts (All)

Silk
Silk Live! Soy Yogurt (All)

Skyr.is
Blueberry
Plain
Vanilla

Stonyfield Farm
Soy Yogurts (All BUT Frozen Yogurt, Oikos Greek Yogurt, YoBaby Plus Fruit & Cereal and YoKids Squeezers)
Yogurts (All BUT Frozen Yogurt, Oikos Greek Yogurt, YoBaby Plus Fruit & Cereal and YoKids Squeezers)

Stop & Shop
Grab'Ums Yogurt To Go - Cotton Candy/Melon ()
Grab'Ums Yogurt To Go - Strawberry/ Blueberry ()
Grab'Ums Yogurt To Go - Tropical Punch/Raspberry ()
Lowfat Blended Blueberry ()
Lowfat Blended Peach ()
Lowfat Blended Raspberry ()
Lowfat Blended Strawberry ()
Lowfat Blended Vanilla ()
Lowfat Fruit On The Bottom - Blueberry ()
Lowfat Fruit On The Bottom - Peach ()
Lowfat Fruit On The Bottom - Raspberry ()
Lowfat Fruit On The Bottom - Strawberry ()
Lowfat Fruit On The Bottom - Strawberry/Banana ()
Nonfat Light Banana ()
Nonfat Light Blueberry ()
Nonfat Light Cherry ()
Nonfat Light Cherry Vanilla ()
Nonfat Light Coffee ()
Nonfat Light Peach ()
Nonfat Light Raspberry ()
Nonfat Light Strawberry ()
Nonfat Light Strawberry/Banana ()
Nonfat Light Vanilla ()
Nonfat Plain ()

Straus Family Creamery ⅄
Yogurt (All)

Tillamook
Yogurt (All)

Wallaby Yogurt Company ⅄
Yogurt (All)

WholeSoy & Co. ⓘ ✔
Apricot Mango Soy Yogurt
Blueberry Soy Yogurt
Cherry Soy Yogurt
Lemon Soy Yogurt
Mixed Berry Soy Yogurt
Peach Soy Yogurt
Plain Soy Yogurt
Raspberry Soy Yogurt
Strawberry Banana Soy Yogurt
Strawberry Soy Yogurt
Vanilla Soy Yogurt

MISCELLANEOUS

Lifeway ⅄
Lifeway Products (All BUT Probiotic Wellness Bars)

Nasoya
Silken Creations Dark Chocolate
Silken Creations Strawberry
Silken Creations Vanilla

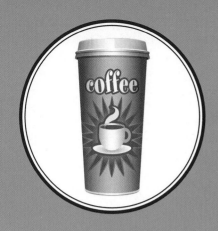

BEVERAGES

BEER

Bard's Tale Beer ✓
  Bard's Gold
Green's ✓
  Discovery Amber Ale
  Endeavour Dubbel Ale
  Quest Tripel Ale
Lakefront Brewery ⓘ ✓
  New Grist

Redbridge ⓘ
  Redbridge Beer
Sprecher Brewing Co. ✓
  Mbege
  Shakparo

CARBONATED DRINKS

7Up
  7Up (All)

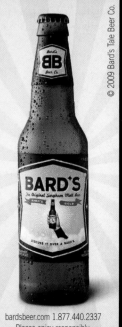

A&W
A&W (All)

Adirondack Beverages
Adirondack Beverages (All)

Barq's
Barq's Root Beer
Caffeine Free Barq's Root Beer
Diet Barq's Red Crème Soda
Diet Barq's Root Beer

Boylan Bottling Co.
Boylan Products (All)

Canada Dry
Canada Dry (All)

Coca-Cola Company, The
Caffeine Free Coca-Cola Classic
Caffeine Free Diet Coke
Cherry Coke
Cherry Coke Zero
Coca-Cola
Coca-Cola Zero
Diet Cherry Coke
Diet Coke
Diet Coke Plus
Diet Coke Sweetened with Splenda
Diet Coke with Lime
Vanilla Coke
Vanilla Coke Zero

Crush
Crush (All)

Diet Rite
Diet Rite (All)

Dr. Pepper
Dr. Pepper (All)

Fanta
Grape
Orange Zero

Fresca
Fresca

Hansen's
Hansen's (All)

Hires
Hires (All)

Hy-Vee
Cherry Cola
Club Soda
Cola
Diet Cola
Diet Dr. Hy-Vee
Diet Orange
Dr. Hy-Vee
Gingerale
Grape
Heee Haw
Lemon Lime
Orange
Root Beer
Seltzer Water
Sour
Strawberry
Tonic Water

IBC
IBC (All)

Izze
Izze Products (All)

Knouse Foods
Sparkling Apple Cider

Kroger
Big K Soft Drinks

Martinelli's
Martinelli's (All)

Meijer
Diet Caffeine-Free Encore Red
Diet Cherry Encore
Diet Encore Blue
Diet Encore Red
Encore Blue
Encore Cherry Red
Encore Red
Red Pop

Mountain Dew
Carbonated Beverages (ALL)

Mug
Carbonated Beverages (All)

Nutrisoda
Nutrisoda (All)

Pepsi
Carbonated Beverages (All)

Publix
Black Cherry Soda
Cherry Cola
Citrus Hit Soda
Club Soda

Cola
Cream Soda
Diet Cola
Diet Ginger Ale
Diet Tonic Water
Ginger Ale
Grape Soda
Lemon Lime Seltzer
Lemon Lime Soda
Orange Soda
Raspberry Seltzer
Root Beer
Tonic Water

RC Cola
RC Cola (All)

Reed's
Apple Ginger Brew
Cherry Ginger Brew
Extra Ginger Brew
Original Ginger Brew
Premium Ginger Brew
Raspberry Ginger Brew

Safeway
Select - Sodas (All Varieties)

Santa Cruz Organic
Santa Cruz Organic (All)

Schweppes
Schweppes (All)

Shasta
Shasta (All Flavors)

Sierra Mist ⅋
Carbonated Beverages (All)

Sonoma Sparkler
Sonoma Sparkler

Sprecher Brewing Co. ✓
Cherry Cola Soda
Cream Soda
Gingerale Soda
Lo-Cal Rootbeer Soda
Orange Cream Soda
Puma Kola Soda
Ravin' Red Soda
Rootbeer Soda

Sprite
Diet Sprite Zero
Sprite

Squirt
Squirt (All)

Stewart's
Stewart's (All)

Stop & Shop
100% Natural Sparkling Apple Juice
(Shelf Stable)

Sundrop
Sundrop (All)

Sunkist
Sunkist (All)

Tropicana Twister Soda ⅋
Tropicana Twister Sodas (All)

Vernors
Vernors (All)

Virgil's
Black Cherry Cream Soda & Diet
Cream Soda & Diet
Orange Cream Soda
Real Cola & Diet
Root Beer & Diet

Welch's
Welch's (All)

CHOCOLATE DRINKS

Yoo-hoo
Yoo-hoo (All)

CIDER (ALCOHOLIC)

Ace Cider ⅋ ✓
Ace Cider (All)

Cider Jack ⅋ ✓
Cider Jack

Fox Barrel ✓
Black Currant Cider
Hard Apple Cider
Pear Cider

J.K. Scrumpy's Orchard Gate Gold
Cider

Magners Irish Cider
Magners Irish Cider

Original Sin Hard Cider
Original Sin Hard Cider

Samuel Smith's Organic Cider
Samuel Smith's Organic Cider

Strongbow ✓
Strongbow

Woodchuck Draft Cider ¥ ✓
Woodchuck Draft Cider - Amber
Woodchuck Draft Cider - Dark & Dry
  802
Woodchuck Draft Cider - Granny Smith
Woodchuck Draft Cider - Pear
Woodchuck Draft Cider - Raspberry

Woodpecker Cider ¥ ✓
Woodpecker

Wyder's Cider ¥ ✓
Wyder's Hard Cider - Apple
Wyder's Hard Cider - Pear
Wyder's Hard Cider - Raspberry

COFFEE DRINKS & MIXES

Caffe D'vita ()
Caffe D'vita (All)

Caribou
Iced Coffee

Chock Full O' Nuts
Coffee Products (All)

DeLallo
Café Espresso
Café Espresso Decaf

Dunkin' Donuts
Coffee (All)

Eight O'Clock Coffee
Coffee (All)

Folgers ¥
Coffees (All)

General Foods International Coffees ᕦ
Café Francais
Café Francais - Dark Mayan Chocolate
Café Francais - French Vanilla Café
Café Francais - Peppermint Mocha
  Limited Edition
Café Francais - Pumpkin Spice
Café Vienna
Café Vienna - Sugar Free
Cappuccino - Café Mocha 100 Calorie
  Packs

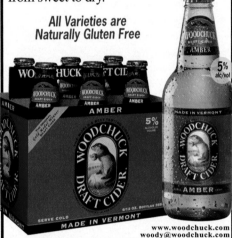

WOODCHUCK
—DRAFT CIDER—

Woodchuck Draft Ciders are handcrafted in small batches at our cidery nestled within the Green Mountains of Vermont. Made with a unique combination of nature's best ingredients, Woodchuck is easy to drink with a variety of styles from sweet to dry.

All Varieties are Naturally Gluten Free

5% alc/vol

AMBER

MADE IN VERMONT

www.woodchuck.com
woody@woodchuck.com

Cappuccino - French Vanilla 100
  Calorie Packs
Cappuccino Coolers - French Vanilla
Cappuccino Coolers - Hazelnut
Cappuccino Coolers - On The Go
  Vanilla Latte Sugar Free
Coffee Drink Mix - Crème Caramel
Coffee House Drink Mix - On The Go
  Café Mocha Sugar Free
Coffee House Drink Mix - On The Go
  Hazelnut Cappuccino Sugar Free
French Vanilla Café
French Vanilla Café - Decaffeinated
French Vanilla Café - Decaffeinated
  Sugar Free
French Vanilla Café - Sugar Free
French Vanilla Nut
Hazelnut Belgian Café
Italian Cappuccino
Orange Cappuccino
Suisse Mocha
Suisse Mocha - Decaffeinated Sugar Free
Suisse Mocha - Sugar Free
Swiss White Chocolate

Viennese Chocolate Café

Great Value (Wal-Mart)
100% Arabica Instant Coffee
100% Arabica Premium Ground Coffee
100% Colombian Naturally
   Decaffeinated Premium Ground
   Coffee
100% Colombian Premium Ground
   Coffee
French Roast 100% Arabica Coffee
Naturally Decaffeinated Instant Coffee

Green Mountain Coffee
Coffees (All)

Harvest Farms (Ingles)
Coffee (All)

Hy-Vee
100% Colombian Coffee
Breakfast Blend Coffee
Coffee
Decaffeinated Coffee
Decaffeinated Instant Coffee
French Roast Coffee
Instant Coffee

Illy
Coffee (All)

JavaSoy Coffee
Coffee Products

Kroger ⓘ
Coffee - Instant
Coffee - Unflavored Ground
Coffee - Whole

Laura Lynn (Ingle's)
Coffee (All)

Luzianne
Dark Roast
Decaf
Liquid Flavoring - Raspberry
Medium Roast

Maxwell House
Breakfast Blend Coffee
Café Collection Cappuccino Coffee
Café Collection Decaffeinated Coffee
   Pods
Café Collection French Roast Coffee
   Pods
Café Collection Hazelnut Coffee Pods

Café Collection House Blend Coffee
   Pods
Coffee Singles - Decaffeinated Instant
   Bags
Coffee Singles - Original Singles
Colombian Supreme Ground Coffee
Dark Roast Coffee
French Roast Ground Coffee
French Roast Vacuum Bags Coffee
Hazelnut Flavored Ground Coffee
Instant Original Decaffeinated Coffee
Lite Ground Coffee
Master Blend Decaffeinated Coffee
Master Blend Ground Coffee
Maxwell House Filter Packs Original
   Coffee
Maxwell House Filter Packs Original
   Decaffeinated Coffee
Original Decaffeinated Ground Coffee
Original Ground Coffee
Original Rich Coffee
Slow Roast Coffee
Slow Roast Ground Coffee
Vanilla Coffee

Meijer
Coffee - Colombian Ground
Coffee - Decaf
Coffee - French Roast
Coffee - French Roast Ground
Coffee - Ground Colombian
Coffee - Ground Lite 50%
Coffee - Ground Lite 50% Decaf
Coffee - Regular

Melitta
Coffee (All)

Millstone
Millstone Coffees

Mountain Blend
Instant Coffee

Nescafé
Classic Instant Coffee
Taster's Choice Instant Coffee (Flavored
   & Non-Flavored)

Newman's Own Organics ⓘ
Coffees (All)

POM Wonderful
POMx Iced Coffee

Publix ()
Coffee (All Varieties)

Rogers Family Coffee Company, The ♒
Coffees

Safeway
Coffee - Decaffeinated Classic Roast
Espresso Coffee Beans
Select - Coffee (Creamy Hazelnut)
Select - Coffee Beverage, Instant
Flavored
Select - Whole Bean Coffees, Flavored

Sanka ✍
Naturally Decaffeinated Coffee

Seattle's Best Coffee
Coffee (All BUT Chocolate Toffee,
Cinnabon, Crème Brulee, Hazelnut
Crème, Javanilla & Decaf Javanilla)

Shamrock Farms
Café Mocha

Starbucks ♒
Doubleshot
Doubleshot Energy
Frappuccino
Iced Coffee

Taster's Choice (Nescafé)
Instant Coffee (Flavored & Non-
Flavored)

Taylors of Harrogate ♒
Coffee (All)

Yuban ✍
100% Arabica Hazelnut Single Serve
Pods
100% Colombian Decaffeinated Single
Serve
100% Colombian Single Serve Pods
Organic Rich Medium Roast Coffee
100% Columbian
Original Coffee 100% Columbian

Creamers & Flavorings

Coffee-Mate
Coffee-Mate Liquid (Flavored & Non-
Flavored)
Coffee-Mate Powder (Flavored & Non-
Flavored)

Cremora
Cremora

Giant
Coffee Cream
Nondairy Creamer

Great Value (Wal-Mart)
Coffee Creamer
French Vanilla Coffee Creamer

Hood
Country Creamer

Hy-Vee
Fat Free French Vanilla Coffee Creamer
(Refrigerated)
Fat Free Hazelnut Coffee Creamer
(Refrigerated)
French Vanilla Coffee Creamer
(Refrigerated)
Hazelnut Coffee Creamer (Refrigerated)

International Delight
International Delight

Laura Lynn (Ingle's)
Non-Dairy Coffee Creamers - Dry (All)

Lucerne (Safeway)
Coffee Creamer - French Vanilla
Coffee Creamer - Original
Coffee Creamer - Powdered
French Vanilla Liquid Creamer
Hazelnut Liquid Creamer
Irish Cream Liquid Creamer
Light Non Dairy Creamer

Luzianne
Liquid Flavoring - Peach Mango

Meijer
Ultra Pasteurized Nondairy Creamer

Nescafé
Ice Java Coffee Syrup (All Flavors)

Publix ()
Coffee Creamer
Fat Free Non-Dairy Creamer
Non-Dairy Creamer (Powder)
Non-Dairy French Vanilla Flavored
Creamer (Powder)
Non-Dairy Lite Creamer (Powder)

Shamrock Farms
Half & Half

Silk
Silk Creamer (All)

Stop & Shop
Fat Free Nondairy Creamer

Torani ⓘ
Syrups (All BUT Classic Caramel, Sugar Free Classic Caramel, Sugar Free French Vanilla & Toasted Marshmallow)

DIET & NUTRITIONAL DRINKS

Boost ⚇
Boost Supplement Drinks (All)

Ensure
Shakes (All)

Gatorade ⟨⟩
Nutrition Shakes

Glucerna
Glucerna Shakes (All Flavors)
Glucerna Snack Shakes (All Flavors)

Hy-Vee
Chocolate Nutritional Supplement
Chocolate Nutritional Supplement Plus
Strawberry Nutritional Supplement
Strawberry Nutritional Supplement Plus
Vanilla Nutritional Supplement
Vanilla Nutritional Supplement Plus

Kroger ⓘ
Active Lifestyle Drink Sticks

Meijer
Chocolate Diabetic Nutritional Drink
Diet Quick Chocolate Extra Thin
Diet Quick Strawberry Extra Thin
Diet Quick Vanilla Extra Thin
Gluco-Burst - Chocolate Diabetic Nutritional Drink
Gluco-Burst - Strawberry Diabetic Nutritional Drink
Gluco-Burst - Vanilla Diabetic Nutritional Drink
Strawberry Diabetic Nutritional Drink
Vanilla Diabetic Nutritional Drink

Rehab
Rehab

Safeway
Nutritional Shake/Drinks (All Flavors, including Plus)
Weight Loss Shakes - Chocolate Royale
Weight Loss Shakes - Milk Chocolate
Weight Loss Shakes - Vanilla

Slim-Fast
Easy to Digest Shake - Chocolate
Easy to Digest Shake - Coffee
Easy to Digest Shake - Vanilla

Vital Jr.
Pediatric Nutritional Products

ENERGY DRINKS

AMP Energy Drink ⚇
AMP Energy Drinks (ALL)

FUZE
Fuze (All Flavors)

Gatorade ⟨⟩
Energy Drink

Hansen's ⚇
Hansen's (All)

Monster Energy
Monster Beverage Products (All)

Red Bull
Red Bull Cola
Red Bull Energy Drink
Red Bull Sugarfree

Red Rain Energy Drinks
Red Rain Energy Drink

Rockstar Energy Drink
Rockstar Energy Drink

Sambazon
Sambazon (All)

SoBe ⚇
SoBe (All)

Turkey Hill ⓘ
Drink Products (All)

FLAVORED OR ENHANCED WATER

Adirondack Beverages ⚇
Adirondack Beverages (All)

Dasani
Essence

Lemon
Plus Cleanse + Restore
Plus Refresh + Revive

Harvest Bay
Coconut Water (All)

Hy-Vee
Black Cherry Water Cooler
Key Lime Water Cooler
Kiwi Strawberry Water Cooler
Mixed Berry Water Cooler
Peach Melba Water Cooler
Peach Water Cooler
Raspberry Water Cooler
Strawberry Water Cooler
White Grape Water Cooler

Kroger ⓘ
Crystal Clear Flavored Waters

Propel ()
Propel

Safeway
Select - Clear Sparkling Water Beverages
(All Flavors)

Smartwater
Smartwater Products (All)

Special K ⅞
Special K2O Protein Water

VIO
Vibrancy Drinks (All)

Vitaminwater
Vitaminwater (All)

Waterplus
Waterplus

HOT COCOA & CHOCOLATE MIXES

Ah!Laska ⅞
Cocoa Mix

Best Friends Cocoa ⅞
Hot Cocoa (All Four Flavors)

Caffe D'vita ()
Caffe D'vita (All)

Ghirardelli ⓘ
Powdered Hot Chocolate

Giant
Hot Cocoa - Mini Marshmallows
Hot Cocoa - Regular

Great Value (Wal-Mart)
Milk Chocolate Hot Cocoa Mix
Milk Chocolate Hot Cocoa Mix w/
Marshmallows

Green Mountain Coffee
Hot Cocoa (All) ()

Hy-Vee
Instant Chocolate Flavored Drink Mix
Instant Hot Cocoa Mix
No Sugar Added Instant Hot Cocoa Mix

Juanitas
Juanitas (All)

Kroger ⓘ
Instant Cocoa

Meijer
Chocolate Flavor Drink Mix
Cocoa Hot Instant Marshmallow
Hot Cocoa Mix
Hot Cocoa Mix No Sugar Added
Hot Cocoa Mix Sugar Free
Hot Cocoa Mix with Marshmallows
Organic Hot Cocoa Regular

Midwest Country Fare (Hy-Vee)
Hot Cocoa Mix
Instant Chocolate Flavored Drink Mix

Safeway
Hot Cocoa Mix - Fat Free
Hot Cocoa Mix - Sugar Free
Hot Cocoa Mix with Marshmallows
Instant Chocolate Drink Mix
Select - Cocoa Mix - European

Stop & Shop
Hot Cocoa - Fat Free No Sugar Added
Hot Cocoa - Light
Hot Cocoa - Mini Marshmallows
Hot Cocoa - Regular

INSTANT BREAKFAST DRINKS

Carnation Instant Breakfast ⓘ
Carnation Instant Breakfast Essentials
(All BUT Chocolate Malt)

Kroger ⓘ
In An Instant Drink Powders

Safeway
Instant Breakfast

Juice Drink Mixes

All-Bran
- Fiber Drink Mixes (All)

Alpine
- Spiced Cider Drink Mix

Celestial Seasonings
- Fruit Punch Go Stix
- Orange Citrus Punch Go Stix
- Triple Berry Go Stix
- Wild Cherry Go Stix

Country Time
- Lemonade Drink Mix
- Lemonade Flavor Drink Mix
- Lemonade Iced Tea Classic Drink Mix
- Lemonade Iced Tea Raspberry Drink Mix
- Lemonade Lite Drink Mix
- On The Go Lemonade Drink Mix Packet
- Pink Lemonade Drink Mix
- Pink Lemonade Flavor Drink Mix
- Pink Lemonade Lite Drink Mix
- Raspberry Lemonade Drink Mix
- Strawberry Lemonade Drink Mix

Crystal Light
- Calcium - Raspberry Peach Sugar Free
- Calcium - Tangerine Strawberry Sugar Free
- Fruit Punch Drink Mix
- Fusion Fruit Punch Fruit Drinks
- Immunity Natural Cherry Pomegranate Drink Mix
- Lemonade Sugar Free
- Liveactive For Digestive Health Mixed Berry Drink Mix
- Liveactive For Digestive Health Raspberry Peach Drink Mix
- On The Go - Energy Wild Strawberry
- On The Go - Fruit Punch Sugar Free
- On The Go - Hydration Lightly Lemon
- On The Go - Immunity Cherry Pomegranate
- On The Go - Raspberry Ice Sugar Free Packets
- On The Go Hunger Satisfaction Natural Strawberry Banana Drink Mix
- On The Go Raspberry Lemonade Sugar Free
- On The Go White Grape Drink Mix
- Pineapple Orange Sugar Free Fruit Drinks
- Pink Lemonade Sugar Free
- Raspberry Ice Sugar Free Fruit Drinks
- Raspberry Lemonade Sugar Free
- Red Tea Natural Mandarin Drink Mix
- Strawberry Kiwi Sugar Free Fruit Drinks
- Strawberry Orange Banana Sugar Free Fruit Drinks
- Sunrise - Classic Orange Sugar Free
- Sunrise - Ruby Red Grapefruit
- Sunrise - Tangerine Strawberry
- White Grape Drink Mix

Giant
- Cherry Drink Mix
- Grape Drink Mix
- Lemonade Drink Mix
- Orange Drink Mix
- Pink Lemonade Drink Mix
- Strawberry Drink Mix
- Sugar Free Drink Mix - Fruit Punch
- Sugar Free Drink Mix - Iced Tea
- Sugar Free Drink Mix - Lemon Lime
- Sugar Free Drink Mix - Lemonade
- Tropical Punch Drink Mix

Hy-Vee
- Splash Cherry Drink Mix
- Splash Grape Drink Mix
- Splash Lemonade Drink Mix
- Splash Orange Drink Mix
- Splash Tropical Fruit Punch Drink Mix

Kool-Aid
- Black Cherry Unsweetened Soft Drink Mix
- Cherry Sugar Free Soft Drink Mix
- Cherry Sugar Sweetened Soft Drink Mix
- Cherry Unsweetened Soft Drink Mix
- Grape Sugar Free Soft Drink Mix
- Grape Sugar Sweetened Soft Drink Mix
- Grape Unsweetened Soft Drink Mix
- Invisible Changin' Cherry Sugar Sweetened Soft Drink Mix
- Invisible Changin' Cherry Unsweetened Soft Drink Mix

Invisible Grape Illusion Sugar Sweetened Soft Drink Mix

Invisible Grape Illusion Unsweetened Soft Drink Mix

Lemonade Sugar Sweetened Soft Drink Mix

Lemonade Unsweetened Soft Drink Mix

Lemon-Lime Unsweetened Soft Drink Mix

On The Go Cherry Soft Drink Mix

On The Go Tropical Punch Soft Drink Mix

Orange Sugar Sweetened Soft Drink Mix

Orange Unsweetened Soft Drink Mix

Pink Lemonade Unsweetened Soft Drink Mix

Singles Cherry Soft Drink Mix

Singles Grape Soft Drink Mix

Singles Orange Soft Drink Mix

Singles Tropical Punch Soft Drink Mix

Soarin' Strawberry Lemonade Unsweetened Soft Drink Mix

Strawberry Sugar Sweetened Soft Drink Mix

Strawberry Unsweetened Soft Drink Mix

Tropical Punch Soft Drink Mix

Tropical Punch Sugar Free Soft Drink Mix

Tropical Punch Sugar Free Twists Soft Drink Mix

Tropical Punch Sugar Sweetened Soft Drink Mix

Tropical Punch Unsweetened Soft Drink Mix

Twists Blastin' Berry Cherry Sugar Free Envelope Soft Drink Mix

Kool-Aid Mad Scientwists ᘓ

Raspberry Reaction Invisible Unsweetened Soft Drink Mix

Wild Watermelon Kiwi Invisible Unsweetened Soft Drink Mix

Kool-Aid Twists ᘓ

Berry Blue Unsweetened Soft Drink Mix

Blastin' Berry Cherry Unsweetened Soft Drink Mix

Ice Blue Raspberry Lemonade Sugar Sweetened Soft Drink Mix

Ice Blue Raspberry Lemonade Unsweetened Soft Drink Mix

Slammin' Strawberry Kiwi Unsweetened Soft Drink Mix

Watermelon Cherry Unsweetened Soft Drink Mix

Kroger ⓘ

Instant Spiced Cider

Meijer

Crystal Quencher - Black Cherry

Crystal Quencher - Key Lime

Crystal Quencher - Kiwi Strawberry

Crystal Quencher - Peach

Crystal Quencher - Raspberry

Crystal Quencher - Tangerine Lime

Crystal Quencher - White Grape

Drink Mix - Breakfast Orange

Drink Mix - Cherry

Drink Mix - Grape

Drink Mix - Lemon Sugar Free

Drink Mix - Lemonade

Drink Mix - Lemonade Stix

Drink Mix - Orange

Drink Mix - Orange Free & Light

Drink Mix - Pink Lemonade

Drink Mix - Pink Lemonade Sugar Free

Drink Mix - Punch

Drink Mix - Raspberry Stix

Drink Mix - Raspberry Sugar Free

Drink Mix - Strawberry

Drink Mix - Strawberry Orange Banana

Strawberry Flavor Drink Mix

Safeway

Spiced Cranberry Apple Cider Mix

Strawberry Star Fruit Drink Mix

Sugar Free Raspberry and Lemonade Drink Mix

South Beach Living ᘓ

On The Go Drink Mix - Natural Strawberry Banana Packets

On The Go Drink Mix - Natural Tropical Breeze Packets

Stop & Shop

Cherry Drink Mix

Grape Drink Mix

Lemonade Drink Mix
Orange Drink Mix
Pink Lemonade Drink Mix
Strawberry Drink Mix
Sugar Free Drink Mix - Fruit Punch
Sugar Free Drink Mix - Iced Tea
Sugar Free Drink Mix - Lemon Lime
Sugar Free Drink Mix - Lemonade
Tropical Punch Drink Mix

Tang

Grape Drink Mix
Jamaica Hibiscus Drink Mix
On The Go Orange Drink Mix
Orange Drink Mix
Orange Kiwi Drink Mix
Orange Pineapple Drink Mix
Orange Strawberry Drink Mix
Orange Sugar Free Drink Mix
Orange with Fruit Pulp Drink Mix
Strawberry with Fruit Pulp Drink Mix
Tangerine Strawberry Drink Mix
Tropical Passionfruit Drink Mix
Wild Berry Drink Mix

Tropicana

Light Lemonade & Punches (All)

JUICES & FRUIT DRINKS

Apple & Eve

Juices (All)

AriZona

Juices (All)

Barsotti's

Freshly Pressed Juices (All)
Freshly Squeezed Juices (All)
Lemonades (All)

Bionaturae

Organic Nectars

Bolthouse Farms ⓘ

Bolthouse Farms Beverages (All BUT Pear Merlot)

Bom Dia

Bom Dia Beverages (All)

Bossa Nova

Superfruit Juices (All)

Campbell's ⓘ

Healthy Request Tomato Juice

Low Sodium Tomato Juice
Organic Tomato Juice
Tomato Juice

Capri Sun

Coastal Cooler Juice Drink
Coastal Cooler/Strawberry Banana Blend Juice Drink
Fruit Punch Juice Drink
Grape Juice Drink
Lemonade Juice Drink
Mountain Cooler Juice Drink
Mountain Cooler Mixed Fruit Juice Drink
Orange Juice Drink
Pacific Cooler Juice Drink
Pacific Cooler Mixed Fruit Blend Juice Drink
Red Berry Juice Drink
Red Berry/Strawberry Raspberry Blend Juice Drink
Splash Cooler Juice Drink
Splash Cooler Mixed Fruit Blend Juice Drink
Strawberry Juice Drink
Strawberry Kiwi Blend Juice Drink
Strawberry Kiwi Juice Drink
Sunrise Berry Strawberry Tangerine Morning Juice Drink
Sunrise Orange Wake Up Juice Drink
Sunrise Tropical Morning Juice Drink
Surfer Cooler Juice Drink
Surfer Cooler Mixed Fruit Blend Juice Drink
Tropical Punch Blend Juice Drink
Tropical Punch Juice Drink
Wild Cherry Blend Juice Drink
Wild Cherry Juice Drink

Capri Sun Roarin' Waters

Grape Fruit Flavored Water Beverage
Strawberry Kiwi Fruit Flavored Water Beverage
Tropical Fruit Flavored Water Beverage
Variety Fruit Flavored Water Beverage
Wild Cherry Fruit Flavored Water Beverage

Capri Sun Sport

Berry Ice All Natural Sports Drink

Lightspeed Lemon Lime with
Electrolytes Sports Drink
Thunder Punch All Natural Sports
Drink
Variety Pk Sports Drink

Ceres
Juices (All)

Clamato
Clamato (All BUT Red Eye)

Country Time (Dr. Pepper/Snapple Group)
Country Time (All)

Country Time ᕦ
Lemonade - Large Ready To Drink
Pouches

Crystal Light ᕦ
Sunrise - Berry Tangerine Morning
Sunrise - Orange Wake Up
Sunrise - Tropical Morning

Dei Fratelli
Dei Fratelli (All BUT Tomato Soup)

Dole ◇
100% Juice Products (All)

Eden Foods ⓘ ✔
Apple Juice - Organic
Cherry Juice Concentrate - Organic
Montmorency Tart Cherry Juice -
Organic

Florida's Natural
Premium Orange Juice
Ruby Red Grapefruit Juice

Fruitworks ⓧ
Juice Drinks (All)

Giant
100% Natural Sparkling Apple Juice
Apple Juice Cocktail From Concentrate
(Shelf-Stable)
Berry Berry Cooler (Shelf-Stable)
Big Apple Cooler (Shelf-Stable)
Cosmic Orange Cooler (Shelf-Stable)
Fruit Punch Juice Drink (Shelf-Stable)
Fruity Punch Cooler (Shelf-Stable)
Goofy Grape Cooler (Shelf-Stable)
Grapefruit Juice (Chilled)
Kids Happy Drinks (Shelf-Stable)
Orange Cranberry Juice (Chilled)

Orange Juice - Added Calcium (Chilled)
Orange Juice - Not Concentrate
(Chilled)
Orange Juice from Concentrate
(Chilled)
Orange Juice with Pulp (Chilled)
Orange Strawberry Juice (Chilled)
Premium Ruby Red Grapefruit Juice -
Not From Concentrate (Chilled)
Prune Juice with Pulp (Shelf-Stable)
Strawberry Kiwi Juice (Shelf-Stable)
Tomato Juice (Shelf-Stable)
Tropical Juice Drink (Shelf-Stable)
Wild Cherry Juice Drink (Shelf-Stable)

Goya
Bitter Orange
Coconut Water
Nectars
Sugar Cane Juice

Great Value (Wal-Mart)
100% Juice Apple (8 Pk)
100% Juice Apple Juice Punch Blend
100% Juice Fruit Punch (8 Pk)
100% Juice Unsweetened Apple Juice
100% Orange Juice
100% Orange Juice From Concentrate
100% Pure Orange Juice
100% Pure Orange Juice with Calcium
Country Style Orange Juice
Fruit Punch
Grape Drink
Grape Punch
Guava Nectar w/Calcium
Kiwi Strawberry Punch
Lemon Berry Punch
Lemon Juice
Light Apple Juice Cocktail w/Splenda
Orange Juice
Orange Juice w/Calcium
Orange Punch
Pineapple Juice
Pineapple Orange Juice
Prune Juice
Strawberry Banana Nectar
Strawberry Banana Nectar w/Calcium
Tomato Juice
Unsweetened Pink Grapefruit Juice

Unsweetened White Grapefruit Juice
Vegetable Juice

Hansen's ⛨
Hansen's (All)

Harvest Farms (Ingles)
Juice (All)

Hawaiian Punch
Hawaiian Punch (All)

Honest Ade ⛨
Honest Ade (All)

Honest Kids ⛨
Honest Kids (All)

Honest Mate ⛨
Honest Mate (All)

Honest Tea ⛨
Honest Tea (All)

Hood
Juices (All)

Hy-Vee
100% Apple Juice From Concentrate
100% Cranberry Juice Blend
100% Cranberry/Apple Juice Blend
100% Cranberry/Raspberry Juice Blend
Cranberry Apple Juice Cocktail From
Concentrate
Cranberry Grape Juice Cocktail From
Concentrate
Cranberry Juice Cocktail From
Concentrate
Cranberry Raspberry Juice from
Concentrate
Cranberry Strawberry Juice Cocktail
from Concentrate
Fruit Punch
Fruit Punch Coolers
No Concentrate Country Style Orange
Juice
No Concentrate Orange Juice
No Concentrate Orange Juice with
Calcium
Not From Concentrate Ruby Red
Grapefruit Juice
Splash Cherry
Splash Grape
Splash Lemonade
Splash Orange
Splash Raspberry

Splash Strawberry
Splash Tropical Punch
Tomato Juice From Concentrate
Tropical Punch Coolers
Vegetable Juice From Concentrate

Italian Volcano
Italian Volcano (All)

Kern's
Horchata Drinks (All)
Nectars (All)

Knouse Foods ⛨
Apple Cider
Apple Juice
Premium Apple Juice

Kool-Aid Bursts ᕲ
Cherry Flavored Soft Drink
Cherry Soft Drink
Grape Flavored Soft Drink
Grape Soft Drink
Lime Soft Drink
Tropical Punch Soft Drink

Kool-Aid Jammers ᕲ
Blue Raspberry Juice Drink
Cherry Juice Drink
Grape Juice Drink
Green Apple Juice Drink
Kiwi-Strawberry Juice Drink
Orange Juice Drink
Tropical Punch Juice Drink

Kroger ⓘ
Fruit Juices
Vegetable Juice

Langer Juice Company
Juices (All)

Laura Lynn (Ingle's)
Juice (All)

Manischewitz
Grape Juice

Martinelli's
Martinelli's (All)

Meijer
Acai and Blueberry Juice Blend (Shelf
Stable)
Acai and Grape Juice Blend (Shelf
Stable)
Apple Juice - Natural (Shelf Stable)

Apple Juice - Not from Concentrate (Shelf Stable)

Apple Juice (Shelf Stable)

Apple Juice from Concentrate (Shelf Stable)

Cherry Juice (Shelf Stable)

Cran Grape Juice Light (Shelf Stable)

Cran/Rasp Juice with 3 Fruit Juices (Shelf Stable)

Cranberry Apple Juice Cocktail (Shelf Stable)

Cranberry Flavored with 2 Fruit Juices (Shelf Stable)

Cranberry Grape Flavored with 2 Juices (Shelf Stable)

Cranberry Grape Juice Cocktail (Shelf Stable)

Cranberry Grape Juice Drink (Shelf Stable)

Cranberry Juice Cocktail (Shelf Stable)

Cranberry Juice Cocktail Light (Shelf Stable)

Cranberry Raspberry 100% (Shelf Stable)

Cranberry Raspberry Juice Cocktail (Shelf Stable)

Cranberry Strawberry Cocktail (Shelf Stable)

Drink - Berry Blend Splash (Shelf Stable)

Drink Cranberry Raspberry (Shelf Stable)

Drink Cranberry Strawberry (Shelf Stable)

Fruit Punch (Shelf Stable)

Fruit Punch Genuine (Shelf Stable)

Fruit Punch Light (Shelf Stable)

Grape Cranberry Juice Cocktail Light (Shelf Stable)

Grape Juice from Concentrate (Shelf Stable)

Grapefruit Juice (Shelf Stable)

Juice - Berry 100% (Shelf Stable)

Juice - Cherry 100% (Shelf Stable)

Juice - Cranapple Cocktail (Shelf Stable)

Juice - Cranberry White Cocktail (Shelf Stable)

Juice - Cranberry White Peach (Shelf Stable)

Juice - Grape (Shelf Stable)

Juice - Grape 100% Genuine (Shelf Stable)

Juice - Grape White (Shelf Stable)

Juice - Punch 100% Genuine (Shelf Stable)

Lemon Juice (Shelf Stable)

Lemon Juice Squeeze Bottle (Shelf Stable)

Light Grape Juice Cocktail with Splenda (Shelf Stable)

Lime Juice (Shelf Stable)

Orange Juice (Shelf Stable)

Orange Premium Carafe (Refrigerated)

Orange Premium High Pulp Carafe (Refrigerated)

Orange Premium with Calcium (Refrigerated)

Orange Premium with Calcium Carafe (Refrigerated)

Orange Reconstituted (Refrigerated)

Orange Reconstituted + Pulp (Refrigerated)

Orange Reconstituted with Calcium (Refrigerated)

Orange with Calcium (Refrigerated)

Organic Apple Juice (Shelf Stable)

Organic Concord Grape Juice (Shelf Stable)

Organic Cranberry Juice (Shelf Stable)

Organic Lemonade (Shelf Stable)

Pink Grapefruit Juice (Shelf Stable)

Pomegranate and Blueberry Blend (Shelf Stable)

Pomegranate and Cranberry Blend (Shelf Stable)

Prune Juice (Shelf Stable)

Raspberry Cranberry Juice Cocktail Light (Shelf Stable)

Ruby Red Grapefruit Cocktail Light (Shelf Stable)

Ruby Red Grapefruit Cocktail Light 22% (Shelf Stable)

Ruby Red Grapefruit Juice Cocktail (Shelf Stable)

Strawberry/Kiwi Splash (Shelf Stable)

Tropical Blend Splash (PGB)
White Cranberry Flavored Juice Blend (Shelf Stable)
White Cranberry Juice Cocktail (Shelf Stable)
White Cranberry Peach Juice Cocktail (Shelf Stable)
White Cranberry Strawberry Juice Cocktail (Shelf Stable)
White Grape Juice Cocktail Concentrate (Shelf Stable)
White Grape Peach Juice Blend (Shelf Stable)
White Grape Raspberry Juice Blend (Shelf Stable)
White Grapefruit Juice (Shelf Stable)

Midwest Country Fare (Hy-Vee)
100% Unsweetened Apple Cider from Concentrate
100% Unsweetened Apple Juice from Concentrate

Minute Maid
Kids + Apple
Lemonade
Light Lemonade
Multi-Vitamin Orange Juice
Pomegranate Blueberry Juice
Pomegranate Lemonade

Mott's
Juice Products (All)

Naked Juice
Naked Juice Products (All BUT Green Machine)

Nantucket Nectars
Nantucket Nectars (All)

Nature Factor ✔
Organic Young Coconut Water

Nature's Promise (Giant)
Organic Cranberry Juice From Concentrate (Shelf Stable)
Pomegranate Juice - Blueberry Blend (Shelf Stable)
Pomegranate Juice - Cranberry Blend (Shelf Stable)
Pomegranate Juice - Regular (Shelf Stable)

Nature's Promise (Stop & Shop)
Organic Cranberry Juice From Concentrate (Shelf Stable)

Nellie & Joe's
Nellie & Joe's (All)

Nestlé Juicy Juice
Juicy Juice (All Flavors)
Juicy Juice Harvest Surprise (All Flavors)

Newman's Own
Gorilla Grape
Grape Juice
Lemon Aided Ice Tea
Lemonade
Lightly Sweetened Lemonade
Limeade
Orange Mango Tango
Organic Lemonade
Pink Lemonade
Razz-Ma-Tazz Raspberry Juice Cocktail

Ocean Spray
Beverages (All)

Odwalla
Juices (All BUT Super Protein Vanilla Al Mondo & Superfood)

Old Orchard
Old Orchard (All)

Orangina
Orangina (All)

POM Wonderful ☷
100% Pomegranate Juice

Publix GreenWise Market ()
100% Organic Apple Juice
Organic Cranberry Juice
Organic Grape Juice
Organic Lemonade
Organic Tomato Juice

Publix ()
Apple Juice
Cranberry Apple Juice Cocktail
Cranberry Juice Cocktail
Deli Old Fashion Lemonade
Grape Juice
Grape-Cranberry Juice Cocktail
Orange Juice From Concentrate
Orange Juice with Calcium From Concentrate

Pineapple Juice
Premium Orange Juice - Calcium Plus (Not from Concentrate)
Premium Orange Juice - Grove Pure (Not from Concentrate)
Premium Orange Juice - Old Fashioned (Not from Concentrate)
Premium Orange Juice - Original (Not from Concentrate)
Premium Ruby Red Grapefruit (Not from Concentrate)
Raspberry Cranberry Juice Cocktail
Ruby Red Grapefruit Juice
Ruby Red Grapefruit Juice from Concentrate
Tomato Juice
White Grape Juice

R.W. Knudsen
R.W. Knudsen Beverages (All BUT Sensible Sippers Juice Boxes)

Raley's
Shelf Stable Juices

ReaLemon
ReaLemon (All)

Red Gold
Tomato Products (All)

Rosenberger's Dairies
Orange Juice

Safeway
Apple Cider
Apple Juice
Apple/Cranberry Juice
Berry Splash
Cranberry Cocktail Juice
Cranberry/Raspberry Juice
Grape/Cranberry Cocktail
Grapefruit Juice
Grapefruit/Tangerine Cocktail Juice
Lemon Juice
Lemonade
Light Cranberry Cocktail Juice
Limeade
Orange Juice
Pink Grapefruit Juice
Prune Juice
Ruby Red Grapefruit Cocktail
Strawberry/Kiwi Splash

Tropical Splash
Vegetable Juice
White Grape Juice
White Grapefruit Juice

Sambazon
Sambazon (All)

Santa Cruz Organic
Santa Cruz Organic (All)

Simply Apple
Simply Apple

Simply Grapefruit
Simply Grapefruit

Simply Lemonade
Simply Lemonade
Simply Lemonade with Raspberry

Simply Limeade
Simply Limeade

Simply Orange Juice
Country Stand Medium Pulp with Calcium
Simply Orange with Mango
Simply Orange with Pineapple

Snapple
Snapple (All)

SoBe
SoBe (All)

Stop & Shop
100% Apple Juice From Concentrate - Regular & Vitamin C Added (Shelf Stable)
100% Berry Juice (Shelf Stable)
100% Cherry Juice (Shelf Stable)
100% Cranberry Juice Blend (Shelf Stable)
100% Grape Cranberry Juice (Shelf Stable)
100% Grape Juice Blend (Shelf Stable)
100% Raspberry Cranberry Juice Blend (Shelf Stable)
100% Unsweetened Grapefruit Juice (Shelf Stable)
100% White Grape Juice (Shelf Stable)
100% White Grapefruit Juice (Shelf Stable)
Apple Juice Cocktail From Concentrate (Shelf Stable)

Artificially Flavored Fruit Drink From Concentrate (Shelf Stable)
Berry Berry Cooler (Shelf Stable)
Big Apple Cooler (Shelf Stable)
Cosmic Orange Cooler (Shelf Stable)
Cran/Apple Juice Cocktail (Shelf Stable)
Cranberry Grape Juice Cocktail (Shelf Stable)
Cranberry Lime Juice Cocktail From Concentrate (Shelf Stable)
Cranberry Raspberry Juice Cocktail (Shelf Stable)
Fruit Punch/Juice Drink (Shelf Stable)
Fruity Punch Cooler (Shelf Stable)
Goofy Grape Cooler (Shelf Stable)
Grape Drink (Shelf Stable)
Grapefruit Juice (Chilled)
Lemon Juice Reconstituted (Chilled)
Lemon Lime Drink (Shelf Stable)
Light Cranberry Juice Cocktail From Concentrate (Shelf Stable)
Lite CranRaspberry Juice Cocktail (Shelf Stable)
Lite Grape Juice Cocktail (Shelf Stable)
Natural Apple Juice - Unsweetened & Added Calcium (Shelf Stable)
Orange Cranberry Juice (Chilled)
Orange Drink (Shelf Stable)
Orange Strawberry Juice (Chilled)
Pink Lemonade (Shelf Stable)
Prune Juice with Pulp (Shelf Stable)
Ruby Red Grapefruit Tangerine Juice (Shelf Stable)
Strawberry Kiwi Juice (Shelf Stable)
Sunrise Valley Orange Juice - Calcium Added
Sunrise Valley Orange Juice - Regular
Tomato Juice (Shelf Stable)
Tropical Carrot/Strawberry/Kiwi Blend (Shelf Stable)
Tropical Juice Drink (Shelf Stable)
Unsweetened Apple Juice with Added Vitamin C (Shelf Stable)
Vegetable Juice From Concentrate (Shelf Stable)
White Cranberry Juice Cocktail (Shelf Stable)

White Cranberry Peach Juice Drink (Shelf Stable)
White Cranberry Strawberry Juice Drink (Shelf Stable)
Wild Cherry Juice Drink (Shelf Stable)
Wildberry Drink (Shelf Stable)

Sunny D
Sunny D (All)

Sunrise Valley (Stop & Shop)
Orange Juice - Calcium Added (Chilled)
Orange Juice - Regular (Chilled)

Sunsweet
Sunsweet (All BUT Chocolate Plum Sweets)

Tang
Watermelon Wallop Juice Drink

Tree Ripe
Juices (All)

Tree Top
Juices (All)

Tropicana
100% Juice Products (All)
Lemonade & Punches (All)

Turkey Hill ⓘ
Drink Products (All)

V8 ⓘ
A-C-E Vitamin Rich
Calcium Enriched Vegetable Juice
Fiber Vegetable Juice
Low Sodium Vegetable Juice
Organic Vegetable Juice
Spicy Hot Vegetable Juice
Splash Berry Blend
Splash Diet Berry Blend
Splash Diet Tropical Blend
Splash Fruit Medley
Splash Mango Peach
Splash Strawberry Kiwi Blend
Splash Tropical Blend
Vegetable Juice
V-Fusion Açai Berry
V-Fusion Goji Raspberry
V-Fusion Light Peach Mango
V-Fusion Light Pomegranate Blueberry
V-Fusion Light Strawberry Banana
V-Fusion Passionfruit Tangerine
V-Fusion Peach Mango

V-Fusion Pomegranate Blueberry
V-Fusion Strawberry Banana
V-Fusion Tropical Orange

Welch's
Welch's (All)

Winn-Dixie ⓘ
Apple Juice - Very Low Sodium

Wyman's
Wyman's (All)

MIXERS

Margaritaville
Margaritaville (All)

Mr. & Mrs. T
Mr. & Mrs. T (All BUT Premium
Bloody Mary Drink & Pina Colada
Mixes)

Rose's
Rose's (All)

Simply Enjoy (Giant)
Cosmopolitan Mixer
Lemon Drop Martini Mixer
Margarita Cocktail Mixer
Mojito Cocktail Mixer
Watermelon Martini Mixer

Simply Enjoy (Stop & Shop)
Cosmopolitan Mixer
Lemon Drop Martini Mixer
Margarita Cocktail Mixer
Mojito Cocktail Mixer
Watermelon Martini Mixer

PROTEIN POWDER

Betty Lou's ✓
Protein Shakes

Bob's Red Mill ⓘ ✓
Soy Protein Powder

Special K ♀
Special K2O Protein Water Mixes

SMOOTHIES & SHAKES

Atkins Nutritionals ()
Ready to Drink Shakes

Cascade Fresh
Cascade Fresh (All)

Lucerne (Safeway)
Smoothies - Light (All Flavors)

Luna ()
Luna Sports Products (All)

Nesquik
MilkShake

Publix ()
Fat Free Light Mixed Berry Yogurt
Smoothie
Fat Free Light Strawberry Yogurt
Smoothie

Sambazon
Sambazon (All)

Special K ♀
Protein Shakes

Stonyfield Farm
Smoothies (All BUT Frozen Yogurt,
Oikos Greek Yogurt, YoBaby Plus
Fruit & Cereal and YoKids Squeezers)

V8 ⓘ
Splash Smoothie - Strawberry Banana
Splash Smoothie - Tropical Colada

SPORTS DRINKS

Clif
Shot Energy Drinks ()

Gatorade ()
Endurance Formula
G2
Thirst Quencher

Luna ()
Luna Sports Products (All)

Meijer
Drink Thirst Quencher Fruit Punch
(Shelf Stable)
Drink Thirst Quencher Lemon Lime
(Shelf Stable)
Drink Thirst Quencher Orange (Shelf
Stable)

POWERade
Grape
Mountain Blast
POWERade with ION4

Safeway

Select - Winners Thirst Quencher, Amazon Freeze
Select - Winners Thirst Quencher, Fruit Punch
Select - Winners Thirst Quencher, Glacier Wave
Select - Winners Thirst Quencher, Lemon
Select - Winners Thirst Quencher, Lemon Ice
Select - Winners Thirst Quencher, Lemon Lime
Select - Winners Thirst Quencher, Orange
Select - Winners Thirst Quencher, Tangerine Freeze
Select - Winners Thirst Quencher, Tropical

TEA & TEA MIXES

Adagio Teas
Teas (All)

Bigelow Tea
Bigelow Tea (All BUT Blueberry Harvest, Chamomile Mango & Cinnamon Spice Herb Teas)

Boston Tea
Tea Products (All)

Caffe D'vita ()
Caffe D'vita (All)

Celestial Seasonings
Acai Mango Zinger
African Orange Mango Red Tea
Antioxidant Supplement Green Tea
Antioxidant Supplement Plum White Tea
Apple Banana Chamomile Tea
Apple Caramel Kiss Cider
Authentic Green Tea
Bengal Spice
Black Cherry Berry
Bluberry Breeze Green Tea
Blueberry Cool Brew Iced Tea
Caffiene Free Herbal Tea
Chamomile

Chocolate Caramel Enchantment Chai
Cinnamon Apple Spice
Cinnamon Apple Tea
Country Peach Passion
Cranberry Apple Zinger
Cranberry Pomengranate Green Tea
Decaf Honey Chamomile Green Tea
Decaf India Spice Chai
Decaf Lemon Mrytle Organic Green Tea
Decaf Mandarin Orchard Green Tea
Decaf Mint Green Tea
Decaf Sweet Coconut Thai Chai
Decaf White Tea
Decaffeinated Green Tea
Devonshire English Breakfast Black Tea
Diet Partner Wellness Tea
Echinacea Complete Care Wellness Tea
Fast Lane Black Tea
Fruit Tea Sampler
Giftable Love Tea - Vanilla Strawberry Rose
Goji Berry Pomengranate Green Tea
Golden Honey Darjeeling Black Tea
Green Tea Sampler
Harvest Apple Spice Cider
Herbal Tea Sampler
Holiday Tea - Candy Cane Lane
Holiday Tea - Nutcracker Sweet
Honey Lemon Diet Tea
Honey Lemon Ginseng Green Tea
Honey Peach Ginger Wellness Tea
Honey Vanilla Apple Cider
Honey Vanilla Chai
Honey Vanilla Chamomile
Imperial White Peach White Tea
India Spice Chai
Lemon Zinger
Lemon Zinger Green Tea
Linden Mint Tea
Madagascar Vanilla Red Tea
Mandarin Orange Spice
Mango Darjeeling Organic Tea
Mint Magic
Morning Thunder
Moroccan Pomengranate Red Tea
Organic Black Tea
Organic Green Tea
Peach Apricot Honeybush Tea

Peach Cool Brew Iced Tea
Peppermint
Perfectly Pear White Tea
Raspberry Cool Brew Iced Tea
Raspberry Gardens Green Tea
Raspberry Zinger
Red Zinger
Safari Spice Red Tea
Sleepytime
Sleepytime Extra Wellness Tea
Sleepytime Throat Tamer Wellness Tea
Sleepytime Vanilla
Sweet Apple Chamomile
Sweet Clementime Chamomile Orangic
   Herb Tea
Tangerine Orange Zinger
Tension Tamer
Tension Tamer Extra Wellness Tea
Throat Soothers Wellness Tea
Tropic of Strawberry
Tropical Acai Berry Green Tea
Tropical Fruit Cool Brew Iced Tea
Tropical Grapefruit Green Tea
True Blueberry
Tummy Mint Wellness Tamer
Tuscany Orange Spice Black Tea
Vanilla Apple White Organic Tea
Vanilla Ginger Green Tea Chai
Victorian Earl Grey Black Tea
Wild Berry Zinger

Crystal Light ◌
Antioxidant Raspberry Green Tea Sugar
   Free Iced Tea
Decaffeinated Lemon Iced Tea
Decaffeinated Sugar Free Iced Tea
Lemon Sugar Free Iced Tea
Metabolism+ Peach Mango Green Tea
   Drink Mix
On The Go - Antioxidant Raspberry
   Green Tea
Peach Iced Tea
Raspberry Sugar Free Iced Tea
Sugar Free Iced Tea

Eden Foods ⓘ ✓
Chamomile Herb Tea - Organic
Genmaicha Tea - Organic

General Foods International Coffees ◌
Chai Latte
Giant
Iced Tea Mix
Great Value (Wal-Mart)
Decaffeinated Tea 100% Natural
Family Size Decaffeinated Tea 100%
   Natural
Family Size Tea 100% Natural
Green Tea with Ginseng And Honey
Green Mountain Coffee
Tea (All)
Harvest Farms (Ingles)
Tea Bags (All)
Hy-Vee
Chai Black Tea
Chamomile Herbal Tea
Cinnamon Apple Herbal Tea
Decaffeinated Green Tea
Decaffeinated Tea Bags
Dream Easy Herbal Tea
Earl Gray Black Tea
English Breakfast Black Tea
Family Size Tea Bags
Green Tea Bags
Green Tea with Pomegranate
Instant Tea
Jasmine Green Tea
Oolong Tea
Orange & Spice Specialty Tea
Peppermint Herbal Tea
Rooibos Red Herbal Tea
Tea Bags
Ineeka ⚇
Ineeka Teas (All)
JFG Tea
Family Tea Bags
Gallon Tea Bags
Tea Bags
Kroger ⓘ
Tea - Bagged
Tea - Instant
Laura Lynn (Ingle's)
Tea Bags (All)
Luzianne
Decaf Tea Bags

Flavored Tea Bags - Lemon
Flavored Tea Bags - Peach
Flavored Tea Bags - Raspberry
Tea Bags

Meijer
Iced Tea Mix
Instant Tea
Tea Bags
Tea Bags - Decaffeinated
Tea Bags - Green
Tea Bags - Green Decaffeinated

Midwest Country Fare (Hy-Vee)
Black Tea

Nestea (Nestlé)
Nestea (All Flavors)

Newman's Own Organics ⓘ
Teas (All)

Numi Organic Tea
Tea (All)

Oregon Chai
Dry Mixes (All BUT Vanilla Dry Mix)
Liquid Concentrates (All)

Orient Emporium Tea Co.
Orient Emporium Teas (All Flavors)

Original Ceylon Tea Company, The
Original Ceylon Tea Company, The (All)

Publix ()
Decaffeinated Tea Bags
Tagless Tea Bags
Tea Bags (All Varieties)

Raley's ☿
Tea Packets

Red Rose
Red Rose Teas (All)

Republic of Tea, The
Teas (All)

Safeway
Iced Tea Mix (All Flavors)
Select - Chai Tea
Select - Herbal Tea, Chamomile
Select - Herbal Tea, Evening Delight
Select - Herbal Tea, Lemon
Select - Herbal Tea, Peppermint
Select - Specialty Tea
Select - Tea, Green
Select - Tea, Orange

Select - Tea, Spice Black
Tea Bags - Decaffeinated

St. Dalfour
Organic Tea ☿

Stash Tea
Teas (All)

Stop & Shop
Iced Tea Mix

Taylors of Harrogate ☿
Tea (All)

Tazo
Teas (All BUT Green Ginger,
Honeybush, Lemon Ginger & Tea
Lemonade)

Tetley ☿
Tetley (All)

Twinings
Teas (All)

Two Leaves and a Bud
Tea (All)

Yogi Tea
Yogi Tea (All BUT Calming, Fasting,
Kava Stress Relief & Stomach Ease
Teas)

TEA DRINKS

AriZona
Teas (All)

Crystal Light ⌇
Peach Sugar Free Iced Tea

Enviga
Berry Sparkling Green Tea
Sparkling Green Tea

FUZE
Fuze (All Flavors)

Gold Peak
Lemon Iced Tea

Great Value (Wal-Mart)
Diet Green Tea with Ginseng And
Honey
Ready To Drink Sweetened Tea
Sugar Free Sweet Iced Tea
Sweet Iced Tea

Hansen's ☿
Hansen's (All)

Honest Tea ☗
   Honest Tea (All)

Hy-Vee
   Diet Green Tea with Citrus
   Green Tea with Citrus
   Honey Lemon Ginseng Green Tea
   Thirst Splashers Raspberry Tea

Inko
   Inko's (All)

ITO EN Shot ()
   Ready-To-Drink Beverage Line (All)

Lipton ☗
   Lipton Brisk
   Lipton Iced Tea
   Lipton Pure Leaf

Luzianne
   Diet Peach Tea (Ready to Drink)
   Lemon Sweet Tea (Ready to Drink)
   Raspberry Sweet Tea (Ready to Drink)
   Sweet Tea (Ready to Drink)

Minute Maid
   Pomegranate Flavored Tea

Natural Fruit Tea ()
   Ready-To-Drink Beverage Line (All)

Nature's Promise (Giant)
   Organic Fair Trade Green Tea - Decaf (Shelf Stable)
   Organic Fair Trade Green Tea - Lemon (Shelf Stable)
   Organic Fair Trade Green Tea - Regular (Shelf Stable)

Nature's Promise (Stop & Shop)
   Organic Fair Trade Green Tea - Decaf (Shelf Stable)
   Organic Fair Trade Green Tea - Lemon (Shelf Stable)
   Organic Fair Trade Green Tea - Regular (Shelf Stable)

Nestea (Coca-Cola Company, The)
   Citrus Green Tea
   Diet Citrus Green Tea
   Diet Lemon
   Diet White Tea Berry Honey
   Lemon Sweet (Hot Fill)
   Red Tea
   Sweetened Lemon Tea
   White Tea Berry Honey

Numi Organic Tea
   Tea (All)

Oi Ocha ()
   Ready-To-Drink Beverage Line (All)

Pacific Natural Foods ⓘ
   Organic Black Tea - Sweetened
   Organic Green Tea - Unsweetened
   Organic Iced Tea - Lemon
   Organic Iced Tea - Peach
   Organic Iced Tea - Raspberry

POM Wonderful ☗
   POMx Tea: The Antioxidant Super Tea

Publix ()
   Deli Iced Tea - Sweetened
   Deli Iced Tea - Unsweetened

Rosenberger's Dairies
   Iced Tea

Santa Cruz Organic
   Santa Cruz Organic (All)

Snapple
   Snapple (All)

SoBe ☗
   SoBe (All)

Teas' Tea ()
   Ready-To-Drink Beverage Line (All)

Turkey Hill ⓘ
   Drink Products (All)

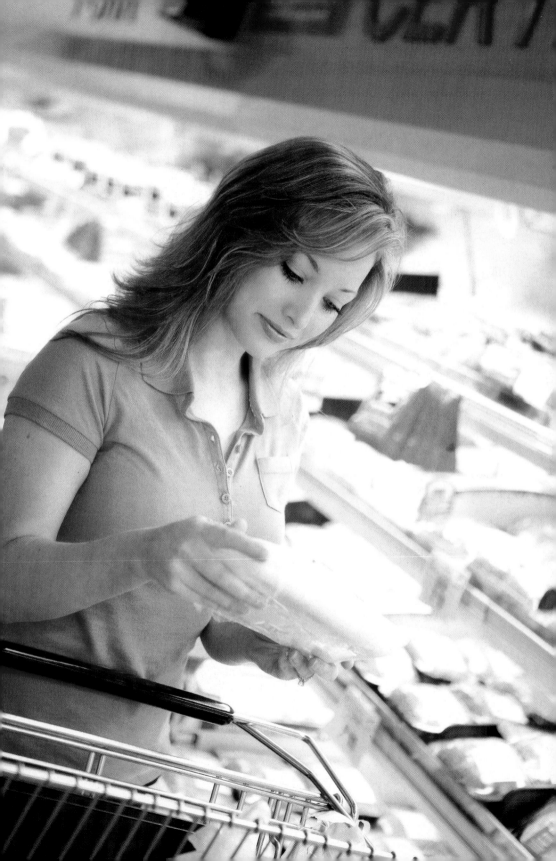

Betty Crocker®

For those of you who said you'd give your right arm, we have some bittersweet news.

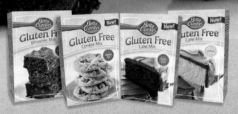

Introducing new Gluten-Free Dessert Mixes.
The wait is over. Now you're free to share and enjoy
the cakes, cookies and brownies you've been missing
with Betty Crocker gluten free dessert mixes.
Available in your neighborhood grocery store.

BAKE LIFE SWEETER™
www.bettycrocker.com/glutenfree

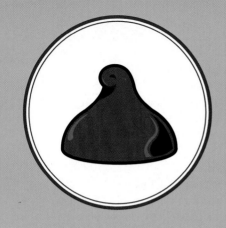

BAKING AISLE

BAKING CHIPS & BARS

Baker's Chocolate ᧰
Baking Chocolate - Bittersweet Squares
Baking Chocolate - Premium White
　Squares
Baking Chocolate - Semi-Sweet
German's Sweet Chocolate Bar
Real Dark Semi-Sweet Dipping
　Chocolate
Real Milk Dipping Chocolate
Semi-Sweet Chocolate Chunks

Enjoy Life Foods ⚕
Chocolate Chips
Semi-Sweet Chocolate Chips

Ghirardelli ⓘ
60% Bittersweet Chocolate Chips
Milk Chocolate Chips
Semi-Sweet Chocolate Chips

Giant
Semi-Sweet Chocolate Chips

Great Value (Wal-Mart)
Semi Sweet Chocolate Chips

Guittard
Guittard (All)

Hershey's
Semi-Sweet Chocolate Bar
Semi-Sweet Chocolate Chips
Unsweetened Baking Chocolate Bar

Hy-Vee
Butterscotch Baking Chips
Milk Chocolate Baking Chips
Mini Semi Sweet Chocolate Chips
Peanut Butter Baking Chips
Semi Sweet Chocolate Chips

Vanilla Flavored White Baking Chips

Kroger ⓘ
Butterscotch Morsels
Chocolate Chunks
Milk Chocolate Chips
Peanut Butter Chips
Semi Sweet Chips
White and Chocolate Bark Coating

Manischewitz
Chocolate Morsels

Meijer
Butterscotch Baking Chips
Chocolate Chips Semi-Sweet
Milk Chocolate Chips
Peanut Butter Chips
White Baking Chips

Midwest Country Fare (Hy-Vee)
Chocolate Flavored Chips

Nestlé Toll House
Milk Chocolate & Peanut Butter Swirled
　Morsels
Milk Chocolate Morsels
Peanut Butter & Milk Chocolate Morsels
Premier White Morsels
Semi-Sweet Chocolate & Premier White
　Swirled Morsels
Semi-Sweet Chocolate Chunks
Semi-Sweet Chocolate Mini Morsels
Semi-Sweet Morsels

Publix ()
Butterscotch Morsels
Milk Chocolate Morsels
Semi-Sweet Chocolate Morsels

Rapunzel
Dark Baking Chocolate (Semisweet)

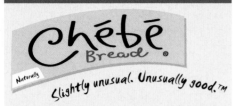
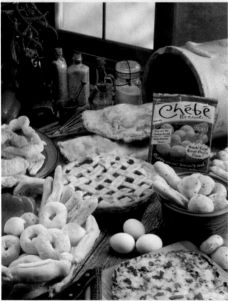
Dark Chocolate Chips, Baking
  Chocolate
Extra Dark Baking Chocolate
  (Bittersweet)
Extra Dark Chocolate Chips 70%
  (Semisweet), Baking Chocolate

Safeway
Butterscotch Chips
Chocolate Chips - Milk Chocolate
Chocolate Chips - Real Chocolate
Chocolate Chips - Semi Sweet
Select - Chocolate Chips

Scharffen Berger
2kg Chocolate Propacks (62%, 70%, 82%
  & 99%) ♼
6 & 9.7 oz. Home Baking Bars (62%,
  70% & 99%) ♼
Cacao Nibs ()
Nibs ()

Stop & Shop
Semi-Sweet Chocolate Chips

BAKING MIXES

1-2-3 Gluten-Free ♼
Aaron's Favorite Rolls Mix
Allie's Awesome Buckwheat Pancakes
  Mix
Chewy Chipless Scrumdelicious Cookie
  Mix
Delightfully Gratifying Poundcake Mix
Deliriously Delicious Devil's Food Cake
  Mix
Devilishly Decadent Brownies Mix
Divinely Decadent Brownies Mix
Lindsay's Lipsmackin' Sugar Cookies
  Mix
Meredith's Marvelous Muffin Mix
Micah's Mouthwatering Corn Bread Mix
Peri's Perfect Chocolate Poundcake Mix
Southern Glory Biscuits Mix
Sweet Goodness Pan Bars Mix
Yummy Yellow Cake Mix

Arrowhead Mills ✓
Bake with Me Gluten-Free Chocolate
  Cupcake Mix

Bake with Me Gluten-Free Vanilla
Cupcake Mix
Gluten-Free Brownie Mix
Gluten-Free Chocolate Chip Cookie
Mix
Gluten-Free Pancake & Waffle Mix
Gluten-Free Pizza Crust Mix
Gluten-Free Vanilla Cake Mix

Betty Crocker 🍸

Gluten-Free Brownie Mix
Gluten-Free Chocolate Chip Cookie
Mix
Gluten-Free Devil's Food Cake Mix
Gluten-Free Yellow Cake Mix

Bob's Red Mill ⓘ ✔

GF Brownie Mix
GF Chocolate Cake Mix
GF Chocolate Chip Cookie Mix
GF Cinnamon Raisin Bread Mix
GF Cornbread Mix
GF Hearty Whole Grain Bread Mix
GF Homemade Bread Mix
GF Pancake Mix
GF Pizza Crust Mix
Wheat-Free Biscuit Mix

Breads From Anna 🍸 ✔

Apple Pancake Muffin Mix
Banana Bread
Banana Bread
Bread Mix
Classic Herb Bread Mix
Cranberry Pancake Muffin Mix
Maple Pancake Muffin Mix
Pie Crust Mix
Pumpkin Bread

Cause You're Special 🍸

Chocolate Chip Cookie Mix
Chocolate Fudge Brownie Mix
Classic Muffin & Quickbread Mix
Classic Sugar Cookie Mix
Famous Pizza Crust Mix
Golden Pound Cake Mix
Hearty Biscuit Mix
Hearty Pancake & Waffle Mix
Homestyle Pie Crust Mix
Homestyle White Bread Mix
Lemon Poppy Seed Muffin Mix

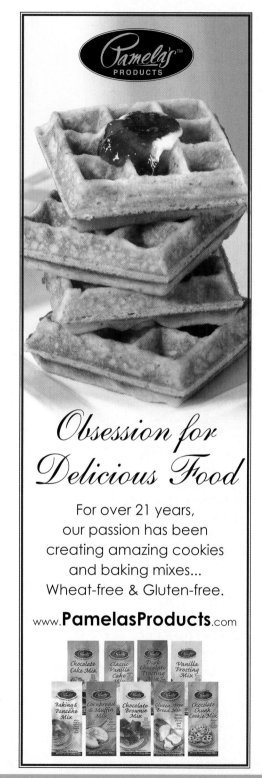

Moist Lemon Cake Mix
Moist Yellow Cake Mix
Rich Chocolate Cake Mix
Sweet Corn Muffin Mix
Traditional French Bread Mix

Chebe ♀ ✓
All-Purpose Bread Mix
Cinnamon Roll-Up Mix
Foccacia Mix
Garlic-Onion Breadstick Mix
Original Chebe Bread Mix
Pizza Crust Mix

Cherrybrook Kitchen ⓘ ✓
Gluten-Free Dreams Chocolate Cake
Gluten-Free Dreams Chocolate Chip
  Cookies
Gluten-Free Dreams Chocolate Chip
  Pancake
Gluten-Free Dreams Fudge Brownie
Gluten-Free Dreams Pancake
Gluten-Free Dreams Sugar Cookie
Gluten-Free Dreams Yellow Cake

Chi-Chi's
Fiesta Sweet Corn Cake Mix

Dowd & Rogers ♀ ✓
Dark Chocolate Brownie Mix
Dark Vanilla Cake Mix
Dutch Chocolate Cake Mix
Golden Lemon Cake Mix

Eagle Brand
Peanut Butter Fudge Dessert Kit

El Torito
Sweet Corn Cake Mix

Food-Tek ⓘ ✓
Gluten-Free Fast & Fresh Line (All)
Gluten-Free Quick-Bake Kids Line (All)

Gillian's Foods ♀
Gillian's Foods (All)

Gluten-Free Pantry, The ♀ ✓
Brown Rice Pancakes And Waffle Mix
Chocolate Chip Cookie & Cake Mix
Chocolate Truffle Brownie Mix
Coffee Cake Mix
Crisp & Crumble Topping Mix
Decadent Chocolate Cake Mix
Favorite Sandwich Bread Mix
French Bread & Pizza Mix

GF Stuffing
Muffin & Scone Mix
Old Fashioned Cake & Cookie Mix
Perfect Pie Crust
Quick Mix
Spice Cake & Gingerbread Mix
Tom's Light Gluten-Free Bread
Whole Grain Bread Mix
Yankee Cornbread & Muffin Mix

Glutino ♀ ✓
All-Purpose Baking Flour
Brown Rice Pancake & Waffle Mix
Chocolate Chip Cookie & Cake Mix
Chocolate Truffle Brownie Mix
Coffee Cake Mix
Crisp & Crumble Topping Mix
Decadent Chocolate Cake Mix
Favorite Sandwich Bread Mix
French Bread & Pizza Mix
Muffin & Scone Mix
Old Fashioned Cake & Cookie Mix
Perfect Pie Crust Mix
Quick Mix
Spice Cake & Gingerbread Mix
Yankee Cornbread Mix

Hodgson Mill
Apple Cinnamon Muffin Mix ♀
Gluten-Free Bread Mix ♀
Gluten-Free Pancake & Waffle Mix ♀
Multi Purpose Baking Mix ♀

Hol-Grain
Chocolate Brownie Mix
Pancake & Waffle Mix

Larrowe's
Instant Buckwheat Pancake Mix

Namaste Foods ♀ ✓
Namaste Foods (All)

Orgran ♀
Orgran (All)

Pamela's Products ♀ ✓
Baking & Pancake Mix
Chocolate Brownie Mix
Chocolate Cake Mix
Chocolate Chunk Cookie Mix
Classic Vanilla Cake Mix
Cornbread & Muffin Mix
Gluten-Free Bread Mix

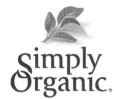

Simply *healthy living.*

Simply *great taste.*

Gluten Free

Our delicious organic, Fair Trade Certified™ baking mixes are made with brown rice containing no wheat, rye or barley & are packed in a GFCO facility. Try all 6 mixes!

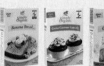

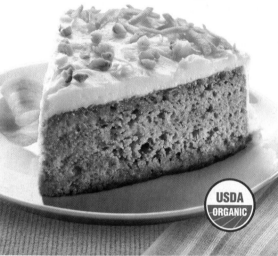

Schar ⛨ ✓
Classic White Bread Mix
Multipurpose Mix

Simply Organic ⛨ ✓
Banana Bread Baking Mix
Carrot Cake Baking Mix
Chai Spice Scone Baking Mix
Cocoa Biscotti Baking Mix
Cocoa Cayenne Baking Mix
Honeypot Ginger Baking Mix

BAKING POWDER

Bob's Red Mill ⓘ ✓
Baking Powder
Clabber Girl
Baking Powder
Davis Baking Powder
Baking Powder
Durkee ⓘ
Baking Powder
Ener-G ⛨
Baking Powder

Hain Pure Foods ✓
Gluten-Free Feather Weight Baking Powder
Hearth Club
Baking Powder
Hy-Vee
Double Acting Baking Powder
Kroger ⓘ
Baking Powder
Royal Baking Powder
Royal Baking Powder
Rumford
Baking Powder
Safeway
Baking Powder

BAKING SODA

Arm & Hammer
Baking Soda
Bob's Red Mill ⓘ ✓
Baking Soda

Durkee ⓘ
Baking Soda

Ener-G ⛑
Calcium Carbonate

Hy-Vee
Baking Soda

Kroger ⓘ
Baking Soda

Meijer
Baking Soda

Stop & Shop
Baking Soda

BREAD CRUMBS & OTHER COATINGS

Ener-G ⛑
Bread Crumbs

Gillian's Foods ⛑
Gillian's Foods (All)

Grandmas ⓘ
Bag N Bake Chicken

Hol-Grain
Brown Rice Bread Crumbs
Chicken Coating Mix

Luzianne
Seafood Coating Mix

Orgran ⛑
Orgran (All)

Schar ⛑ ✔
Bread Crumbs

Shake 'n Bake ᨒ
Seasoned Coating Mix - Barbecue Glaze
with Shaker Bag

Sunbird ⓘ
Tempura Batter

Taste of Thai, A
Peanut Bake

Williams ⓘ
Bag-N-Bake Chicken

COCOA POWDER

Ah!Laska ⛑
Unsweetened Bakers Cocoa

Ghirardelli ⓘ
Baking Cocoa Powder

Guittard
Guittard (All)

Hershey's
Cocoa

Hy-Vee
Baking Cocoa

Kroger ⓘ
Baking Cocoa

Scharffen Berger
Cocoa Powder ⟨⟩
Sweetened Cocoa Powder ⟨⟩

Stop & Shop
Baking Cocoa

COCONUT

Baker's Coconut ᨒ
Angel Flake Sweetened Coconut

Great Value (Wal-Mart)
Sweetened Flaked Coconut

Kroger ⓘ
Coconut - Regular
Coconut - Sweetened

Let's Do...Organic ✔
Organic Coconut Flakes
Organic Reduced Fat Shredded Coconut
Organic Shredded Coconut

Publix ⟨⟩
Coconut Flakes

Raley's ⛑
Coconut Flakes
Shredded Coconut

Safeway
Sweetened Coconut

CORN SYRUP

Brer Rabbit ⓘ
Syrup - Full
Syrup - Light

Karo ⛑
Beehive
Crown
Lily White
Syrups (All)

Meijer
Syrup - Lite Corn

CORNMEAL

Arrowhead Mills ✓
Blue Corn Meal
Yellow Corn Meal
Bob's Red Mill ⓘ ✓
GF Cornmeal
Goya
Corn Meal ◌
Pinol (Ground Toasted Corn)
Pinolillo
Hodgson Mill
Organic Yellow Corn Meal - Plain ⓘ
White Corn Meal - Plain ⓘ
Yellow Corn Meal - Plain ⓘ
Publix ◌
Plain Yellow Corn Meal
Safeway
Yellow Corn Meal ◌

EXTRACTS AND FLAVORINGS

Butter Buds ⛉
Butter Buds
DeLallo
Lemon Juice Plus
Lime Juice
Durkee ⓘ
Liquid Extracts (All)
Liquid Flavorings (All)
Hy-Vee
Imitation Vanilla
Kroger ⓘ
Extracts
Flavorings
McCormick
Extracts (All)
Meijer
Imitation Vanilla
Vanilla Extract
Midwest Country Fare (Hy-Vee)
Imitation Vanilla Flavor

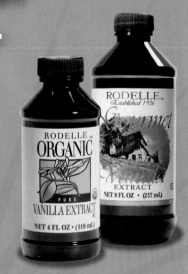

ALWAYS READ LABELS

Molly McButter ()
  Molly McButter Products
Nielsen-Massey
  Nielsen-Massey (All)
Publix ()
  Almond Extract
  Lemon Extract
  Vanilla Extract
Rodelle
  Almond Extract
  Anise Extract
  Bourbon Vanilla Beans
  Gourmet Vanilla Extract
  Lemon Extract
  Organic Pure Vanilla Extract
  Pure Vanilla Extract
  Vanilla Flavor (Alcohol Free)
  Vanilla Paste
Spice Islands ⓘ
  see Durkee
  Specialty - Vanilla Bean
Tone's ⓘ
  see Durkee
TryMe
  TryMe Liquid Smoke
Wright's Liquid Smoke ⓘ
  Liquid Smoke - Hickory
  Liquid Smoke - Mesquite

Flax Meal

Arrowhead Mills ✓
  Flax Seed Meal
Bob's Red Mill ⓘ ✓
  Flaxseed Meal - Brown
  Organic Flaxseed Meal - Brown
  Organic Golden Flaxseed Meal
Hodgson Mill
  Brown Milled Flax Seed ⚇
  Organic Golden Milled Flax Seed ⚇
  Travel Flax Brown Milled Flax Seed ⓘ
  Travel Flax Organic Golden Milled Flax
    Seed ⓘ

Flours & Flour Mixes

Arrowhead Mills ✓
  Buckwheat Flour
  Gluten-Free All Purpose Baking Mix
  Long Grain Brown Rice Flour
  Millet Flour
  Soy Flour
  White Rice Flour
Bob's Red Mill ⓘ ✓
  Almond Meal/Flour
  Black Bean Flour
  Brown Rice Flour
  Fava Bean Flour
  Garbanzo Bean Flour
  Garbanzo/Fava Bean Flour
  GF All Purpose Baking Flour
  GF Corn Flour
  Green Pea Flour
  Hazelnut Meal/Flour
  Millet Flour
  Millet Grits/Meal
  Organic Amaranth Flour
  Organic Brown Rice Flour
  Organic Coconut Flour
  Organic Quinoa Flour
  Organic White Rice Flour
  Potato Flour
  Sorghum Flour
  Sweet White Rice Flour
  Tapioca Flour
  Teff Flour
  White Bean Flour
  White Rice Flour
Diamond K ⚇
  Diamond K Rice Flour
Dowd & Rogers ⚇ ✓
  California Almond Flour
  Italian Chestnut Flour
Ener-G ⚇
  Brown Rice Flour
  Corn Mix
  Gluten-Free Gourmet Blend
  Potato Flour
  Potato Mix
  Potato Starch Flour
  Rice Mix

Sweet Rice Flour
Tapioca Flour
White Rice Flour

Fearn Natural Foods ⓘ
Brown Rice Baking Mix
Rice Baking Mix
Rice Flour

Gillian's Foods ⛌
Gillian's Foods (All)

Gluten-Free Pantry, The ⛌ ✓
Beth's All Purpose Baking Flour

Goya
Mandioca ⟨⟩
Masarepa ⟨⟩
Rice Flour ⟨⟩
Yuca Flour ⟨⟩

Hodgson Mill
Brown Rice Flour ⓘ
Buckwheat Flour ⓘ
Organic Soy Flour ⓘ
Soy Flour ⓘ

Kokuho Rose ⛌
Kokuho Rose Rice Flour

Lundberg Family Farms
Rice Flours & Grinds

Mochiko ⛌
Mochiko Blue Star Sweet Rice Flour

Orgran ⛌
Orgran (All)

Pocono
Buckwheat Flour

Tom Sawyer ⛌
All Purpose Gluten-Free Flour

FOOD COLORING

Durkee ⓘ
Food Coloring (All)

Hy-Vee
Assorted Food Coloring

Kroger ⓘ
Food Colors

Safeway
Food Coloring - Assorted

Spice Islands ⓘ
see Durkee

Tone's ⓘ
see Durkee

FROSTING

Cherrybrook Kitchen ⓘ ✓
Gluten-Free Dreams Chocolate Frosting
Gluten-Free Dreams Ready to Spread
    Vanilla Frosting
Gluten-Free Dreams Vanilla Frosting

Dr. Oetker ⟨⟩
Organic Icing Mix - Chocolate
Organic Icing Mix - Chocolate Fudge
Organic Icing Mix - Vanilla

Duncan Hines
Chocolate Buttercream
Classic Chocolate
Classic Vanilla
Cream Cheese
Dark Chocolate Fudge
Fluffy White
Lemon Supreme
Milk Chocolate
Strawberry Cream
Vanilla Butter Cream
Whipped Chocolate
Whipped Cream Cheese
Whipped Vanilla

Food-Tek ⓘ ✓
Gluten-Free Quick-Bake Line (All)

Pamela's Products ⛌ ✓
Confetti Frosting Mix
Dark Chocolate Frosting Mix
Vanilla Frosting Mix

Pillsbury
Frosting (All BUT Coconut Pecan)

Publix ⟨⟩
Buttercream Icing (Bakery)
Cream Custard (Natilla) (Bakery)

HONEY

Great Value (Wal-Mart)
Clover Honey

Harvest Farms (Ingles)
Honey (All)

Hy-Vee
Clover Honey
Honey
Squeeze Bear Honey

Laura Lynn (Ingle's)
Honey (All)

Meijer
Honey
Honey Squeeze Bear
Honey Squeeze Bottles

Publix GreenWise Market ()
Organic Honey

Publix ()
Clover Honey
Orange Blossom Honey
Wildflower Honey

Raley's ⚇
Honey

Safeway
Creamed Honey
Pure Honey

St. Dalfour
Honey ⚇

Wholesome Sweeteners ⚇
Organic Amber & Raw Honey

MARSHMALLOWS

Great Value (Wal-Mart)
Marshmallow Creme
Marshmallows
Miniature Flavored Marshmallows
Miniature Marshmallows

Hy-Vee
Colored Miniature Marshmallows
Marshmallows
Miniature Marshmallows

Jet-Puffed ⌒
Chocomallows Marshmallows
Marshmallows
Marshmallows Creme
Mini Variety Marshmallows
Miniature Choco Mallows
Marshmallows
Miniature Marshmallows
Miniature Marshmallows Funmallows

Miniature Strawberry Mallows
Marshmallows
Starmallows Vanilla Marshmallows
Strawberrymallows Marshmallows
Toasted Coconut Marshmallows

Kroger ⓘ
Colored Marshmallows
Large Marshmallows
Marshmallow Cream
Miniature Marshmallows

Manischewitz
Marshmallows

Marshmallow Fluff
Marshmallow Fluff

Meijer
Marshmallows - Mini
Marshmallows - Mini Flavored
Marshmallows - Regular

Publix ()
Marshmallows

Safeway
Marshmallows - Large
Marshmallows - Mini

MILK, CONDENSED

Eagle Brand
Sweetened Condensed Milk

Great Value (Wal-Mart)
Fat Free Sweetened Condensed Milk
Sweetened Condensed Milk

Hy-Vee
Sweetened Condensed Milk

La Lechera
Sweetened Condensed Milk

Meijer
Milk - Sweetened Condensed

Nestlé Carnation
Sweetened Condensed Milk

Raley's ⚇
Condensed Milk

Safeway
Sweetened Condensed Milk

Milk, Evaporated

Great Value (Wal-Mart)
Evaporated Milk
Fat Free Evaporated Skimmed Milk

Hy-Vee
Evaporated Milk
Fat Free Evaporated Milk

Meijer
Milk - Evaporated Lite Skimmed
Milk - Evaporated Small
Milk - Evaporated Tall

Nestlé Carnation
Evaporated Milk
Fat Free Evaporated Milk
Low Fat Evaporated Milk

PET Evaporated Milk
PET Evaporated Milk

Raley's ♀
Evaporated Milk

Safeway
Evaporated Milk

Milk, Instant or Powdered

Giant
Instant Nonfat Dry Milk

Hy-Vee
Instant Non Fat Dry Milk

Kroger ⓘ
Milks - Powdered

Meijer
Milk - Instant

Nestlé Carnation
Instant Nonfat Dry Milk

Publix ⟨⟩
Instant Nonfat Dry Milk

Safeway
Instant Milk

Stop & Shop
Instant Nonfat Dry Milk

Molasses

Brer Rabbit ⓘ
Molasses - Blackstrap
Molasses - Full
Molasses - Mild

Crosby's ♀
Molasses

Dixie Crystals
Sugar Products (All)

Dynasty
Bead Molasses

Grandma's Molasses ⓘ
Original
Robust

Holly Sugar
Sugar Products (All)

Imperial Sugar
Sugar Products (All)

Savannah Gold
Sugar Products (All)

Wholesome Sweeteners ♀
Organic Blackstrap Molasses

Oil & Oil Sprays

Annie's Naturals
Basil Flavored Olive Oil
Dipping Oil Herb Flavored Olive Oil
Roasted Garlic Flavored Extra Virgin
Olive Oil
Roasted Pepper Flavored Olive Oil

B.R. Cohn
Extra Virgin Olive Oils

Bella Tavola (Ingles)
Olive Oils (All)

Bertolli
Olive Oils (All)

Bionaturae ♀
Organic Olive Oil

Blue Plate
Oil

Bragg
Bragg (All)

Colavita
Olive Oils (All)

Crisco
Crisco (All BUT Cooking Spray with
Flour)

DeLallo
Basil Flavored Dipping Oil
Extra Light Olive Oil
Extra Virgin Olive Oil
Garlic Flavored Dipping Oil
Grapeseed Oil
Lemon Flavored Dipping Oil
Pure Olive Oil
Red Pepper Flavored Dipping Oil

Dynasty
Chili Oil
Sesame Oil
Stir Fry Oil

Eden Foods ⓘ ✓
Hot Pepper Sesame Oil
Olive Oil - Extra Virgin - Spanish
Safflower Oil - Organic
Sesame Oil - Extra Virgin - Organic
Soybean Oil - Organic
Toasted Sesame Oil

Emeril's ⓘ
Buttery Cooking Spray
Canola Oil Cooking Spray

Enova
Enova Oil

Filippo Berio ⚱
Extra Light-Tasting
Extra Virgin
Olive Oil
Organic Extra Virgin Olive Oil

Giant
Blended Oil
Canola Oil
Extra Light Olive Oil
Grill Spray
Peanut Oil
Pure Olive Oil
Soybean Oil

Goya
Olive Oil

Grand Selections (Hy-Vee)
100% Pure & Natural Olive Oil
Extra Virgin Olive Oil
Olive Oil Lemon

Great Value (Wal-Mart)
Canola Oil Blend
Extra Virgin Olive Oil

Light Tasting Olive Oil
Olive Oil
Pure Canola Oil
Pure Corn Oil, Bilingual
Pure Vegetable Oil

Harvest Bay
Coconut Oil (All)

Harvest Farms (Ingles)
Olive Oils (All)

House Of Tsang
Hot Chili Sesame Oil
Mongolian Fire Oil
Sesame Oil
Wok Oil

Hy-Vee
100% Pure Canola Oil
100% Pure Corn Oil
100% Pure Vegetable Oil
Natural Blend Oil

Kroger ⓘ
Canola Oil
Corn Oil
Olive Oil
Sunflower Oil
Vegetable Oil

Lapas ◇
Organic Olive Oil

Laura Lynn (Ingle's)
Cooking Oils (All)
Olive Oils (All)

Lee Kum Kee ⓘ
Blended Sesame Oil
Pure Sesame Oil

Lucini
Olive Oil (All)

Manischewitz
Cooking Sprays (All Varieties)
Vegetable Oil

Mazola
Oils (All)
Sprays (All)

Meijer
Cooking Spray - Butter
Cooking Spray - Olive Oil Extra Virgin
Cooking Spray - Vegetable Oil
Oil - Blended Canola/Vegetable

Oil - Canola
Oil - Corn
Oil - Olive
Oil - Olive 100% Pure-Italian Classic
Oil - Olive Extra Virgin
Oil - Olive Extra Virgin-Italian Classic
Oil - Olive Infused Garlic & Basil Italian
Oil - Olive Infused Roasted Garlic-Italian
Oil - Olive Infused Spicy Red Pepper Italian
Oil - Olive Milder Tasting
Oil - Peanut
Oil - Sunflower
Oil - Vegetable
Olive-Italian Select Premium Extra Virgin

Midwest Country Fare (Hy-Vee)
100% Pure Vegetable Oil
Vegetable Oil

Montebello ()
Organic Olive Oil

Newman's Own Organics ⓘ
Olive Oil

Nunez de Prado ()
Organic Olive Oil

O Olive Oil ⓘ
O Olive Oil (All)

Olivado
Specialty Oils (All)

Publix ()
Butter Flavored Cooking Spray
Canola Oil
Corn Oil
Garlic Flavored Cooking Spray
Lemon Flavored Cooking Spray
Olive Oil
Olive Oil Cooking Spray
Original Canola Cooking Spray
Peanut Oil
Vegetable Oil

Rapunzel
Canola Oil
Hazelnut Oil
Safflower Oil
Sesame Oil
Spanish Olive Oil

Sunflower Oil

Safeway
Cooking Spray - Butter Flavored Oils

Simply Enjoy (Giant)
Flavored Extra Virgin Olive Oil - Basil
Flavored Extra Virgin Olive Oil - Garlic
Flavored Extra Virgin Olive Oil - Lemon
Flavored Extra Virgin Olive Oil - Orange
Flavored Extra Virgin Olive Oil - Pepper
Regional Extra Virgin Olive Oil - Apulian
Regional Extra Virgin Olive Oil - Sicilian
Regional Extra Virgin Olive Oil - Tuscan
Regional Extra Virgin Olive Oil - Umbrian

Simply Enjoy (Stop & Shop)
Extra Virgin Olive Oil - Apulian
Extra Virgin Olive Oil - Sicilian
Extra Virgin Olive Oil - Umbrian
Extra Virgin Olive Oil -Tuscan
Flavored Extra Virgin Olive Oil - Basil
Flavored Extra Virgin Olive Oil - Garlic
Flavored Extra Virgin Olive Oil - Lemon
Flavored Extra Virgin Olive Oil - Orange
Flavored Extra Virgin Olive Oil - Pepper

Smart Balance
Smart Balance (All)

Stop & Shop
Blended Oil
Butter Flavored Cooking Spray
Canola Cooking Spray
Canola Oil
Corn Oil
Extra Light Olive Oil
Garlic Flavored Cooking Spray
Grill Spray
Olive Oil Cooking Spray
Pure Olive Oil
Soybean Oil
Vegetable Cooking Spray
Vegetable Oil

Villa Flor ()
Organic Olive Oil

Winn-Dixie ⓘ
Extra Virgin Olive Oil

RICE SYRUP

Lundberg Family Farms
Rice Syrup - Eco-Farmed Sweet Dreams
Rice Syrup - Organic Sweet Dreams

SHORTENING & OTHER FATS

Crisco
Crisco (All BUT Cooking Spray with Flour)
Empire Kosher
Rendered Chicken Fat
Great Value (Wal-Mart)
Animal Vegetable Shortening
Vegetable Shortening (All)
Hy-Vee
Vegetable Oil Shortening
Vegetable Shortening - Butter Flavor
Laura Lynn (Ingle's)
Shortening
Meijer
Shortening
Midwest Country Fare (Hy-Vee)
Pre-Creamed Shortening
Publix ⟨⟩
Vegetable Shortening
Stop & Shop
Meat Fat/Vegetable Shortening
Vegetable Shortening

SPICE MIXES & PACKETS

Ac'cent ⓘ
Flavor Enhancers (All)
Andy's Seasoning ⓘ
Seasoned Salt
Bone Suckin' Sauce ✓
Bone Suckin' Seasoning & Rub
Bragg
Bragg (All)
Cajun King
Char-Grill Seasoning Mix

Cajun's Choice
Blackened Seasoning
Cajun Shrimp Mix
Creole Seasoning
Gumbo File'
Jambalaya Mix
Shrimp/Crab/Crawfish Boil
Cali Fine Foods ⚱ ✓
Dill Delight Seasoning
Garlic Gusto Seasoning
Herb Medley Seasoning
Spicy Fiesta Seasoning
Sweet & Spicy BBQ Seasoning
Casa Fiesta
Taco Seasoning Mix
Chi-Chi's
Fiesta Restaurante Seasoning Mix
Chugwater Chili
Steak Rub
Durkee ⓘ
Apple Pie Spice
Chicken & Rib Rub
Chicken Seasoning
Chili Powder
Crazy Dave's (All)
Curry Powder
Garlic Pepper
Garlic Salt
Italian Seasoning
Jamaican Jerk Seasoning
Lemon & Herb
Lemon Pepper
Lime Pepper
Mr. Pepper
Onion Salt
Oriental 5-Spice
Pickling Spice
Pizza Seasoning
Poultry Seasoning
Pumpkin Pie Spice
Rosemary Garlic Seasoning
Salt-Free Garden Seasoning
Salt-Free Garlic & Herb
Salt-Free Lemon Pepper
Salt-Free Original All-Purpose
Salt-Free Veg. Seasoning
Six Pepper Blend

Smokey Mesquite Seasoning
Spaghetti/Pasta Seasoning
Spicy Spaghetti Seasoning
Steak Seasonings (All)

Dynasty
Chinese Five Spices

Emeril's ⓘ
Bam It Salad Seasoning
Chicken Rub
Essence - Bayou Blast
Essence - Italian
Essence - Original
Essence - Southwest
Fish Rub
Garlic Parmesan Essence for Bread
Rib Rub
Steak Rub
Turkey Rub

Fischer & Wieser ⓘ
Just Add Avocados Guacamole Starter

Goya
Adobo Goya
Chili Powder
Garlic Salt
Jamaican Curry Powder
Salad and Vegetable Seasoning
Sazón Goya
Sofrito

Grandmas ⓘ
Chili Package
Spaghetti

Hy-Vee
Chicken Grill Seasoning
Chili Powder
Garlic Salt
Italian Seasoning
Lemon Pepper
Steak Grilling Seasoning
Taco Mix

Johnny's Fine Foods ⓘ
Crab Boil
Dill Ranch
Game Seasoning
Garlic Salt
Great Caesar Garlic Spread & Seasoning
Hunter's Blend
Jamaica Me Crazy Lemon Pepper

Jamaica Me Crazy Salad Seasoning
Jamaica Me Crazy Seasoned Pepper
Jamaica Me Crazy Seasoned Sea Salt
Jamaica Me Hot 'n Crazy Sea Salt
Jamaica Me Steak Seasoning
Johnny's Seasoning Salt (Original)
Lamb & Game Seasoning
Northwest Style Steak Seasoning
Pasta Elegance
Pork & Chicken Seasoning
Salad Elegance
Salmon Seasoning
Seafood Seasoning
Seasoned Tenderizer
Vegetable Elegance

Konriko
Chipotle Seasoning
Creole Seasoning
Greek Seasoning
Gulf Coast Seasoning Blend
Jalapeno Seasoning
Mojo Seasoning

Lawry's
Seasoned Salt

Louisiana Fish Fry ()
Blackened Fish Seasoning
Cajun Seasoning
Chinese Red Pepper Seasoning
Crawfish Crab and Shrimp Boil
Fish Fry All Natural
Fish Fry New Orleans Style with Lemon
Fish Fry Seasoned

Luzianne
Cajun Seasoning

Mayacamas ✓
Chicken Fettuccine Sauce
Cream Pesto Sauce
Pesto Sauce
Skillet Toss - Black Olive Pesto
Skillet Toss - Dried Tomato
Skillet Toss - Garden Style
Skillet Toss - Green Olive Pesto
Skillet Toss - Seafood
Skillet Toss - Spicy

Meijer
Chili Powder
Garlic Salt

Mild Taco
Onion Salt
Seasoned Salt
Spaghetti Mix
Taco Seasoning

Mexene
Chili Powder Seasoning

Midwest Country Fare (Hy-Vee)
Chili Powder
Garlic Salt
Italian Seasoning
Season Salt

Morton
Garlic Salt
Hot Salt
Nature's Seasons Seasoning Blend
Seasoned Salt

Mrs. Dash
Seasoning Blends (All) () ⵜ

Old Bay
Old Bay Seasoning

Ortega ⓘ
Chipotle Mix
Guacamole Mix
Jalapeno & Onion Mix
Taco 40% Less Sodium Mix
Taco Meat Mix

Oven Fry ⌇
Fish Fry For Fish Seasoned Coating

Publix ()
Adobo Seasoning with Pepper
Adobo Seasoning Without Pepper
Chili Powder
Garlic Powder with Parsley
Garlic Salt
Italian Seasonings
Lemon & Pepper
Seasoned Salt
Taco Seasoning Mix

Robert Rothschild Farm
Caribbean Jerk Rub
Chop House Steak & Beef Rub
Fennel Herb Pork & Beef Rub
Limon Pepper Meat, Fish, Poultry Rub

Safeway
Fajita Seasoning Mix

Spice Hunter ⓘ
Spice Blends (All)

Spice Islands ⓘ
Grilling Gourmet & World Flavors (All)
Grinder Blends (All)
see Durkee
Specialty - Beau Monde
Specialty - Fines Herbs
Specialty - Garlic Pepper Seasoning
Specialty - Italian Herb Seasoning
Specialty - Summer Savory

Spike ⓘ
5Herb Magic!
Garlic Magic!
Hot 'n Spicy Magic!
Onion Magic!
Original Magic!
Salt Free Magic!
Vegit Magic!

Sunbird ⓘ
Beef & Broccoli
Chinese Chicken Salad
Chop Suey
Chow Mein
Fried Rice
General Tso's Chicken
Honey Sesame Chicken
Honey Teriyaki
Hot & Spicy Fried Rice
Hot & Spicy Kung Pao
Hot & Spicy Szechwan
Lemon Chicken Stir Fry
Mongolian Beef
New Hot & Sour Soup
Oriental Vegetable Stir Fry
Phad Thai
Spare Rib
Spicy Orange Beef
Stir Fry
Sweet & Sour
Thai Chicken
Thai Fried Rice
Thai Red Curry
Thai Spicy Beef
Thai Stir Fry

Swanson (Williams Food) ⓘ
Swanson Chicken Salad

Tone's ⓘ
see Durkee

Tradiciones ⓘ
Carne Adovada
Chimichurri
Green Mole
Guajillo Enchilada
Red Mole

TryMe
Tiger Seasoning

Wagners ⓘ
Hollandaise

Wick Fowler's
Taco Seasoning

Williams ⓘ
Chili Makins
Chili with Onions
Chipotle Chili
Chipotle Taco
Country Store Chili Soup
Country Store Tortilla Soup
Fancy Chili
Original Chili
Taco
Tex-Mex Chili
Tex-Mex Taco - Hot
White Chicken Chili

SPICES

DeLallo
Dipping Seasoning Spices

Durkee ⓘ
Allspice
Alum
Anise Seed
Basil
Bay Leaves
Caraway Seed
Cardamom
Cayenne Pepper
Celery Flakes
Celery Seed
Chives
Cilantro
Cinnamon
Cloves

Coriander
Cream of Tartar
Crushed Red Pepper
Cumin
Dill Seed/Weed
Fennel
Garlic Minced
Garlic Powder
Ginger
Hickory Smoke Salt
Mace
Marjoram
Meat Tenderizer
Mint Leaves
MSG
Mustard
Nutmeg
Onion Powder
Onion, Minced
Orange Peel
Oregano
Paprika
Parsley
Pepper - Black/White (All)
Pepper - Green Bell
Poppy Seed
Rosemary
Sage
Sesame Seed
Tarragon
Thyme
Turmeric

Eden Foods ⓘ ✓
Sea Salt - French
Sea Salt - Portuguese

Giant
Iodized Salt
Plain Salt

Goya
Achiotina (Annatto in Lard)
All Spice
Anis Seed
Bay Leaf
Camomile Manzanilla
Comino Molido
Crushed Peppers
Cumin Seed

Flor de Tilo
Garlic Powder
Ground Black Pepper
Ground Cinnamon
Ground Cumin
Ground Oregano
Ground Pepper
Onion Powder
Oregano Leaf
Paprika
Star Anis
Stick Cinnamon
Whole Black Pepper
Whole Cloves

Great Value (Wal-Mart)
Iodized Salt

Hy-Vee
Basil Leaf
Bay Leaves
Black Pepper
Chopped Onion
Dill Weed
Garlic Powder
Ground Cinnamon
Ground Cloves
Ground Mustard
Iodized Salt
Meat Tenderizer
Oregano Leaf
Paprika
Parsley Flakes
Plain Salt
Red Crushed Pepper
Rosemary
Salt & Pepper Shaker Set
Seasoned Salt
Thyme

Johnny's Fine Foods (i)
Popcorn Salt

Kroger (i)
Salt

Litehouse
Freeze Dried Cilantro
Freeze-Dried Basil
Freeze-Dried Chives
Freeze-Dried Dill
Freeze-Dried Garlic

Freeze-Dried Oregano
Freeze-Dried Parsley
Freeze-Dried Red Onion
Freeze-Dried Salad Herb Blend

Manischewitz
Salt

McCormick
Single Ingredient Herbs (All)
Single Ingredient Spices (All)

Meijer
Black Pepper
Cinnamon
Garlic Powder
Minced Onion
Oregano Leaves
Paprika
Parsley Flakes
Salt Iodized
Salt Plain

Midwest Country Fare (Hy-Vee)
Chopped Onion
Cinnamon
Garlic Powder
Ground Black Pepper
Onion Powder
Parsley Flakes
Pure Ground Black Pepper

Morton
Canning & Pickling Salt
Coarse Kosher Salt
Iodized Table Salt
Lite Salt Mixture
Plain Table Salt
Popcorn Salt
Salt & Pepper Shakers
Salt Substitute
Sea Salt (Fine and Coarse)
Smoke Flavored Sugar Cure
Sugar Cure (Plain)
Tender Quick

No Salt
No Salt Salt Substitute

NU-Salt
NU-Salt

Polaner (i)
Ready To Use Wet Spices - Basil
Ready To Use Wet Spices - Garlic

Ready To Use Wet Spices - Jalapenos
Publix ◊
Black Pepper
Cinnamon
Garlic Powder
Ground Ginger
Ground Red Pepper
Minced Onion
Onion Powder
Paprika
Parsley Flakes
Salt
Whole Bay Leaves
Whole Black Pepper
Whole Oregano
Spice Hunter ⓘ
Herbs
Spices
Spice Islands ⓘ
Salt-Free (All)
see Durkee
Specialty - Crystallized Ginger
Specialty - Old Hickory Smoked Salt
Specialty - Saffron
Stop & Shop
Iodized Salt
Plain Salt
Tone's ⓘ
see Durkee

SPRINKLES

Kroger ⓘ
Rainbow Sprinkles
Sugar Sprinkles
Let's Do... ✔
Carnival Sprinkelz
Chocolatey Sprinkelz
Confetti Sprinkelz
Safeway
Sprinkles - Easter
Sprinkles - Halloween
Sprinkles - Holiday
Sprinkles - Sand Sugar Party
Sprinkles - Valentines

STARCHES

Argo ⛨
Corn Starch
Benson's
Corn Starch
Bob's Red Mill ⓘ ✔
Arrowroot Starch
Cornstarch
Potato Starch
Canada
Corn Starch
Clabber Girl
Cornstarch ⓘ
Durkee ⓘ
Arrowroot
Hodgson Mill
Pure Corn Starch ⓘ
Hy-Vee
Cornstarch
Kingsford
Corn Starch
Kroger ⓘ
Corn Starch
Let's Do...Organic ✔
Organic Cornstarch
Organic Tapioca Starch
Manischewitz
Potato Starch
Meijer
Corn Starch
Rumford
Cornstarch ⓘ
Safeway
Corn Starch

SUGAR & SUGAR SUBSTITUTES

Billington's ⛨
Dark Brown Molasses Sugar
Demerara Sugar
Light Muscovado Sugar
Natural Sugar Crystals
C&H Sugar
C&H Sugar (All)

Dixie Crystals
Sugar Products (All)

Domino
Sugars (All)

Equal
Equal

Florida Crystals
Sugar Products (All)

Giant
Granulated Sugar
Sucralose

Great Value (Wal-Mart)
Altern No Calorie Sweetener
Calorie Free Sweetener
Confectioners Powdered Sugar
Extra Fine Granulated Sugar
Light Brown Sugar
Pure Cane Sugar

Holly Sugar
Sugar Products (All)

Imperial Sugar
Sugar Products (All)

Ingles Markets
Brown Sugar (All)
Confectioners Sugar (All)
Crystal Granulated Sugar (All)

Kroger ⓘ
Dark Brown Sugar
Granulated Sugar
Light Brown Sugar
Powdered Sugar
Sugar Substitutes

Laura Lynn (Ingle's)
Brown Sugar (All)
Confectioners Sugar (All)
Granulated Sugar (All)

Meijer
Sugar
Sugar - Confectioners
Sugar - Dark Brown
Sugar - Light Brown

Midwest Country Fare (Hy-Vee)
Granulated Sugar
Light Brown Sugar
Powdered Sugar

NatraTaste ⚕
NatraTaste
NatraTaste Gold

Nielsen-Massey
Nielsen-Massey (All)

Nutrasweet ⚕
NutraSweet (All)

Publix ()
Dark Brown Sugar
Granulated Sugar
Light Brown Sugar
Powdered - 10X Sugar
Powdered - 4X Sugar

Safeway
Aspartame Sweetener
Sugar - Brown, Granulated & Powdered

Savannah Gold
Sugar Products (All)

Splenda
Brown Sugar Blend
Flavor Accents - Lemon
Flavor Accents - Raspberry
Flavor Blends For Coffee - Caramel
Flavor Blends For Coffee - Cinnamon
  Spice
Flavor Blends For Coffee - French
  Vanilla
Flavor Blends For Coffee - Hazelnut
Flavor Blends For Coffee - Mocha
Mini
No Calorie Sweetener (Packets, Café
  Sticks and Granulated)
Splenda with Fiber
Sugar Blend

Stevia Extract in the Raw ⚕
Stevia Extract in the Raw

Stop & Shop
Granulated Sugar
Sucralose
Sweet Measure

Sugar in the Raw
Sugar In The Raw

Sweet 'N Low ⚕
Sweet 'n Low

Truvia
Truvia

Wholesome Sweeteners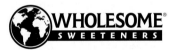

- Dark Brown Sugar
- Evaporated Cane Juice (All Types)
- Light Brown Sugar
- Organic Agave Syrups
- Organic Cane Syrups, Inverts & Blends (All Types)
- Organic Evaporated Cane Juice (All Types)
- Organic Sucanat (All Types)
- Turbinado Sugar, Sucanat (All Types)

WHOLE GRAINS

Alter Eco Fair Trade
- Quinoa (Black, Red & White) ✓

Arrowhead Mills ✓
- Buckwheat Groats
- Flax Seed
- Golden Flax Seed
- Hulled Millet
- Quinoa

Bob's Red Mill ⓘ ✓
- Flaxseed (Brown)

- GF Rolled Oats
- GF Steel Cut Oats
- Hulled Millet
- Organic Amaranth Grain
- Organic Buckwheat Berries
- Organic Buckwheat Groats
- Organic Buckwheat Kernels - Kasha
- Organic Flaxseed - Brown
- Organic Golden Flaxseed
- Organic Quinoa Grain
- Teff Grain

Eden Foods ⓘ ✓
- Buckwheat - Organic
- Millet - Organic
- Quinoa - Organic
- Red Quinoa - Organic

Pocono
- Cream of Buckwheat
- Kasha
- Whole Buckwheat Groats

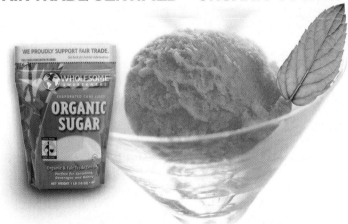

WHOLESOME® SWEETENERS

FAIR TRADE CERTIFIED™ ORGANIC SUGARS

Fair Trade Certified™ Organic & Natural Sugars, Syrups, Nectars & Honey.

Wholesome Sweeteners products are Gluten-Free.
For a copy of Wholesome Sweeteners' Gluten-Free Statement, please email info@OrganicSugars.biz.

www.OrganicSugars.biz · 1.800.680.1896 · info@OrganicSugars.biz

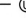

Yeast

Bakipan
- Active Dry Yeast (ADY)
- Bread Machine Yeast
- Instant Yeast

Bob's Red Mill ✓
- Yeast - Active Dry
- Yeast - Nutritional T6635 Lg Flake

Bragg
- Bragg (All)

Fleischmann's Yeast
- Fleischmann's Yeast (All)

Gayelord Hauser
- Brewers Yeast

Hodgson Mill
- Active Dry Yeast ⓘ
- Fast Rise Yeast ⓘ

Kroger ⓘ
- Yeast Packets

Red Star Yeast
- Active Dry Yeast (ADY)
- Bread Machine Yeast
- Quick Rise Yeast

SAF
- Active Dry Yeast (ADY)
- Bread Machine Yeast
- Perfect Rise

Miscellaneous

Bob's Red Mill ⓘ ✓
- GF Corn Grits/Polenta
- Guar Gum
- Organic Textured Soy Protein
- Rice Bran
- Soy Lecithin
- Textured Vegetable Protein (TVP)
- Xanthan Gum

Certo
- Liquid Fruit Pectin

Ener-G
- Rice Bran
- Xanthan Gum

Fearn Natural Foods ⓘ
- Lecithin Granules
- Liquid Lecithin

- Soya Granules
- Soya Powder
- Soya Protein Isolate

Let's Do…Organic ✓
- Organic Tapioca Granules
- Organic Tapioca Pearls

MCP
- Premium For Homemade Jams & Jellies Fruit Pectin

Sure.Jell
- Fruit Pectin - Premium For Homemade Jams & Jellies
- Fruit Pectin - Premium For Lower Sugar Recipes
- Jam Pectin - No Cook

Williams ⓘ
- Jel Ease - Pectin

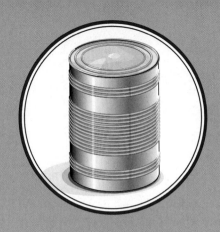

CANNED AND PACKAGED FOODS

Asian Specialty Items

Eden Foods ⓘ ✔
Shiro Miso - Organic
Wasabi Powder

Beans, Baked

B&M Baked Beans ⓘ
B&M Baked Beans (All)

Bush's Best
Bush's Best (All BUT Chili Beans, Chili Magic Chili Starter & Homestyle Chili Lines)

Eden Foods ⓘ ✔
Baked Beans with Sorghum & Mustard - Organic

Giant
Brown Sugar & Bacon Baked Beans
Pork & Beans
Vegetarian Baked Beans

Great Value (Wal-Mart)
Pork & Beans

HealthMarket (Hy-Vee)
Organic Baked Beans
Organic Maple & Onion Baked Beans

Heinz ⓘ
Vegetarian Beans

Hormel
Kid's Kitchen - Beans & Wieners

Hy-Vee
Home Style Baked Beans
Maple Cured Bacon Baked Beans
Onion Baked Beans
Original Baked Beans
Pork & Beans

Laura Lynn (Ingle's)
Baked Beans (All)
Pork & Beans

Meijer
Baked Beans Organic
Pork and Beans

Midwest Country Fare (Hy-Vee)
Pork & Beans

Publix ⟨⟩
Baked Beans
Pork & Beans

Safeway
Pork & Beans

Stop & Shop
Brown Sugar & Bacon Baked Beans
Homestyle Baked Beans
Vegetarian Baked Beans

Winn-Dixie ⓘ
Baked Beans
Baked Beans with Bacon & Onion

Beans, Other

Arrowhead Mills ✔
Adzuki Beans
Garbanzo Beans
Green Lentils
Red Lentils
Split Peas, Green

Bush's Best
Bush's Best (All BUT Chili Beans, Chili Magic Chili Starter & Homestyle Chili Lines)

DeLallo
Black Beans
Butter Beans
Cannellini Beans
Chick Peas
Chili Beans in Sauce
Great Northern Beans
Imported Lupini Beans
Light Red Kidney Beans
Navy Beans
Pinto Beans
Romano Beans

Eden Foods ⓘ ✓
Adzuki Beans - Organic
Black Beans - Organic
Black Eyed Peas -Organic
Black Soybeans - Organic
Butter Beans (Baby Lima) - Organic
Cajun Rice & Small Red Beans - Organic
Cannellini (White Kidney) Beans -
   Organic
Caribbean Black Beans
Caribbean Rice & Black Beans - Organic
Curried Rice & Lentils - Organic
Garbanzo Beans (Chick Peas) - Organic
Great Northern Beans - Organic
Kidney Beans - Organic
Mexican Rice & Black Beans - Organic
Moroccan Rice & Garbanzo Beans -
   Organic
Navy Beans - Organic
Pinto Beans - Organic
Rice & Garbanzo Beans - Organic
Rice & Kidney Beans - Organic
Rice & Lentils - Organic
Rice & Pinto Beans - Organic
Small Red Beans - Organic
Spanish Rice & Pinto Beans - Organic

Fantastic World Foods
Instant Black Beans

Furmano's ⚕
Bean Products (All)

Giant
Black Beans
Kidney Beans - Dark & Light Red
Kidney Beans - No Added Salt
Kidney Beans - Regular

Organic Black Beans
Organic Garbanzo Beans
Organic Light Kidney Beans
Pink Beans
Pinto Beans
Red Beans
Romano Beans

Goya
Blue-Labeled Canned Beans

Grand Selections (Hy-Vee)
Fancy Cut Green Beans
Fancy Whole Green Beans

Great Value (Wal-Mart)
Baby Lima Beans
Black Beans
Chick Peas (Garbanzos), Bilingual
Great Northern Beans
Large Lima Beans
Lentils
Light Red Kidney Beans
Mayocoba Beans, Bilingual
Navy Beans
Pink Beans, Bilingual
Pinto Beans
Small Red Beans
Southern Ranch Beans

HealthMarket (Hy-Vee)
Organic Black Beans
Organic Cut Green Beans
Organic Dark Red Kidney Beans
Organic French Cut Green Beans
Organic Garbanzo Beans
Organic Pinto Beans

Hy-Vee
Baby Lima Beans
Black Beans
Black-Eyed Peas
Butter Beans
Chili Style Beans
Dark Red Kidney Beans
Garbanzo Beans Chick Peas
Great Northern Beans
Large Lima Beans
Lentils
Light Red Kidney Beans
Navy Beans
Pinto Beans

Red Beans
Red Kidney Beans

Joan of Arc ⓘ
Black Beans
Butter Beans
Garbanzo Beans
Great Northern Beans
Light & Dark Red Kidney Beans
Pinto Beans
Red Beans

Kroger ⓘ
Unseasoned Beans - Canned
Unseasoned Beans - Dry

Meijer
Beans - Mexican Style
Black Beans
Black Beans Organic
Blackeye Peas
Butter Beans
Garbanzo Beans
Garbanzo Beans - Organic
Great Northern Beans
Kidney Beans - Dark Red
Kidney Beans - Dark Red Organic
Kidney Beans - Light Red
Lima Beans
Pinto Beans
Pinto Beans - Organic
Red Beans

Midwest Country Fare (Hy-Vee)
Chili Style Beans

Ortega ⓘ
Fat Free Refried Beans

Publix GreenWise Market ⓞ
Organic Black Beans
Organic Dark Red Kidney Beans
Organic Garbanzo Beans
Organic Pinto Beans
Organic Soy Beans

Publix ⓞ
Green Lima Beans
Kidney Beans - Dark Red

Safeway
Black Beans
Black-Eyed Beans
Chick Peas
Dark Kidney Beans

Light Kidney Beans
Mexican Style Chili Beans
Pinto Beans

Stop & Shop
Black Beans
Black Eyed Peas
Chick Peas
Kidney Beans - Light & Dark Red
Lima Beans
Pink Beans
Pinto Beans
Red Beans
Romano Beans

Teasdale 🏅 ✓
Black Beans
Chili
Dark Red Kidney Beans
Garbanzo Beans
Pinto Beans
Small Red Beans

Winn-Dixie ⓘ
Ford Hook Lima Beans
Garbanzo Beans

BEANS, REFRIED

Amy's Kitchen ⓘ ✓
Refried Beans with Green Chiles
Refried Black Beans
Refried Black Beans - Light in Sodium
Traditional Refried Beans
Traditional Refried Beans - Light in
    Sodium
Vegetarian Refried Beans

Casa Fiesta
Refried Beans

Eden Foods ⓘ ✓
Refried Black Beans - Organic
Refried Black Soy & Black Beans -
    Organic
Refried Kidney Beans - Organic
Refried Pinto Beans - Organic
Spicy Refried Black Beans - Organic
Spicy Refried Pinto Beans - Organic

Fantastic World Foods
Instant Refried Beans

HealthMarket (Hy-Vee)
Organic Refried Beans

Hy-Vee
Black Refried Beans
Fat Free Refried Beans
Traditional Refried Beans
Vegetarian Refried Beans

Laura Lynn (Ingle's)
Refried Beans (All)

Meijer
Fat Free Refried Beans
Refried Beans
Refried Beans - Fat Free
Refried Beans - Organic Black Bean
Refried Beans - Organic Black Bean/
Jalapeno
Refried Beans - Organic Roasted Chili/
Lime
Refried Beans - Organic Traditional
Refried Beans - Vegetarian

Ortega ⓘ
Refried Regular Beans

Safeway
Refried Beans

Taco Bell 〰
Fat Free Refried Beans
Vegetarian Blend Refried Beans

BOUILLON

Better than Bouillon ⚱
Beef Base
Chicken Base
Chili Base
Clam Base
Ham Base
Lobster Base
Low Sodium Chicken Base
Mushroom Base
Organic Beef Base
Organic Chicken Base
Organic Mushroom Base
Organic Vegetable Base
Turkey Base
Vegan No Beef Base
Vegan No Chicken Base
Vegetable Base

Edward & Sons ✓
Garden Veggie Bouillon Cubes
Low Sodium Veggie Bouillon Cubes
Not-Beef Bouillon Cubes
Not-Chick'n Bouillon Cubes

Giant
Beef Flavored Bouillon Cubes - Instant
Beef Flavored Bouillon Cubes - Regular
Chicken Flavored Bouillon Cubes -
Instant
Chicken Flavored Bouillon Cubes -
Regular

Goya
Consomme-Chicken Bouillon
Cubitos - Beef Bouillon
Cubitos - Chicken Bouillon
Ham Flavored Concentrate

Herb-Ox Bouillon
Beef
Chicken
Garlic Chicken
Vegetable

Laura Lynn (Ingle's)
Bouillon Cubes (All)
Instant Bouillon (All)

Lee Kum Kee ⓘ
Chicken Bouillon Powder
Kum Chun Chicken Bouillon Powder

Rapunzel
Vegetable Bouillon No Salt Added/Low
Sodium ◇
Vegetable Bouillon with Herbs ◇
Vegetable Bouillon with Sea Salt ◇

Stop & Shop
Beef Flavored Bouillon Cubes - Instant
Beef Flavored Bouillon Cubes - Regular
Chicken Flavored Bouillon Cubes -
Instant
Chicken Flavored Bouillon Cubes -
Regular

BROTH & STOCK

College Inn ⓘ
Beef Sirloin Bold Stock
Garden Vegetable Variety
Organic Beef Broth

White Wine & Herb Culinary Chicken
Broth

DeLallo
Clam Juice Broth

Emeril's ⓘ
Beef Stock
Chicken Stock
Vegetable Stock

Giant
Beef Broth
Chicken Broth

Great Value (Wal-Mart)
Beef Broth Ready To Serve
Chicken Broth Ready To Serve

Imagine ✔
Beef Flavored Broth
Free Range Chicken Broth
Low Sodium Beef Flavored Broth
Low Sodium Chicken Broth
Low Sodium Vegetable Broth
No-Chicken Broth
Vegetable Broth

Ingles Markets
Aseptic Chicken Broths (All)

Kitchen Basics ✔
Beef Stock (All)
Chicken Stock (All)
Clam Stock (All)
Ham Stock (All)
Pork Stock (All)
Seafood Stock (All)
Turkey Stock (All)
Vegetable Stock (All)

Meijer
Broth - Chicken
Broth Chicken (First Line)

Nature's Promise (Giant)
All Natural Beef Broth
Organic Chicken Broth
Organic Vegetable Broth

Nature's Promise (Stop & Shop)
All Natural Beef Broth
Organic Chicken Broth
Organic Vegetable Broth

Pacific Natural Foods ⓘ
Natural Beef

Natural Free Range Chicken
Organic Beef
Organic Free Range Chicken
Organic Low Sodium Chicken
Organic Low Sodium Vegetable
Organic Mushroom
Organic Vegetable

Papa Charlie's ⓘ
Italian Style Seasoned Broth

Rachael Ray ◇
Beef Stock
Chicken Stock

Safeway
Chicken Broth

Shelton's
Chicken Broth Fat Free
Chicken Broth Original
Organic Chicken Broth Fat Free
Organic Chicken Broth Original

Stop & Shop
Beef Broth
Chicken Broth

Swanson ⓘ
Beef Stock (Aseptic)
Chicken Broth (Aseptic & Canned)
Chicken Broth with Garlic (Canned)
Chicken Stock (Aseptic)
Natural Goodness Chicken Broth
(Aseptic & Canned)
Vegetarian Broth (Canned)

Valley Fresh
Broth

CHILI & CHILI MIXES

Amy's Kitchen ⓘ ✔
Black Bean Chili
Medium Chili
Medium Chili - Light in Sodium
Medium Chili with Vegetables
Spicy Chili
Spicy Chili - Light in Sodium

Bean Cuisine
Bean Soups Bag - Chili

Bush's Best
- Bush's Best (All BUT Chili Beans, Chili Magic Chili Starter & Homestyle Chili Lines)

Carroll Shelby Chili
- Original Texas Chili Kit

Chugwater Chili
- Chili Blend

Del Monte ⓘ
- Harvest Selection "Heat & Eat" Chili & Beans

Hormel
- Chili with Beans - Chunky
- Chili with Beans - Hot
- Chili with Beans - Regular

Hy-Vee
- Chili with Beans
- Hot Chili with Beans

Juanitas
- Juanitas (All)

Meijer
- Chili with Beans (Regular)
- Chili with No Beans (Regular)

Safeway
- Healthy Advantage - Vegetarian Chili

Shelton's
- Chicken Chili Mild
- Chicken Chili Spicy
- Turkey Chili Mild
- Turkey Chili Spicy

Texas Pete
- Chili No Bean ⓘ
- Hot Dog Chili ⓘ

Wick Fowler's
- 2-Alarm Chili Kit
- False Alarm Chili Kit
- One Step Wick Fowler Chili

COCONUT MILK

Goya
- Coconut Milk
- Cream of Coconut

Let's Do…Organic ✓
- Organic Creamed Coconut

Native Forest ✓
- Organic Coconut Milk
- Organic Light Coconut Milk

Taste of Thai, A
- Coconut Milk
- Lite Coconut Milk

Thai Kitchen ⓘ
- Coconut Milk Lite
- Coconut Milk Lite Organic
- Premium Coconut Milk
- Premium Coconut Milk Organic

CRANBERRY SAUCE

Hy-Vee
- Jellied Cranberry Sauce
- Whole Berry Cranberry Sauce

Laura Lynn (Ingle's)
- Cranberry Sauce (All)

Ocean Spray
- Sauces (All)

Publix ◌
- Whole Cranberry Sauce

Safeway
- Cranberry Sauce - Jellied
- Cranberry Sauce - Whole

Stop & Shop
- Cranberry Sauce - Jellied
- Cranberry Sauce - Whole Berry

FRUIT

Del Monte ⓘ
- Canned/Jarred Fruits

DeLallo
- San Martino Peach Halves in Lite Syrup
- San Martino Pear Halves

Dole ◌
- Canned Fruit (All)
- Fruit Bowls (All)
- Fruit in Jars (All)

Giant
- Apricots - Heavy Syrup
- Apricots - Island in Light Syrup
- Bartlett Pear Halves - Heavy Syrup
- Bartlett Pear Halves - Juice

Bartlett Pear Halves - Light Syrup
Bartlett Pear Halves - Pear Juice
Bartlett Pear Halves - Splenda
Blueberries in Syrup
Fruit Cocktail - Heavy Syrup
Fruit Cocktail - Pear Juice
Fruit Cocktail - Splenda
Fruit Mix in Heavy Syrup
Peaches - Heavy Syrup
Peaches - Pear Juice
Peaches - Yellow Cling
Red Tart Pitted Cherries in Water
Sweet Cherries in Heavy Syrup - Dark
Sweet Cherries in Heavy Syrup - Light
Very Cherry Fruit Mix in Light Syrup
Whole Plums in Heavy Syrup

Great Value (Wal-Mart)
Bartlett Pear Halves In Heavy Syrup
Bartlett Sliced Pears In Heavy Syrup
Blackberries
Blueberries
Crushed Pineapple
Fruit Cocktail In Heavy Syrup
Fruit Cocktail Sweetened w/Splenda
Fruit Selections Crushed Pineapple
Fruit Selections Diced Peaches & Pears In Strawberry & Raspberry Light Syrup
Fruit Selections Diced Peaches In Light Syrup
Fruit Selections Diced Peaches In Strawberry & Banana Light Syrup
Fruit Selections Diced Peaches w/ Splenda
Fruit Selections Mandarin Oranges In Light Syrup
Fruit Selections Mixed Fruit In Light Syrup
Fruit Selections Mixed Fruit w/Splenda
Fruit Selections Pineapple Chunks
Fruit Selections Pineapple Slices
Fruit Selections Pineapple Tidbits In Pineapple Juice
Fruit Selections Tropical Fruit Mix In Light Syrup
Fruit Slices
Jellied Cranberry Sauce

Maraschino Cherries
Maraschino Cherries w/Stems
No Sugar Added Bartlett Pear Halves
No Sugar Added Chunky Mixed Fruits
No Sugar Added Fruit Cocktail
No Sugar Added Yellow Cling Peach Halves
No Sugar Added Yellow Cling Sliced Peaches
Orange Slices
Peaches & Pears In Cherry Gel
Pineapple Chunks
Pineapple Slices
Red Raspberries
Sliced Peaches
Tidbit Pineapple
Triple Cherry Fruit Mix In Light Syrup
Tropical Fruit Salad
Whole Berry Cranberry Sauce
Whole Segment Mandarin Oranges In Light Syrup
Whole Strawberries
Yellow Cling Peach Halves In Heavy Syrup
Yellow Cling Sliced Peaches Sweetened w/Splenda

Harvest Farms (Ingles)
Canned Fruits (All)

Hy-Vee
Bartlett Pear Halves
Bartlett Pear Slices
Chunk Pineapple
Crushed Pineapple
Diced Peaches
Fruit Cocktail
Fruit Mix
Lite Bartlett Pear Halves
Lite Chunk Mixed Fruit
Lite Diced Peaches
Lite Fruit Cocktail
Lite Unpeeled Apricot Halves Sweetened with Splenda
Lite Yellow Cling Peach Halves
Lite Yellow Cling Peach Slices
Mandarin Oranges
Mandarin Oranges in Light Syrup

Mandarin Oranges in Orange Gel Fruit Cups
Natural Lite Diced Bartlett Pears
Peaches in Strawberry Gel Fruit Cups
Pineapple in Lime Gel Fruit Cups
Pumpkin
Purple Plums
Sliced Pineapple
Unpeeled Apricot Halves
Yellow Cling Peach Halves
Yellow Cling Peach Slices

Knouse Foods ⚥
Dutch Baked Apples
Fried Apples
Red Tart Pitted Cherries
Sliced Apples
Spiced Apple Rings
Spiced Crab Apples

Kroger ⓘ
Fruit - Canned

Laura Lynn (Ingle's)
Canned Fruits (All)

Libby's
Libby's 100% Pure Pumpkin

Meijer
Apricot Halves Unpeeled in Pear Juice
Fruit Cocktail in Heavy Syrup
Fruit Cocktail in Pear Juice Lite
Fruit Cocktail Juice
Fruit Cocktail Juice Easy Open
Fruit Mix Juice
Fruit Salad Tropical
Grapefruit Sections in Juice
Grapefruit Sections in Syrup
Mandarin Oranges Light Syrup
Peaches - Cling Halves in Heavy Syrup
Peaches - Cling Halves in Juice Lite
Peaches - Cling Halves Pear Juice Lite
Peaches - Cling Sliced in Heavy Syrup
Peaches - Cling Sliced in Juice
Peaches - Cling Slices Pear Juice Lite
Peaches - Yellow Sliced in Heavy Syrup
Pear Halves - Lite
Pear Slices in Heavy Syrup
Pears - Halves in Heavy Syrup
Pears - Halves in Juice Lite
Pears - Slices in Juice Lite

Pineapple - Crushed Heavy Syrup
Pineapple - Crushed in Juice
Pineapple - Sliced Heavy Syrup
Pineapple - Sliced in Juice
Pineapple Chunks - Heavy Syrup
Pineapple Chunks in Juice
Pineapple Juice
Pumpkin

Midwest Country Fare (Hy-Vee)
Bartlett Pear Halves in Light Syrup
Crushed Pineapple
Fruit Cocktail
Lite Peach Halves
Lite Peach Slices
Pineapple Chunks
Pineapple Slices
Pineapple Tidbits

Native Forest ✓
Organic Mango Chunks
Organic Papaya Chunks
Organic Pineapple Chunks
Organic Pineapple Crushed
Organic Pineapple Slices
Organic Tropical Fruit Salad

Publix ()
Apricot Halves - Unpeeled in Heavy Syrup
Bartlett Pears in Heavy Syrup (Halves and Slices)
Chunky Mixed Fruit in Heavy Syrup
Fruit Cocktail in Heavy Syrup
Lite Bartlett Pear Halves in Pear Juice
Lite Chunky Mixed Fruit in Pear Juice
Lite Fruit Cocktail in Pear Juice
Lite Yellow Cling Peaches in Pear Juice (Halves and Slices)
Mandarin Oranges in Light Syrup
Pineapple (All Styles)
Yellow Cling Peaches in Heavy Syrup (Halves and Slices)

Raley's ⚥
Canned Pineapple

S&W ⓘ
Canned/Jarred Fruits (All)

Safeway
Canned Pumpkin
Mixed Fruit & Peel

Red Tart Pitted Cherries
Sliced Peaches

Stop & Shop
Apricots - Heavy Syrup & Splenda
Bartlett Pear Halves - Heavy Syrup,
Light Syrup, Pear Juice & Splenda
Fruit Cocktail - Heavy Syrup, Pear Juice
& Splenda
Fruit Mix in Heavy Syrup
Island Apricots in Light Syrup
Peaches - Yellow Cling, Pear Juice &
Heavy Syrup (Whole & Slices)
Very Cherry Fruit Mix in Light Syrup
Whole Plums in Heavy Syrup

Wyman's
Wyman's (All)

MEALS & MEAL STARTERS

Allergaroo ⅋
Chili Mac
Spaghetti
Spyglass Noodles
Annie's Homegrown
Rice Pasta & Cheddar ⅋
Bob Evans ()
Cheddar Mashed Potatoes
Garlic Mashed Potatoes
Glazed Apples
Mashed Sweet Potatoes
Original Mashed Potatoes
Sausage Chili
Slow Roasted Beef Pot Roast with Gravy
Texas Mashed Potatoes
Turkey Breast with Gravy
Casa Fiesta
Taco Dinners
DeBoles ✓
Rice Pasta & Cheese
Rice Shells & Cheddar
Del Monte ⓘ
Harvest Selections "Heat & Eat" Santa
Fe Style Rice & Beans
DeLallo
Instant Polenta
Dinty Moore
Microwave Meals - Rice with Chicken

Microwave Meals - Scalloped Potatoes
& Ham
Gluten-Free & Fabulous ⅋ ✓
Bon Appetit! Quinoa with Marinara
Macaroni & Cheese
Homestyle Meals
Homestyle Meals Shredded Beef in BBQ
Sauce
Hormel
Beef Tamales
Compleats Microwave Meals - BBQ Beef
& Beans
Compleats Microwave Meals - Chicken
& Rice
Compleats Microwave Meals - Sweet &
Sour Rice
Refrigerated Entrées - Beef Roast Au Jus
Refrigerated Entrées - Italian Style Beef
Roast
Refrigerated Entrées - Pork Roast Au Jus
Refrigerated Entrées - Turkey Stroganoff
Ian's Natural Foods ⅋ ✓
Wheat and Gluten-Free Recipe Pasta
Dinner Kit

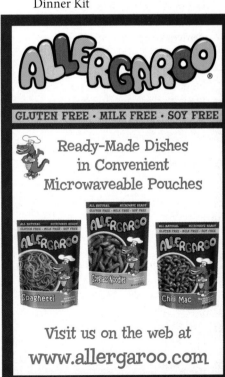

Wheat and Gluten-Free Recipe Pizza Dinner Kit

Juanitas
Juanitas (All)

Luzianne
Creole Dinner Kit
Jambalaya Dinner Kit

Orgran
Orgran (All)

Ortega ⓘ
Pizza Grande Dinner Kit
Taco Kit

Oscar Mayer Lunchables ∿
Cheese Dip & Salsa Cracker Stackers/ Nachos

Publix ()
Carrot Salad (Deli)
Chicken Salad (Deli)
Chicken Tarragon Salad (Deli)
Chunky Chicken Salad (Deli)
Cranberry Orange Relish Salad (Deli)
Egg Salad (Deli)
Garlic Redskin Smashed Potatoes (Deli)
German Potato Salad (Deli)
Greek Potato Salad (Deli)
Ham Salad (Deli)
Homestyle Potato Salad (Deli)
Marshmallow Delight Salad (Deli)
New York Style Potato Salad (Deli)
Santa Fe Turkey Salad (Deli)
Southern Style Potato Salad (Deli)

Road's End Organics ✓
GF Alfredo Chreese Mix
GF Cheddar Chreese Mix
Organic GF Alfredo Mac & Chreese
Organic GF Cheddar Penne & Chreese

Safeway
Classic Potato Salad (Deli Counter) ()
Deviled Egg Potato Salad (Deli Counter) ()
Mustard Potato Salad (Deli Counter) ()
Old Fashioned Potato Salad (Deli Counter) ()
Select - Cheese Fondue

Simply Potatoes
Simply Potatoes (All)

St. Dalfour
Gourmet on the Go - Three Beans ⓘ

Gourmet on the Go - Wild Salmon ⓘ

Sunbird ⓘ
Asian Skillet Classics - Sweet & Sour Pork

Taco Bell ∿
Taco Dinner - Sauce & Taco Shells
Ultimate Nachos! Home Originals - Refried Beans, Cheese Sauce, Tortilla Chips & Salsa

Taste of China, A
Szechuan Noodles

Taste of India, A
Spiced Rice with Raisins

Taste of Thai, A
Chicken & Rice
Coconut Ginger Noodles
Pad Thai For Two
Pad Thai Noodles
Peanut Noodles
Red Curry Noodles
Yellow Curry Noodles

Tasty Bite
Agra Peas & Greens
Bengal Lentils
Bombay Potatoes
Jaipur Vegetables
Jodhpur Lentils
Kashmir Spinach
Kerala Vegetables
Madras Lentils
Massaman Vegetables
Paneer Makhani
Peas Paneer
Punjab Eggplant
Satay Vegetables
Spinach Dal
Spinach Soy

Thai Kitchen ⓘ
Noodle Carts - Pad Thai
Noodle Carts - Roasted Garlic
Noodle Carts - Thai Peanut
Noodle Carts - Toasted Sesame
Stir-Fry Rice Noodle Meal Kit - Lemongrass & Chili
Stir-Fry Rice Noodle Meal Kit - Original Pad Thai

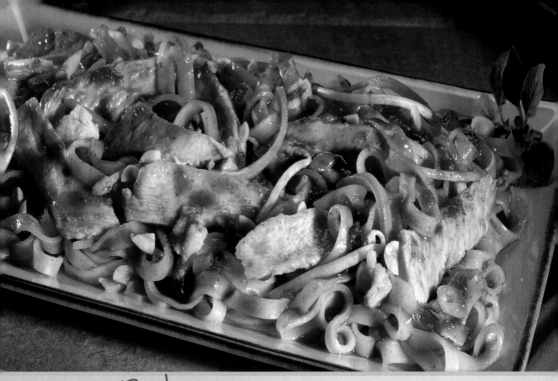

Real ^Pad Thai. Real Easy.

It's easy to make delicious, restaurant-style Pad Thai meals with A Taste Of Thai®. Microwave a Quick Meal for one in minutes, or add a few simple ingredients to create an authentic Thai classic for two or more! Enjoy the same exotic food you used to go out for, right at home! **For any size family!**

Reduced Sodium ~~~ Gluten Free

for you

for two

for the whole crew

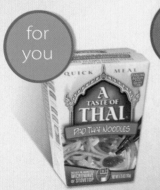
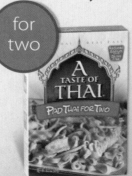
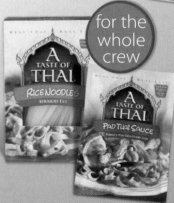

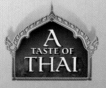

Look for **A Taste of Thai®** in the Asian aisle, or call 800-243-0897. Free recipes at **atasteofthai.com**

Stir-Fry Rice Noodle Meal Kit - Thai
Peanut
Take-Out Boxes - Ginger & Sweet Chili
Take-Out Boxes - Original Pad Thai
Take-Out Boxes - Thai Basil & Chili

Meat

Giant
Premium Chunk Chicken Breast in
Water
Great Value (Wal-Mart)
Potted Meat Product
Vienna Sausage
Hormel
Black Label - Canned Hams
Breast of Chicken Chunk Meats
Chicken Chunk Meats
Corned Beef
Corned Beef Hash
Dried Beef
Ham Chunk Meats
Turkey Chunk Meats
Kroger ⓘ
Chicken - Canned
Chicken - Pouch
Laura Lynn (Ingle's)
Canned Chicken (All)
Canned Tuna (All)
Corned Beef Hash
Meijer
Chicken Chunk White
Corned Beef Hash
Safeway
Corned Beef Hash
SPAM
Classic
Less Sodium
Lite
Oven Roasted Turkey
Smoke Flavored
Stop & Shop
Premium Chunk Chicken Breast in
Water
Thrifty Maid ⓘ
Corned Beef

Underwood ⓘ
Deviled Ham Spread
Valley Fresh
Chicken
Turkey

Pie Fillings

Comstock
Pie Fillings
Giant
Blueberry Fruit Filling
Cherry Pie Filling
Lite Cherry Pie Filling
Spiced Apple Pie Filling
Great Value (Wal-Mart)
Apple Pie Filling
Blueberry Pie Filling
Cherry Pie Filling
No Sugar Added Apple Pie Filling w/
Splenda
No Sugar Added Cherry Pie Filling w/
Splenda
Hy-Vee
100% Natural Pumpkin
More Fruit Apple Pie Filling Or Topping
More Fruit Cherry Pie Filling Or
Topping
Knouse Foods 🏅
Apple Pie Filling
Apricot Pie Filling
Banana Crème Pie Filling
Blackberry Pie Filling
Blueberry Pie Filling
Cherries Jubilee Pie Filling
Cherry Pie Filling
Chocolate Crème Pie Filling
Coconut Crème Pie Filling
Dark Sweet Cherry Pie Filling
Key Lime Pie Filling
Lemon Crème Pie Filling
Lemon Pie Filling
Lite Apple Pie Filling
Lite Cherry Pie Filling
Peach Pie Filling
Pineapple Pie Filling
Raisin Pie Filling

Strawberry Glaze Pie Filling
Strawberry Pie Filling
Vanilla Crème Pie Filling

Kroger ⓘ
Canned Pie Filling

Libby's
Libby's Easy Pumpkin Pie Mix

Meijer
Pie Filling - Apple
Pie Filling - Blueberry
Pie Filling - Cherry
Pie Filling - Cherry Lite
Pie Filling - Peach

Midwest Country Fare (Hy-Vee)
Apple Pie Filling
Cherry Pie Filling

Wilderness
Pie Fillings

SEAFOOD, OTHER

Bubbies ♗
Bubbies (All)

Chicken of the Sea
Chicken of The Sea (All BUT Crab-Tastic! Imitation Crab, Smoked Teriyaki Oysters, Tuna Salad Kits, Tuna Salad Lunch Solutions Cup with Crackers, Tuna Snax in Original, Lemon Pepper, & Tomato Basil Flavors in Cup)

Crown Prince ♗
Anchovy Fillets
Anchovy Paste
Boiled Baby Clams
Brisling Sardines in Mustard
Brisling Sardines in Olive oil
Brisling Sardines in Water
Clam Juice
Crab Meat
Kippers
Pink Salmon
Skinless Boneless Pink Salmon
Skinless Boneless Sardines in Olive Oil
Skinless Boneless Sardines in Water
Smoked Baby Clams in Olive Oil
Smoked Coho Salmon

Smoked Oysters in Olive Oil
Whole Boiled Oysters

DeLallo
Chopped Sea Clams
Flat Fillet Anchovies
Minced Sea Clams
San Martino Crabmeat

Giant
Filet of Mackerel
Portuguese Sardines

Goya
Octopus
Sardines

Great Value (Wal-Mart)
Crab Meat
Lightly Smoked Sardines In Oil
Smoked Oysters (China)
Smoked Oysters (South Korea)
Tiny Shrimp

Hy-Vee
Alaska Pink Salmon
Alaska Red Salmon

King Oscar ⓘ
King Oscar (All BUT Brisling Sardines with Balsamic Vinegar and Gourmet Chipotle Sauce)

Kroger ⓘ
Salmon - Canned
Sardines - Canned

Meijer
Salmon - Pink
Salmon - Sockeye Red

Strub's ()
Strub's (All)

SEAFOOD, TUNA

Bumble Bee
Canned Seafood Products (All)

Chicken of the Sea
Chicken of The Sea (All BUT Crab-Tastic! Imitation Crab, Smoked Teriyaki Oysters, Tuna Salad Kits, Tuna Salad Lunch Solutions Cup with Crackers, Tuna Snax in Original, Lemon Pepper, & Tomato Basil Flavors in Cup)

Crown Prince
Albacore Tuna No Salt Added
Albacore Tuna Regular
Tongol Tuna No Salt Added
Tongol Tuna Regular
Yellowfin Tuna in Olive Oil

Great Value (Wal-Mart)
Chunk Light Tuna In Water
Premium Chunk Light Tuna In Water
Solid White Albacore Tuna In Water

Hy-Vee
Chunk Light Premium Tuna in Water
Chunk White Albacore Premium Tuna in Water
Light Chunk Tuna in Water

Kroger ⓘ
Tuna - Canned
Tuna - Pouch

Midwest Country Fare (Hy-Vee)
Light Tuna Chunks Packed in Water

Safeway
Chunk Light Tuna
Select - Tuna, Tongol

StarKist Tuna ⓘ
Starkist Tuna (All BUT Crackers in Lunch To-Go)
Starkist Tuna Creations (All BUT Herb & Garlic and Tomato Pesto Albacore)
Starkist Tuna Fillets (All BUT Teriyaki)

SOUPS & SOUP MIXES

Amy's Kitchen ⓘ ✔
Black Bean Vegetable Soup
Chunky Tomato Bisque
Chunky Tomato Bisque - Light in Sodium
Chunky Vegetable Soup
Corn Chowder
Cream of Tomato Soup
Cream of Tomato Soup - Light in Sodium
Fire Roasted Southwestern Vegetable Soup
Lentil Soup
Lentil Soup - Light in Sodium
Lentil Vegetable Soup
Lentil Vegetable Soup - Light in Sodium
Potato Leek Soup
Split Pea Soup
Split Pea Soup - Light in Sodium
Thai Coconut Soup
Tuscan Bean & Rice Soup

Bean Cuisine
Bean Soups Bag - Island Black Bean
Bean Soups Bag - Lots of Lentil
Bean Soups Bag - Louisiana Cajun
Bean Soups Bag - Santa Fe Corn Chowder
Bean Soups Bag - Southwest Tortilla
Bean Soups Bag - Thick As Fog Split Pea
Bean Soups Bag - Thirteen Bean Bouillabaisse
Bean Soups Bag - White Bean Provencal

Bear Creek
Cheddar Broccoli
Cheddar Potato
Chili
Clam Chowder
Creamy Potato
Creamy Wild Rice
Navy Bean
Split Pea
Tortilla

Dr. McDougall's Right Foods
Black Bean & Lime Big Cup
Light Sodium Split Pea
Pad Thai Noodle Big Cup
Tamale Big Cup
Tortilla Big Cup

Eden Foods ⓘ ✔
Genmai (Brown Rice) Miso - Organic

Ener-G
Cream of Mushroom Soup

Fantastic World Foods
Baja Black Bean Soup Cup

Blarney Stone Simmer Soup
Buckaroo Bean Chili Soup Cup
Creamy Potato Leek Soup Cup
Creamy Potato Simmer Soup
Great Lakes Cheddar Broccoli Soup Cup
Split Pea Soup Cup
Summer Vegetable Rice Soup Cup

Gold's
Borscht
Lo-Calorie Borscht
Russian Style Borscht
Schav
Unsalted Borscht

Hormel
Microwave Bean & Ham Soup
Microwave Chicken with Vegetables & Rice Soup

Imagine ✓
Creamy Acorn Squash & Mango Soup
Creamy Broccoli Soup
Creamy Butternut Squash Soup
Creamy Corn & Lemongrass Soup
Creamy Portobello Mushroom Soup
Creamy Potato Leek Soup
Creamy Sweet Pea Soup
Creamy Sweet Potato Soup
Creamy Tomato Basil Soup
Creamy Tomato Soup
Light in Sodium Broccoli Soup
Light in Sodium Creamy Garden Tomato Soup
Light in Sodium Creamy Harvest Corn Soup
Light in Sodium Creamy Red Bliss Potato & Roasted Garlic Soup
Light in Sodium Sweet Potato Soup

Juanitas
Juanitas (All)

Laura Lynn (Ingle's)
Chicken & Rice Soup

Manischewitz
Borscht (All)
Chicken Soup
Clear Chicken Consomme
Condensed Clear Chicken Soup
Hearty Bean Cello Soup Mix
Schav

Split Pea Soup Mix w/Seasoning Cello Soup Mix

Mayacamas ✓
Dark Mushroom Soup
French Onion Soup
Lentil Soup
Potato Leek Soup
Tomato Soup

Meijer
Chicken (Aseptic)
Condensed Chicken with Rice Soup
Homestyle Chicken with Rice Soup

Midwest Country Fare (Hy-Vee)
Onion Soup

Miso-Cup ✓
Japanese Restaurant Style
Original Golden Vegetable
Reduced Sodium
Savory Seaweed
Traditional with Tofu

Orgran ⚉
Orgran (All)

Pacific Natural Foods ⓘ
Buttery Sweet Corn
Cashew Carrot Ginger
Creamy Roasted Carrot
Curried Red Lentil
Organic Creamy Butternut Squash
Organic Creamy RRP & Tomato
Organic Creamy Tomato
Organic French Onion
Organic Light Sodium Creamy Butternut Squash
Organic Light Sodium RRP & Tomato
Organic Savory Chicken & Wild Rice
Organic Spicy Black Bean with Chicken Sausage
Organic Spicy Chicken Fajita
Organic Split Pea with Ham & Swiss Cheese

Publix ()
Broccoli and Cheddar Soup (Deli)
Chicken Tortilla Soup (Deli)
Potato Cheddar and Bacon Soup (Deli)
Spring Vegetable Soup (Deli)

Robert Rothschild Farm
- Creamy Tomato Vodka Soup with Sweet Basil
- Potato Soup

Safeway
- Chicken with Rice Soup
- Condensed Homestyle Chicken with Wild Rice Soup
- Onion Soup Mix
- Select - Signature Soup, Autumn Harvest Butternut Squash
- Select - Signature Soup, Baked Potato
- Select - Signature Soup, Fajita Chicken & Toasted Corn Chowder
- Select - Signature Soup, Fiesta Chicken Tortilla
- Select - Signature Soup, Rosemary Chicken & White Bean
- Select - Soup Cups, Black Bean ()
- Select - Soup Cups, Potato Leek ()
- Select - Soup Cups, Split Pea ()
- Select - Soup Cups, Tex Mex ()
- Select - Soup Mix, Black Bean & Rice ()
- Select - Soup Mix, Tortilla Con Queso ()

Simply Asia ()
- Rice Noodle Soup Bowls - Garlic Sesame
- Rice Noodle Soup Bowls - Sesame Chicken
- Rice Noodle Soup Bowls - Spring Vegetable

Stop & Shop
- Condensed Chicken with Rice Soup
- Ready To Serve Chunky Vegetable Soup

Taste of Thai, A
- Coconut Ginger Soup Mix

Thai Kitchen ⓘ
- Coconut Ginger Soup (Can)
- Hot & Sour Soup (Can)
- Instant Rice Noodle Soup - Bangkok Curry
- Instant Rice Noodle Soup - Garlic & Vegetable
- Instant Rice Noodle Soup - Lemongrass & Chili
- Instant Rice Noodle Soup - Spring Onion
- Instant Rice Noodle Soup - Thai Ginger
- Rice Noodle Soup Bowls - Lemongrass & Chili
- Rice Noodle Soup Bowls - Mushroom
- Rice Noodle Soup Bowls - Roasted Garlic
- Rice Noodle Soup Bowls - Spring Onion
- Rice Noodle Soup Bowls - Thai Ginger

STEWS

Dinty Moore
- Beef Stew
- Chicken Stew
- Microwave Meals - Beef Stew

Juanitas
- Juanitas (All)

TOMATO PASTE

Contadina ⓘ
- Flavored Tomato Paste (All BUT Italian Tomoto Paste with Italian Seasonings)
- Tomato Paste

Del Monte ⓘ
- Tomatoes & Tomato Products (All BUT Spaghetti Sauce Flavored with Meat)

DeLallo
- Tomato Paste

Giant
- Tomato Paste

Great Value (Wal-Mart)
- Tomato Paste

Hy-Vee
- Tomato Paste

Meijer
- Tomato Paste Domestic
- Tomato Paste Organic

Nature's Promise (Giant)
- Organic Tomato Paste

Nature's Promise (Stop & Shop)
- Organic Tomato Paste

Publix GreenWise Market ()
- Organic Tomato Paste

Publix ()
- Tomato Paste

Safeway
Canned Tomato Products (All)

Stop & Shop
Tomato Paste

TOMATOES

Bionaturae ⛾
Organic Tomatoes

Cara Mia
Cara Mia (All)

Cento
Canned Tomatoes (All)

Contadina ⓘ
Crusted Tomatoes (All)
Diced Tomatoes (All)
Stewed Tomatoes (All)
Tomato Puree
Tomato Sauces (All)
Whole Tomatoes

Cucina Antica
Tomato Sauces

Dei Fratelli
Dei Fratelli (All BUT Tomato Soup)

Del Monte ⓘ
Tomatoes & Tomato Products (All BUT
Spaghetti Sauce Flavored with Meat)

DeLallo
Crushed Tomatoes in Light Puree
Diced Tomatoes in Juice
Fire Roasted Diced Tomatoes
Imported Italian Crushed Tomatoes
Imported Italian Diced Tomatoes
Imported Italian Whole Peeled
Tomatoes
Imported Organic San Marzano
Tomatoes
Imported San Marzano Tomatoes
Imported Sun Roasted Cherry Tomatoes
Italian Organic Crushed Tomatoes
Italian Organic Diced Tomatoes
Italian Organic Whole Peeled Tomatoes
Italian Stewed Tomatoes
Pear Tomatoes in Juice
Sun Dried Tomatoes in Olive Oil
Tomato Puree
Tomato Sauce

Whole Tomatoes in Juice

Eden Foods ⓘ ✓
Crushed Tomatoes - Organic
Crushed Tomatoes with Basil - Organic
Crushed Tomatoes with Onion & Garlic
- Organic
Diced Tomatoes
Diced Tomatoes with Basil - Organic
Diced Tomatoes with Green Chilies -
Organic
Diced Tomatoes with Roasted Onion -
Organic
Whole Tomatoes - Organic
Whole Tomatoes with Basil - Organic

Furmano's ⛾
Tomato Products (All)

Great Value (Wal-Mart)
Chili Ready Tomatoes
Concentrated Crushed Tomatoes
Crushed Tomatoes In Puree
Diced Tomatoes In Tomato Juice
Italian Diced Tomatoes
Italian Stewed Tomatoes w/Basil, Garlic,
& Oregano
No Salt Added Diced Tomatoes
No Salt Added Tomato Sauce
Pear Tomato Strips w/Basil In Puree
Petite Diced Tomatoes
Sliced Stewed Tomatoes In Tomato Juice
Tomato Puree
Tomato Sauce
Whole Tomatoes In Tomato Juice

Harvest Farms (Ingles)
Canned Tomatoes (All)

Hy-Vee
Crushed Tomatoes
Diced Tomatoes
Diced Tomatoes - Chili Ready
Diced Tomatoes with Chilies
Diced Tomatoes with Roasted Garlic &
Onions
Italian Style Diced Tomatoes
Italian Style Stewed Tomatoes
Mild Diced Tomatoes & Green Chilies
Original Diced Tomatoes & Green
Chilies
Petite Cut Diced Tomatoes

Petite Cut Diced Tomatoes with Garlic & Olive Oil
Petite Cut Diced Tomatoes with Sweet Onion
Petite Diced Tomatoes
Stewed Tomatoes
Tomato Sauce
Whole Peeled Tomatoes

Laura Lynn (Ingle's)
Canned Tomatoes (All)

Mediterranean Organics 🍽
Mediterranean Organics (All)

Meijer
Diced Tomatoes Chili Ready
Diced Tomatoes in Italian
Diced Tomatoes in Juice
Diced Tomatoes Organic
Stewed Tomatoes
Stewed Tomatoes Italian
Stewed Tomatoes Mexican
Tomato Puree
Tomato Sauce
Tomato Sauce - Organic
Tomatoes - Diced with Green Chiles
Tomatoes - Petite Diced
Tomatoes - Whole Peeled
Tomatoes - Whole Peeled No Salt
Tomatoes Crushed in Puree
Tomatoes with Basil, Organic

Midwest Country Fare (Hy-Vee)
Tomato Sauce

Nature's Promise (Giant)
Organic Crushed Tomatoes with Basil
Organic Diced Tomatoes
Organic Whole Peeled Tomatoes

Nature's Promise (Stop & Shop)
Organic Crushed Tomatoes with Basil
Organic Diced Tomatoes
Organic Tomato Sauce
Organic Whole Peeled Tomatoes

Publix GreenWise Market ⟨⟩
Organic Crushed Tomatoes
Organic Diced Tomatoes - Basil, Garlic & Oregano
Organic Diced Tomatoes - Regular

Publix ⟨⟩
Tomato Sauce

Tomatoes - Crushed
Tomatoes - Diced with Green Chilies
Tomatoes - Diced with Roasted Garlic & Onion
Tomatoes - Peeled Whole
Tomatoes - Sliced, Stewed

Red Gold
Tomato Products (All)

S&W ⓘ
Canned Vegetables (All)

Safeway
Canned Tomato Products (All)

Stop & Shop
Crushed Tomatoes - Italian Seasoning
Crushed Tomatoes - No Added Salt
Crushed Tomatoes - Regular
Diced Tomato - Italian Seasonings
Diced Tomato - No Salt Added
Diced Tomato - Regular
Stewed Tomatoes - Italian Seasonings
Stewed Tomatoes - Mexican Style
Stewed Tomatoes - No Salt Added
Stewed Tomatoes - Regular
Tomato Puree
Tomato Sauce - Regular & No Added Salt
Whole Peeled Tomatoes - Regular & No Added Salt

Thrifty Maid ⓘ
Petite Diced Tomatoes

VEGETABLES

Allens
Canned Items (All) 🍽

Bruce's Yams
Cut Yams
Whole Yams

Cara Mia
Cara Mia (All)

Casa Fiesta
Whole Green Chilies

Colavita
Vegetables in Oil (All)

Del Monte ⓘ
Canned Vegetables

DeLallo

Artichoke Bruschetta
Artichoke Hearts
Artichoke Quarters
Capanota
Chopped Garlic in Oil
Imported Whole Clove Garlic in Oil
Italian Garlic Mushrooms
Marinated Artichoke Hearts
Mild Giardiniera
Minced Garlic in Water
Olive Bruschetta
Portabella Mushrooms with Roasted Peppers
Roasted Garlic in Oil
Roasted Pepper Bruschetta
Sun Dried Tomato Bruschetta
Whole Hearts of Palm

Giant

Beets - No Salt Added
Beets - Regular
Black Eyed Peas
Carrots
Chick Peas
Corn - Cream Style
Corn - Mexican
Corn - No Added Salt
Corn - Whole Kernel
Cut Sweet Potatoes - Light Syrup
Cut Sweet Potatoes - Regular
Golden Cut Wax Beans
Green Beans - French
Lima Beans
Spinach - No Salt Added
Spinach - Regular
Succotash
Sweet Peas
Whole Potatoes - No Salt Added
Whole Potatoes - Regular

Goya

Artichoke Hearts
Blue-Labeled Canned Peas
Canned Hominy

Grand Selections (Hy-Vee)

Crisp & Sweet Whole Kernel Corn
Fancy Cut Green Beans
Fancy Whole Green Beans

Young, Early June Premium Peas

Great Value (Wal-Mart)

Asparagus Cuts & Tips
Blackeye Peas
Collard Greens
Cream Style Corn
Crinkle Cut Carrots
Diced Potatoes
French Style Green Beans
Golden Sweet Whole Kernel Corn
Green Beans
Green Split Peas
Italian Cut Green Beans
Minced Garlic
Mustard Greens
No Salt Added Cut Green Beans
No Salt Added French Style Green Beans
No Salt Added Golden Sweet Whole Kernel Corn
No Salt Added Sweet Peas
Nopalitos Sliced Tender Cactus, Bilingual
Peas & Carrots
Pieces & Stems Mushrooms
Pieces & Stems Mushrooms (China)
Pieces & Stems Mushrooms (Vietnam)
Sliced Beets
Sliced Carrots
Sliced Mushrooms
Sliced New Potatoes
Sliced Pickled Beets
Sweet Corn
Sweet Peas
Turnip Greens
White Hominy
Whole Green Beans
Whole Kernel Golden Corn
Whole Leaf Spinach
Whole New Potatoes
Whole Spear Asparagus

Harvest Farms (Ingles)

Canned Vegetables (All)

HealthMarket (Hy-Vee)

Organic Sweet Peas
Organic Whole Kernel Corn

Hy-Vee
- Blue Lake Cut Green Beans
- Blue Lake French Style Green Beans
- Blue Lake Whole Green Beans
- California Blend
- Cream Style Corn
- Cut Green Beans
- Diced Green Chilies
- Fancy Diced Beets
- Fancy Sliced Beets
- Green Split Peas
- Mushrooms - Stems & Pieces
- Sliced Carrots
- Sliced Hot Jalapenos
- Sliced Mushrooms
- Sliced Water Chestnuts
- Sweet Peas
- Whole Green Chilies
- Whole Kernel Corn
- Whole Kernel White Sweet Corn

Kroger ⓘ
- Plain Canned Vegetables

Laura Lynn (Ingle's)
- Canned Sweet Potatoes/Yams (All)
- Canned Vegetables (All)

Meijer
- Asparagus Cuts & Tips
- Beets - Harvard Sweet Sour
- Beets - Sliced
- Beets - Sliced, No Salt
- Beets - Sliced, Pickled
- Beets - Whole Medium
- Beets - Whole Pickled
- Carrots - Sliced
- Carrots - Sliced, No Salt
- Chilies - Diced Mild Mexican Style
- Corn - Cream Style
- Corn - Golden Sweet Organic
- Corn - Whole Kernel Crisp and Sweet
- Corn - Whole Kernel Golden
- Corn - Whole Kernel Golden No Salt
- Corn - Whole Kernel White
- Green Beans - Cut
- Green Beans - Cut Blue Lake
- Green Beans - Cut No Salt
- Green Beans - Cut Organic
- Green Beans - Cut Veri Green

- Green Beans - French Style
- Green Beans - French Style Blue Lake
- Green Beans - French Style No Salt
- Green Beans - French Style Organic
- Green Beans - French Style Veri Green
- Green Beans - Whole
- Hominy - White
- Kale Greens (Chopped)
- Mixed Vegetables
- Mushrooms - Sliced
- Mushrooms - Stems & Pieces
- Mushrooms - Stems & Pieces No Salt
- Mushrooms - Whole
- Mustard Greens (Chopped)
- Peas & Sliced Carrots
- Pimentos - Pieces
- Pimentos - Sliced
- Small Peas
- Spinach
- Spinach - Cut Leaf
- Spinach - No Salt
- Sweet Peas
- Sweet Peas - No Salt
- Sweet Peas - Organic
- Sweet Potatoes Cut - Light Syrup
- Turnip Greens, Chopped
- Wax Beans Cut
- White Potatoes - Sliced
- White Potatoes - Whole

Midwest Country Fare (Hy-Vee)
- Cream Style Golden Corn
- Cut Green Beans
- Mushrooms & Stems
- No Salt Added Mushrooms & Stems
- Sweet Peas
- Whole Kernel Golden Corn

Native Forest ✓
- Artichoke Hearts - Marinated
- Artichoke Hearts - Quartered
- Artichoke Hearts - Whole
- Green Asparagus Cuts & Tips
- Green Asparagus Spears
- Organic Baby Corn
- Organic Bamboo Shoots
- Organic Hearts of Palm

Nature's Promise (Giant)
- Organic Corn

Organic Cut Green Beans
Organic Sweet Peas

Nature's Promise (Stop & Shop)
Organic Corn
Organic Cut Green Beans
Organic Sweet Peas

Princella Sweet Potatoes
Canned Items (All)

Publix GreenWise Market ()
Organic Green Beans
Organic Sweet Peas
Organic Whole Kernel Corn

Publix ()
Beets
Carrots
Corn - Cream Style Golden
Corn - Whole Kernel Golden Sweet
Green Beans
Green Beans - Veggi-Green
Mixed Vegetables
Potatoes - White
Spinach
Sweet Peas
Sweet Peas - Small

Raley's
Canned Mushroom
Canned Peas
Peas & Carrots

Royal Prince Sweet Potatoes
Canned Items (All)

S&W (i)
Canned Vegetables (All)
Pickled Beets

Sabrett
Onions

Safeway
Button Sliced Mushrooms
Cream Style Corn
Green Beans
Lima Beans
No Salt Whole Kernel Corn
White Hominy

Stop & Shop
Beets - Sliced
Beets - Whole
Carrots
Cut Sweet Potatoes in Light Syrup

Golden Cut Wax Beans
Green Beans - French Style & No Added
 Salt
Mexican Style Corn
Mixed Vegetables - Regular & No Added
 Salt
Peas - No Salt Added
Peas and Carrots
Spinach - Regular & No Added Salt
Sweet Peas
Whole Kernel Corn
Whole Potatoes - Regular & No Added
 Salt

Teasdale ✓
Hominy

Thrifty Maid (i)
Cream Style Golden Sweet Corn

Trappey (i)
Okra

Winn-Dixie (i)
Golden Medium Carrots
Green Beans
Whole Corn

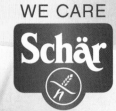
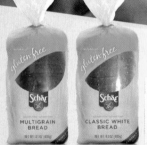
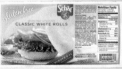

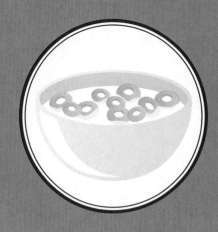
©iStockphoto.com/Mei-Yan Irene Chan

BREAD, CEREAL, PASTA, etc.

BREAD

Ener-G ☷
Brown Rice English Muffins with Flax
Brown Rice Hamburger Buns
Brown Rice Loaf
Egg Free Raisin Loaf
English Muffins
Four Flour Loaf
Hi Fiber Loaf
Light Brown Rice Loaf
Light Tapioca Loaf
Light White Rice Flax Loaf
Light White Rice Loaf
Papas Loaf
Raisin Loaf with Egg
Rice Starch Loaf
Seattle Brown Loaf
Seattle Hamburger Buns
Seattle Hot Dog Buns
Tapioca Dinner Rolls
Tapioca Hamburger Buns
Tapioca Hot Dog Buns
Tapioca Loaf (Thin Sliced)
White Rice Flax Loaf
White Rice Hamburger Buns
White Rice Loaf
Yeast Free Brown Rice Loaf
Yeast Free Sweet Loaf
Yeast Free White Rice Loaf

Enjoy Life Foods ☷
Cinnamon Raisin Bagels
Classic Original Bagels

Food for Life ⓘ ☷ ✔
Wheat & Gluten-Free Raisin Pecan
Bread
Wheat & Gluten-Free Rice Almond
Bread
Wheat & Gluten-Free Rice Pecan Bread
Wheat & Gluten-Free White Rice Bread
Wheat & Gluten-Free Whole Grain
Brown Rice Bread
Whole Grain Bhutanese Red Rice Bread
Yeast Free, Wheat and Gluten-Free
Multi Seed Rice Bread

Foods by George ☷
English Muffins - Cinnamon Currant
English Muffins - No-Rye Rye
English Muffins - Plain

French Meadow Bakery
Gluten-Free Italian Rolls
Gluten-Free Pizza Crust

Gillian's Foods ☷
Gillian's Foods (All)

Glutino ☷ ✔
Premium Cinnamon & Raisin Bagels
Premium Cinnamon & Raisin Bread
Premium English Muffins
Premium Fiber Bread
Premium Flax Seed Bread
Premium Harvest Corn Bread
Premium Plain Bagels
Premium Poppy Seed Bagels
Premium Sesame Bagels

Mariposa Baking Company ☷
Bagels
Pumpkin Bread

Schar ☷ ✔
Ciabatta Parbaked Rolls
Classic White Bread
Classic White Rolls

Barbara's® Multigrain and Honey Rice Puffins® Are Now Gluten Free!

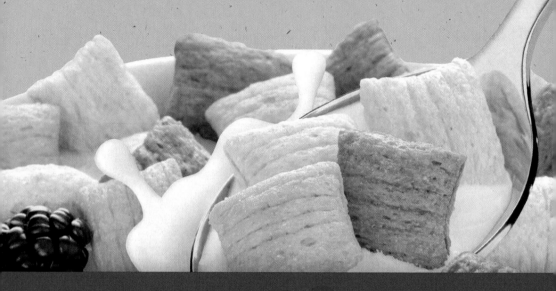

All Natural Since 1971
BARBARA'S®

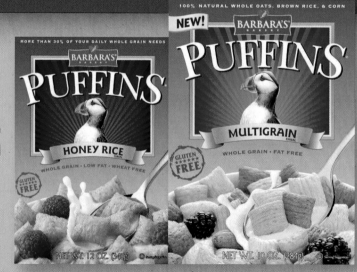

100% Natural Barbara's Puffins® Honey Rice and Multigrain cereals are packed with whole-grain gluten-free goodness and a delicate sweetness the whole family will love.

MORE THAN 30% OF YOUR DAILY WHOLE GRAIN NEEDS

BARBARA'S BAKERY

PUFFINS CEREAL

HONEY RICE

WHOLE GRAIN · LOW FAT · WHEAT FREE

GLUTEN FREE

NET WT. 12 OZ. (340g)

100% NATURAL WHOLE OATS, BROWN RICE, & CORN

NEW! **BARBARA'S** BAKERY

PUFFINS

MULTIGRAIN CEREAL

WHOLE GRAIN · FAT FREE

GLUTEN FREE

NET WT. 10 OZ. (284g)

PuffinsCereal.com

Hearty Grain Bread

Italian Breadsticks

Multigrain Bread

CEREAL & GRANOLA

Arrowhead Mills ✓

Maple Buckwheat Flakes

Rice & Shine Cereal

Sweetened Rice Flakes

Yellow Corn Grits

Bakery on Main

Apple Raisin Walnut Gluten-Free Granola

Cranberry Orange Cashew Gluten-Free Granola

Extreme Fruit & Nut Gluten-Free Granola

Nutty Maple Cranberry Gluten-Free Granola

Rainforest Gluten-Free Granola

Barbara's Bakery

Barbara's Classics - Brown Rice Crisps ⓘ

Barbara's Classics - Corn Flakes ⓘ

Puffins Honey Rice ✓

Puffins Multigrain ✓

Bob's Red Mill ⓘ ✓

Brown Rice Farina

GF Mighty Tasty Hot Cereal

Organic Brown Rice Farina

Organic Creamy Buckwheat Cereal

Soy Grits

Chex ♀

Chocolate Chex (Verify Gluten-Free Written On Package)

Cinnamon Chex (Verify Gluten-Free Written On Package)

Corn Chex (Verify Gluten-Free Written On Package)

Honey Nut Chex (Verify Gluten-Free Written On Package)

Rice Chex (Verify Gluten-Free Written On Package)

Strawberry Chex (Verify Gluten-Free Written On Package)

Cocoa Pebbles ⌇

Cocoa Pebbles

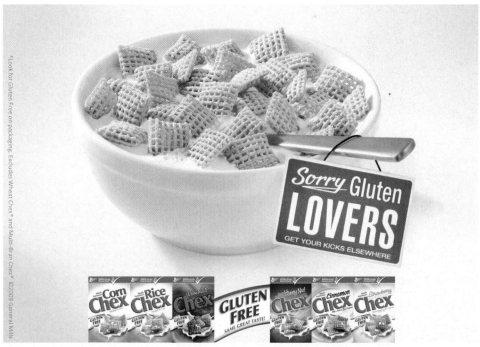

*Look for Gluten Free on packaging. Excludes Wheat Chex® and Multi-Bran Chex® ©2009 General Mills

Sorry Gluten **LOVERS** GET YOUR KICKS ELSEWHERE

Chex® Cereal has gone gluten free. So now you can get the **same great taste** without all the gluten. And with six delicious flavors,* even the gluten lovers could fall in love.

Cream of Rice ⓘ
  Cream of Rice
Enjoy Life Foods ⚇
  Cinnamon Crunch Granola
  Cranapple Crunch Granola
  Very Berry Crunch Granola
EnviroKidz ⓘ ✓
  Amazon Frosted Flakes
  Gorilla Munch
  Koala Crisp
  Leapin Lemurs
  Peanut Butter Panda Puffs
Erewhon
  Aztec Crunchy Corn & Amaranth ✓
  Brown Rice Cream
  Cocoa Crispy Brown Rice ✓
  Corn Flakes ✓
  Crispy Brown Rice - Gluten-Free ✓
  Crispy Brown Rice with Mixed Berries ✓
  Rice Twice ✓
  Strawberry Crisp ✓
Fruity Pebbles ⌇
  Fruity Pebbles

Glutenfreeda ⚇ ✓
  Oatmeal (All)
Glutino ⚇ ✓
  Cereal - Apple & Cinnamon
  Cereal - Honey Nut
Laura Lynn (Ingle's)
  Quick Cooking Grits
Lundberg Family Farms
  Hot Cereal - Purely Organic
Malt-O-Meal ◊
  Fruity Dyno-Bites
Meijer
  Grits Buttered Flavored Instant
  Grits Quick
Nature's Path ⓘ ✓
  Crispy Rice
  Fruit Juice Cornflakes
  Honey'd Cornflakes
  Mesa Sunrise Flakes
  Whole O's
New Morning
  Cocoa Crispy Rice ✓

Why is Gluten-Free Cereal so Hard to Find?

When you first learned about what gluten-free meant, you probably quickly realized that bread and cookies were off limits, but cereal? Before I went gluten-free, my favorite cereals were Rice Krispies and Frosted Flakes. From years of perusing the box at the breakfast table, I knew the former was made mostly of rice, and the latter of corn. Hey, Rice Krispies even has "rice" in the name! So, I never imagined I'd have to give them up.

It turns out I'm not alone. I've talked to many others who were shocked at how limited the cereal selection became once they went gluten-free.

Blame the barley malt. Many cereals, like Rice Krispies and Frosted Flakes, use "malt flavoring," which is derived from barley (and barley, as you know, is not gluten-free).

On the bright side, more companies than ever are now reformulating their cereals with people like us in mind. Our cereal list is as big as ever, and we're truly grateful.

Orgran ♀
- Multigrain Os with Quinoa
- Puffed Amaranth Breakfast Cereal

Safeway
- Cocoa Astros Cereal ()
- Fruity Nuggets Cereal ()
- Puffed Corn Cereal ()

Winn-Dixie ⓘ
- Corn Flakes
- Crispy Rice Cereal

PASTA & NOODLES

Ancient Harvest
- Gluten-Free Pasta ♀

Andean Dream ♀
- Quinoa Pasta - Fusilli
- Quinoa Pasta - Macaroni
- Quinoa Pasta - Spaghetti

Annie Chun's ♀
- Maifun Rice Noodles
- Pad Thai Rice Noodles

Bionaturae ♀
- Gluten-Free Organic Pastas ✓

DeBoles ✓
- Corn Elbows
- Corn Spaghetti
- Multi Grain Penne
- Multi Grain Spaghetti
- Rice Angel Hair
- Rice Fettuccine
- Rice Lasagna
- Rice Penne
- Rice Spaghetti
- Rice Spirals

Dynasty
- Maifun Rice Stick Noodles
- Saifun Bean Thread Noodles

Eden Foods ⓘ ✓
- Bifun (Rice) Pasta
- Kuzu Pasta
- Mung Bean (Harusame) Pasta

Ener-G ♀
- White Rice Lasagna
- White Rice Macaroni
- White Rice Small Shells

- White Rice Spaghetti
- White Rice Vermicelli

Gillian's Foods ♀
- Gillian's Foods (All)

Glutino ♀ ✓
- Fusilli
- Macaroni
- Spaghetti

Hodgson Mill
- Gluten-Free Brown Rice Angel Hair with Milled Flaxseed ♀
- Gluten-Free Brown Rice Elbows with Milled Flaxseed ♀
- Gluten-Free Brown Rice Linguine with Milled Flaxseed ♀
- Gluten-Free Brown Rice Penne with Milled Flaxseed ♀
- Gluten-Free Brown Rice Spaghetti with Milled Flaxseed ♀

Lundberg Family Farms
- Elbow
- Penne
- Rotini
- Spaghetti

Manischewitz
- Passover Noodles

Mrs. Leeper's
- Gluten-Free Pasta

Namaste Foods ♀ ✓
- Namaste Foods (All)

Notta Pasta
- Fettuccine
- Linguine
- Spaghetti

Orgran ♀
- Orgran (All)

Schar ♀ ✓
- Anellini
- Fusilli
- Multigrain Penne Rigate
- Penne
- Spaghetti
- Tagliatelle

Taste of Thai, A
- Rice Noodles
- Thin Rice Noodles

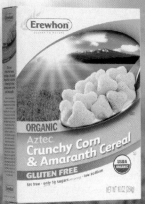
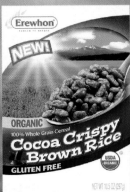
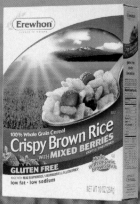
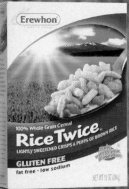
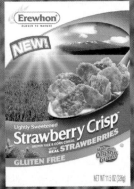
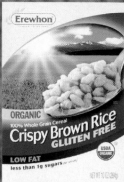
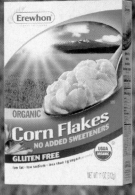

Eat our gluten-free cereal because you want to, not because you have to.

All of our cereals are made from the purest, finest, natural ingredients – organically grown whenever possible. Available wherever natural foods are sold. For nutritional information visit www.usmillsllc.com.

Vermicelli Rice Noodles
Wide Rice Noodles

Thai Kitchen ⓘ
Stir-Fry Rice Noodles
Thin Rice Noodles

Tinkyada 🏅
Brown Rice Elbow
Brown Rice Fettuccini
Brown Rice Fusilli
Brown Rice Grand Shells
Brown Rice Lasagna
Brown Rice Little Dreams
Brown Rice Penne
Brown Rice Shells
Brown Rice Spaghetti
Brown Rice Spirals
Organic Brown Penne
Organic Brown Rice Elbow
Organic Brown Rice Lasagna
Organic Brown Rice Spaghetti
Organic Brown Rice Spirals
Spinach Brown Rice Spaghetti
Vegetable Brown Rice Spirals
White Rice Spaghetti

PIZZA CRUST

Gillian's Foods 🏅
Gillian's Foods (All)

Glutino 🏅 ✓
Premium Pizza Crusts

Rustic Crust ✓
Napoli Herb Gluten-Free Pizza Crust

Schar 🏅 ✓
Pizza Crusts

POLENTA

DeCecco
Polenta

San Gennaro Foods 🏅
Basil Garlic Polenta
Sun Dried Tomato Garlic Polenta
Traditional Polenta

POTATOES, INSTANT & MIXES

Edward & Sons ✓
Chreesy Mashed Potato Mix
Organic Home Style Mashed Potato Mix
Organic Roasted Garlic Mashed Potato Mix

Great Value (Wal-Mart)
Au Gratin Potatoes
Instant Mashed Potatoes
Scalloped Potatoes In Creamy Sauce

Honest Earth ⓘ
Baby Reds
Creamy Mashed
Yukon Golds

Hungry Jack
Instant Mashed Potatoes

Hy-Vee
Four Cheese Mashed Potatoes
Mashed Potatoes Real Russet Potatoes
Roasted Garlic Mashed Potatoes
Sour Cream & Chive Mashed Potatoes

Idahoan ⓘ
Au Gratin
Baby Reds
Baby Reds Garlic & Parmesan
Butter & Herb
Creamy Home Style
Four Cheese
Original Flakes
Real
Roasted Garlic
Romano Cheese
Scalloped
Southwest
Yukon Golds

Kroger ⓘ
Plain Instant Potatoes

Manischewitz
Homestyle Potato Latke Mix
Mini Potato Knish Mix
Potato Kugel Mix
Potato Pancake Mix
Sweetened Potato Pancake Mix

Meijer
Potatoes - Hash Browns
Potatoes - Instant Mashed

Safeway

Herb/Butter Instant Mashed Potatoes
Instant Potatoes
Roasted Garlic Instant Mashed Potatoes
Select - Potato Cups, Buttermilk Ranch ()
Select - Potato Cups, Roasted Garlic ()
Select - Potato Cups, Sour Cream Chive ()
Select - Potato Cups, Three Cheese
  Broccoli ()
Select - Roasted Rosemary Wedges
Select - Signature Broccoli Cheddar Au
  Gratin

Winn-Dixie ⓘ

Creamy Idaho Mashed Potatoes

RICE & RICE MIXES

Annie Chun's ⚇
Rice Express Products (All)

Arrowhead Mills ✔
Brown Rice, Basmati
Brown Rice, Long Grain

Botan Calrose
Botan Calrose Rice

Carolina Rice
Authentic Spanish Rice
Basmati Rice
Brown Rice (Whole Grain)
Gold (Parboiled)
Jasmine Rice
Long Grain & Wild Rice
Saffron Yellow Rice
White Rice

DeCecco
Rices

Dynasty
Jasmine Rice

Eden Foods ⓘ ✔
Wild Rice

Fantastic World Foods
Arborio Rice
Basmati Rice
Jasmine Rice

Giant
Rice - Brown
Rice - Instant White

Glutino ⚇ ✔
Whole Grain Brown Rice with
  Prebiotics
Whole Grain Brown Rice with
  Prebiotics HOMESTYLE

GoGo Rice
Organic Brown Rice
Organic Rice Medley
Organic White Rice
Sushi Rice with Seaweed Wraps

Goya
Canilla Long Grain Rice
Medium Grain Rice

Great Value (Wal-Mart)
Brown Rice
Enriched Long Grain Rice, Extra Fancy
Parboiled Rice

Hy-Vee
Boil-In-Bag Rice
Enriched Extra Long Grain Rice
Enriched Long Grain Instant Rice
Extra Long Grain Rice
Instant Brown Rice
Natural Long Grain Brown Rice
Spanish Rice (Canned)

Kokuho Rose ⚇
Kokuho Rose (medium grain)

Konriko
Aix-En Provence Brown Rice
Artichoke Brown Rice Mix
Hot 'n Spicy Brown Rice Pilaf
Original Brown Rice
Quick-Cook Brown Rice
Wild Pecan Rice

Laura Lynn (Ingle's)
Instant Rice (All)

Lotus Foods
Heirloom Rices (All)

Louisiana Fish Fry ()
Dirty Rice Mix
Jambalaya Mix

Lundberg Family Farms
Heat & Eat Organic Brown Rice Bowls -
  Countrywild Brown
Heat & Eat Organic Brown Rice Bowls -
  Long Grain Brown

Heat & Eat Organic Brown Rice Bowls - Short Grain
Rice (All Varieties)
Risotto - Butternut Squash
Risotto - Cheddar Broccoli
Risotto - Creamy Parmesan
Risotto - Garlic Primavera
Risotto - Italian Herb
Risotto - Organic Alfredo
Risotto - Organic Florentine
Risotto - Organic Porcini Mushroom
Risotto - Organic Tuscan

Mahatma
Authentic Spanish Rice
Basmati Rice
Jasmine Rice
Parboiled Rice
Yellow Rice

Manischewitz
Lentil Pilaf Mix

Meijer
Rice - Brown
Rice - Instant
Rice - Instant Boil in a Bag
Rice - Instant Brown
Rice - Long Grain
Rice - Medium Grain

Midwest Country Fare (Hy-Vee)
Pre-Cooked Instant Rice

Minute Rice
Boil-in-Bag Rice
Brown Rice
Ready to Serve Brown & Wild Rice
Ready to Serve Brown Rice
Ready to Serve Chicken Rice Mix
Ready to Serve White Rice
Ready to Serve Yellow Mixed Rice
White Rice

Nishiki
Nishiki Rice

Ortega ⓘ
Saffron Yellow Rice
Spanish Rice

Publix ◌
Long Grain Brown Rice
Long Grain Enriched Rice
Medium Grain White Rice
Precooked Instant Boil in Bag
Precooked Instant Brown Rice
Precooked Instant White Rice
Yellow Rice Mix

RiceSelect ⓘ ✓
Chef's Originals Smokey Cowboy Beans & Rice
Jasmati Rice
Kasmati Rice
Organic Garden Vegetable Rice Mix
Organic Roasted Chicken Herb Rice Mix
Organic Three Cheese Rice Mix
Organic Toasted Almond Pilaf
Organic Wild Mushroom & Herb Rice Mix
Risotto (Arborio)
Royal Blend Rice
Sonoran Mexican Rice
Texmati Brown Rice
Texmati Light Brown Rice
Texmati White Rice

Safeway
Instant Rice
Rice - Enriched Calrose
Rice - Long Grain
Rice - White
Risotto - Cheese ◌
Select - Basmati Rice

Sho-Chiku-Bai ⓨ
Sho-Chiku-Bai Sweet Rice

Stop & Shop
Instant Brown Rice
Organic Long Grain Rice - Brown
Organic Long Grain Rice - White

Success Rice
Jasmine Rice
White Rice
Whole Grain Brown Rice

Taste of China, A
Sweet & Sour Rice

Taste of India, A
Masala Rice

Taste of Thai, A
Coconut Ginger Rice
Garlic Basil Rice
Jasmine Rice
Yellow Curry Rice

Tasty Bite
Basmati Rice
Beans Masala & Basmati Rice
Brown Rice
Jasmine Rice
Long Grain Rice
Mexican Fiesta Pilaf
Peas Paneer & Basmati Rice
Pesto Pilaf
Spinach Dal and Basmati Rice
Sprouts Curry and Basmati Rice
Tandoori Pilaf
Vegetable Supreme and Basmati Rice

Thai Kitchen ⓘ
Jasmine Rice Mixes - Green Chili & Garlic
Jasmine Rice Mixes - Jasmine Rice
Jasmine Rice Mixes - Lemongrass & Ginger
Jasmine Rice Mixes - Roasted Garlic & Chili
Jasmine Rice Mixes - Spicy Thai Chili
Jasmine Rice Mixes - Sweet Chili & Onion
Jasmine Rice Mixes - Thai Yellow Curry

Ukrop's
Caribbean Rice and Beans (Deli)
Jasmine Rice (Deli)

Uncle Ben's
Boil-In-Bag Rice
Fast & Natural Whole Grain Instant Brown Rice
Instant Rice
Original Converted Brand Rice
Ready Rice - Original Long Grain Rice
Ready Whole Grain Rice - Whole Grain Brown
Whole Grain Brown Rice

TACO SHELLS

Casa Fiesta
Taco Shells

Giant
Taco Shells

Hy-Vee
Taco Shells

Meijer
Taco Shells

Mission Foods
Corn Products (All)

Ortega ⓘ
Hard Shells - White
Hard Shells - Yellow
Tostada Shells

Safeway
Jumbo Taco Shells
White Corn Taco Shells

Taco Bell ⌇
Taco Shells
Taco Shells - Home Originals Nacho
Taco Shells - Home Originals Ranch

TORTILLAS & WRAPS

Food for Life ⓘ ⚕ ✓
Organic Sprouted Whole Kernel Flourless Corn Tortillas
Whole Grain Brown Rice Tortillas

Goya
Corn Tortillas

Great Value (Wal-Mart)
Corn Tortillas

Hy-Vee
White Corn Tortilla

La Tortilla Factory ✓
Smart & Delicious Dark Teff Wraps ⓘ
Smart & Delicious Ivory Teff Wraps ⓘ

Sonoma All Natural Dark Teff Wraps ⓘ
Sonoma All Natural Ivory Teff Wraps ⓘ
Sonoma Yellow Corn Tortillas ♀

Manny's
Corn Tortillas

Mission Foods
Corn Products (All)

Winn-Dixie ⓘ
Corn Tortilla (24 Count)

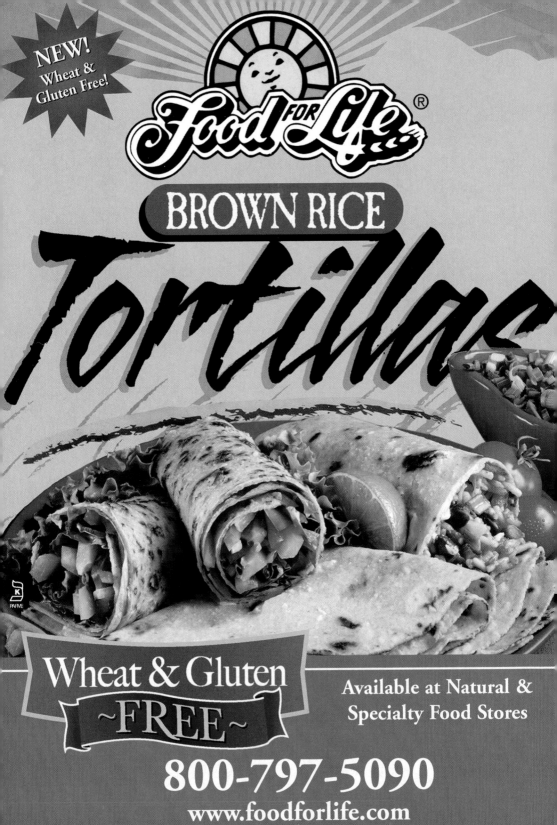

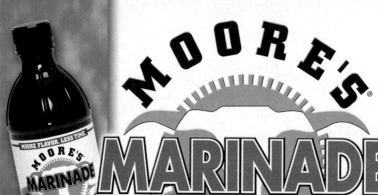
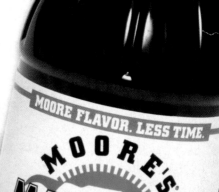

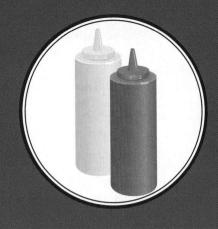

©istockphoto.com/Cheryl Graham

CONDIMENTS, SAUCES & DRESSINGS

ASIAN SAUCES, MISC.

A.1. ✐
Teriyaki (UPC 5440000555)

Dynasty
Chinese Style BBQ Sauce
Golden Plum Sauce
Hoisin Sauce
Plum Sauce

Earth Family ✓
Asian Sauce

Eden Foods ⓘ ✓
Mirin (Rice Cooking Wine)
Ume Plum Vinegar

Gold's
Hot & Spicy Duck Sauce
Oriental Garlic Duck Sauce
Squeeze Wasabi Sauce
Sweet and Sour Duck Sauce

Jack Daniel's Sauces ⓘ
EZ Marinader - Teriyaki Variety

Kikkoman
Manjo Aji Mirin

Kraft ✐
Sweet 'n Sour Sauce

Lee Kum Kee ⓘ
Chili Garlic
Choy Sun Oyster Flavored Sauce
Duck Sauce
Gold Label Plum Sauce
Plum Stir-Fry & Dipping Sauce

Marukan
Citrus Ponzu Dressing

Moore's ♟ ✓
Moore's Teriyaki Marinade

Organicville
Organicville (All)

Premier Japan ✓
Organic Wheat-Free Hoisin
Organic Wheat-Free Teriyaki

Taste of Thai, A
Fish Sauce
Green Curry Paste
Pad Thai Sauce
Panang Curry Paste
Peanut Satay Sauce
Peanut Sauce Mix
Red Curry Paste
Yellow Curry Paste

Tasty Bite
Good Korma Simmer Sauce
Pad Thai Simmer Sauce
Rogan Josh Simmer Sauce
Satay Partay Simmer Sauce
Tikka Masala Simmer Sauce

Thai Kitchen ⓘ
Fish Sauce
Green Curry Paste
Green Curry Simmer Sauce
Original Pad Thai Sauce
Panang Curry Simmer Sauce
Peanut Satay Sauce
Red Curry Paste
Red Curry Simmer Sauce
Yellow Curry Simmer Sauce

ASIAN, SOY & TAMARI SAUCES

Eden Foods ⓘ ✓
Tamari Soy Sauce - Brewed in U.S. - Organic
Tamari Soy Sauce - Imported, Organic

Hy-Vee
Soy Sauce

San-J ⓘ ✓
Organic Wheat Free Reduced Sodium Tamari (Platinum Label)
Organic Wheat Free Tamari (Gold Label)

BACON BITS

Garrett County Farms
Salt Cured Bacon Bits

Great Value (Wal-Mart)
Imitation Bacon Bits

Hormel
Bacon Bits, Pieces & Crumbs

Oscar Mayer ⌇
Real Bacon Bits

Wellshire Farms ✓
Salt Cured Bacon Bits

BARBEQUE SAUCE

Annie's Naturals
Organic Hot Chipotle
Organic Original Recipe
Organic Smokey Maple
Organic Sweet & Spicy

Arriba!
Arriba! (All)

Bone Suckin' Sauce ✓
Bone Suckin' Sauce - Hiccuppin' Hot
Bone Suckin' Sauce - Hot
Bone Suckin' Sauce - Hot Thicker Style
Bone Suckin' Sauce - Regular
Bone Suckin' Sauce - Thicker Style

Fischer & Wieser ⓘ
Elly May's Wild Mountain Honey BBQ Sauce
Plum Chipotle BBQ Sauce
Southern Style BBQ Sauce

Follow Your Heart ⓘ ⛶
Unforgettable Balsamic Barbecue Sauce - Mild
Unforgettable Balsamic Barbecue Sauce - Spicy

Giant
BBQ Sauce - Hickory Smoke
BBQ Sauce - Honey
BBQ Sauce - Original

Gold's
Barbecue Sauce with Horseradish
New England Barbecue Sauce

Heinz ⓘ
Chicken & Rib BBQ Sauce
Garlic BBQ Sauce
Honey Garlic BBQ Sauce
Original BBQ Sauce

Homestyle Meals
Original BBQ Sauce
Smoked Chipotle BBQ Sauce

Hy-Vee
Hickory BBQ Sauce
Honey Smoke BBQ Sauce
Original BBQ Sauce

Jack Daniel's Sauces ⓘ
Hickory Brown Sugar BBQ Sauce
Honey Smokehouse BBQ Sauce
Original #7 BBQ Sauce
Spicy BBQ Sauce

Kraft Barbecue Sauce ⌇
Char Grill Barbecue Sauce
Hickory Barbecue Sauce
Hickory Smoke Barbecue Sauce
Hickory Smoke Onion Bits Barbecue Sauce
Honey Barbecue Sauce
Honey Hickory Smoke Barbecue Sauce
Honey Mustard Barbecue Sauce
Honey Roasted Garlic Barbecue Sauce
Hot Barbecue Sauce
Light Original Barbecue Sauce
Mesquite Smoke Barbecue Sauce
Original Barbecue Sauce
Spicy Honey Barbecue Sauce
Sweet Recipes Honey Barbecue Sauce
Thick 'n Spicy Brown Sugar Barbecue Sauce

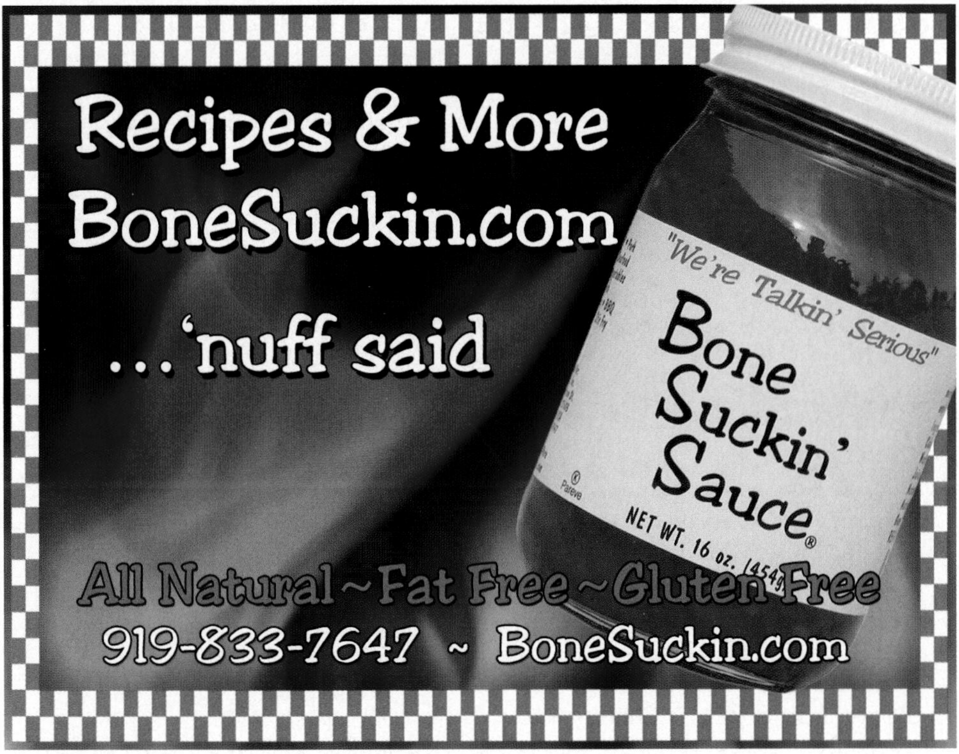

- Thick 'n Spicy Hickory Smoke Barbecue Sauce
- Thick 'n Spicy Honey Barbecue Sauce
- Thick 'n Spicy Original Barbecue Sauce

Midwest Country Fare (Hy-Vee)
- Hickory BBQ Sauce
- Honey BBQ Sauce
- Original BBQ Sauce

Organicville
- Organicville (All)

Publix
- BBQ Sauce (Deli)
- Hickory BBQ Sauce
- Honey BBQ Sauce
- Original BBQ Sauce

Safeway
- Select - BBQ Sauce, Hickory Smoked
- Select - BBQ Sauce, Honey Mustard
- Select - BBQ Sauce, Honey Smoked
- Select - BBQ Sauce, Original

Sprecher Brewing Co. ✔
- Rootbeer BBQ Sauce

Stop & Shop
- BBQ Sauce - Hickory Smoke
- BBQ Sauce - Original

Stubb's ⓘ
- Honey Pecan Bar-B-Q Sauce

Sweet Baby Ray's ⓘ
- Sweet Baby Ray's Barbeque Sauce (All)

Ukrop's
- Honey BBQ Sauce (Deli)
- Tomato BBQ Sauce (Deli)

Walden Farms
- Walden Farms (All)

Chocolate Syrup

Giant
- Chocolate Syrup

Hershey's
- Chocolate Syrup

Hy-Vee
- Chocolate Syrup

Meijer
- Syrup - Chocolate

Midwest Country Fare (Hy-Vee)
- Chocolate Flavored Syrup

Nesquik
Syrup (All Flavors)

Publix ()
Chocolate Syrup

Safeway
Chocolate Syrup

Stop & Shop
Chocolate Syrup

Winn-Dixie ⓘ
Real Chocolate Flavor Syrup

CHUTNEYS

Native Forest ✓
Organic Hot Mango Chutney
Organic Mango Passion Chutney
Organic Papaya Chutney
Organic Pineapple Chutney

Robert Rothschild Farm
Hot Peach & Apple Chutney
Pomegranate Cranberry Chutney
Pomegranate Cranberry Chutney with
Onions

COCKTAIL & SEAFOOD SAUCE

Cains
Cocktail Sauce

Captains Choice (Safeway)
Cocktail Sauce

Crosse & Blackwell
Crosse & Blackwell (All BUT Branston
Pickle Relish, Fish & Chip Vinegar,
and Plum Pudding)

Giant
Seafood Cocktail Sauce

Gold's
Cocktail Sauce

Heinz ⓘ
Cocktail Sauce

Heluva Good ⛉
Cocktail Sauce

Hy-Vee
Cocktail Sauce For Seafood

Ken's ⓘ
Blue Label Cocktail Sauce

Green Label Cocktail Sauce

Kraft ⌒
Cocktail Sauce
Hot & Spicy Cocktail Sauce

Legal
Seafood Cocktail

Louisiana Fish Fry ()
Cocktail Sauce
Seafood Sauce

Robert Rothschild Farm
Raspberry Seafood Sauce

Safeway
Cocktail Sauce

Stop & Shop
Seafood Cocktail Sauce

Texas Pete
Seafood Sauce ⛉

TryMe
Oyster & Shrimp Sauce

Ukrop's
Cocktail Sauce (Deli)

CROUTONS

Ener-G ⛉
Plain Croutons

Gillian's Foods ⛉
Gillian's Foods (All)

Gluten-Free Pantry, The ⛉ ✓
Olive Oil & Garlic Croutons

Mariposa Baking Company ⛉
Croutons

DESSERT SYRUPS, SAUCES & GLAZES

Giant
Strawberry Syrup

Hy-Vee
Strawberry Syrup

Litehouse
Blueberry Glaze
Peach Glaze
Strawberry Glaze
Sugar Free Strawberry Glaze

Marie's
Fruit Glazes (All)

Mrs. Richardson's
Mrs. Richardson's Toppings (All)

Robert Rothschild Farm
Cherry Almond Gourmet Sauce
Cinnamon Bun Caramel Dessert Sauce
& Dip
Old-Fashioned Caramel Sauce
Old-Fashioned Hot Fudge Sauce
Red Raspberry Gourmet Sauce

Santa Cruz Organic
Santa Cruz Organic (All)

Smucker's
Butterscotch Sundae Syrup
Caramel Sundae Syrup
Chocolate Sundae Syrup
Magic Shell Topping - Caramel
Magic Shell Topping - Chocolate
Magic Shell Topping - Chocolate Fudge
Spoonable Topping (All BUT 3
Musketeers & Milky Way)
Strawberry Sundae Syrup

DIP & DIP MIXES - SAVORY

Arriba!
Arriba! (All)

Cabot
Cabot's Products (All)

Cantaré Foods
Olive Tapenade Spreads

Chi-Chi's
Con Queso
Nacho Cheese Snackers

Chugwater Chili
Dip/Dressing Mix

Creamland Dairies ()
Dips

EatSmart
Sweet Salsa Dip
Three Bean Dip

Emerald Valley Kitchen
Emerald Valley Kitchen (All)

Fritos ⓘ
Bean Dip
Chili Cheese Dip
Hot Bean Dip

Jalapeno & Cheddar Flavored Cheese
Dip
Mild Cheddar Flavor Cheese Dip

Garden Fresh Gourmet ⅋
Guacamoles (All)
Specialty Dips (All)

Giant
French Onion Dip
Ranch Dip
Refrigerated Veggie Dip
Salsa Dip

Grande ⓘ
Salsa Con Queso Dip
Tres Bean Dip

Great Value (Wal-Mart)
Homestyle Pimento Spread

Guiltless Gourmet
Bean Dips (All) ⅋

Heluva Good ⅋
Bacon Horseradish
Bodacious Onion
Buttermilk Ranch
Creamy Salsa
Dinosaur BBQ
Fat Free French Onion
French Onion
Jalapeno Cheddar
New England Clam
Ranch
White Cheddar Bacon

Hy-Vee
Bacon & Cheddar Sour Cream Dip
French Onion Sour Cream Dip
Ranch & Dill Sour Cream Dip
Salsa Sour Cream Dip
Toasted Onion Sour Cream Dip
Vegetable Party Sour Cream Dip

Kraft Dips ⌇
Bacon & Cheddar
Creamy Ranch
French Onion
Green Onion
Green Onion
Guacamole Flavor

Lay's ⓘ
Creamy Ranch Dip
French Onion Dip

French Onion Flavored Dry Dip Mix
Green Onion Flavored Dry Dip Mix
Ranch Flavored Dry Dip Mix

Litehouse
Avocado Dip
Dilly Dip
Garden Ranch Dip
Onion Dip
Organic Ranch Dip
Ranch Dip
Ranch Veggie Dippers
Southwest Ranch Dip

Lucerne (Safeway)
Avocado Dip
Bacon Onion Dip
Clam Dip
French Onion Dip
Green Onion Dip
Guacamole Dip
Ranch Dip

Marie's
Dips (All)

O-Ke-Doke ⓘ
Cheddar Cheese Dip
Salsa Con Queso Dip

Publix ()
French Onion Sour Cream Dip
Green Onion Sour Cream Dip
Guacamole Sour Cream Dip

Purity Dairies
Milk and Cultured Products (All)

Ricos ✔
Cheese (All)

Road's End Organics ✔
Mild Nacho Chreese Dip
Spicy Nacho Chreese Dip

Robert Rothschild Farm
Artichoke Spinach Dip with Cream
    Cheese
Black Bean Dip
Blackberry Honey Mustard Pretzel Dip
Buffalo Bleu Cheese Dip
Champagne Garlic Honey Mustard
    Pretzel Dip
Dirty Martini Cheeseball Dip
Emerald Isle Onion Dill Horseradish
    Dip

Green Chile/Hatch Pepper Dip
Jalapeno Pepper Dip
Onion Blossom Horseradish Dip
Peppermint Dip
Red Pepper & Onion Dip & Relish
Raspberry Honey Mustard Pretzel Dip
Roasted Pineapple Habanero Dip
Sesame Honey Mustard Pretzel Dip
Southwest Dip
Sun-Dried Tomato Vegetable Dip
Sweet Heat Pretzel Dip
Toasted Garlic Horseradish Dip

Sauces 'n Love ⛊
Sauces 'n Love (All)

Snyder's of Hanover ⓘ
Salsa Con Queso Dip
Tres Bean Dip

Stop & Shop
Refrigerated French Onion Dip
Refrigerated Ranch Dip
Refrigerated Veggie Dip

Taco Bell 〰
Bean Con Queso - Home Originals
Chili Con Queso - Home Originals with
    Meat

Tostitos ⓘ
Creamy Southwestern Ranch Dip
Creamy Spinach Dip
Monterey Jack Queso
Spicy Nacho Cheese Dip
Spicy Queso Supreme
Zesty Bean & Cheese Dip

Ukrop's
Bruschetta (Deli)
Buffalo Chicken Dip (Deli)
Charleston Shrimp Spread (Deli)
Garlic Herb Dip (Deli)
Seven-Layered Dip (Deli)
Special Sauce (Deli)
Spinach Artichoke Dip (Deli)

Utz ⛊ ✔
Cheddar & Jalapeno Dip
Mild Cheddar Cheese Dip

Walden Farms ⛊
Walden Farms (All)

DIP & DIP MIXES - SWEET

Litehouse
100 Calorie Chocolate Dip
Chocolate Caramel
Chocolate Dip
Chocolate Yogurt Fruit Dip
Low Fat Caramel
Original Caramel
Strawberry Yogurt Fruit Dip
Toffee Caramel
Vanilla Yogurt Fruit Dip

Marie's
Dips (All)

Robert Rothschild Farm
Chocolate Fudge Pretzel Dip
Ginger Bread Cream Cheese Dip
Raspberry Chocolate Pretzel Dip
Strawberries & Cream Dip

Ukrop's
Fruit Dip (Deli)
Hawaiian Pineapple Nut Spread (Deli)

FRUIT BUTTERS & CURDS

Dickinson's
Dickinson's (All)

Eden Foods ⓘ ✓
Apple Butter - Organic
Apple Cherry Butter - Organic
Cherry Butter, Montmorency Tart -
Organic

Fischer & Wieser ⓘ
Texas Pecan Apple Butter
Texas Pecan Peach Butter

Giant
Apple Butter

Great Value (Wal-Mart)
Spiced Apple Butter

Knouse Foods ⓤ
Apple Butter

Laura Lynn (Ingle's)
Apple Butter

Manischewitz
Apple Butter

Robert Rothschild Farm
Key Lime Curd & Tart Filling
Lemon Curd & Tart Filling
Pumpkin Curd & Tart Filling

Santa Cruz Organic
Santa Cruz Organic (All)

GRAVY & GRAVY MIXES

Imagine ✓
Roasted Turkey
Savory Beef

Mayacamas ✓
Brown Gravy
Chicken Gravy
Savory Herb Gravy
Turkey Gravy

Orgran ⓤ
Orgran (All)

Road's End Organics ✓
Organic Golden Gravy Mix
Organic Savory Herb Gravy Mix
Organic Shiitake Gravy Mix

HORSERADISH

Boar's Head
Condiments (All)

Bubbies ⓤ
Bubbies (All)

Gold's
Hot Horseradish
Red Horseradish
Squeeze Horseradish Sauce
White Horseradish

Heinz ⓘ
Horseradish Sauce

Heluva Good ⓤ
Horseradish

Hy-Vee
Prepared Horseradish

Kaneku
Horseradish Powder

Kraft ⌒
Horseradish Sauce

Lou's Famous
Creamy Horseradish

Manischewitz
- Horseradish (All)

Robert Rothschild Farm
- Horseradish Sauce
- Raspberry Cranberry Horseradish Sauce

Strub's ()
- Strub's (All)

Thummann's
- Condiments (All)

HOT SAUCE

A.1. 🌀
- Bold & Spicy with Tabasco

Arriba!
- Arriba! (All)

Butcher's Cut (Safeway)
- Jazz N Spicy Buffalo Wing Sauce

Cholula Hot Sauce
- Cholula (All)

Fischer & Wieser ⓘ
- Blackberry Chipotle Sauce
- Blueberry Chipotle Sauce
- Mango Ginger Habanero Sauce
- Original Roasted Raspberry Chipotle Sauce, The
- Papaya Lime Serrano Sauce
- Pomegranate & Mango Chipotle Sauce

Frank's RedHot
- Buffalo Wing Sauce
- Chile 'n Lime Hot Sauce
- Original RedHot Sauce
- Xtra Hot RedHot Sauce

Giant
- Chili Sauce
- Hot Sauce

Great Value (Wal-Mart)
- Chili Sauce
- Louisiana Hot Sauce

Heinz ⓘ
- Chili Sauce

Huy Fong
- Chili Garlic Sauce
- Sambal Oelek
- Sriracha Hot Chili Sauce

Hy-Vee
- Chili Sauce

Juanitas
- Juanitas (All)

Laura Lynn (Ingle's)
- Hot Sauce (All)
- Jalapeno Sauce (All)

Lee Kum Kee ⓘ
- Sambal Oelek Chili Sauce
- Sriracha Chili Sauce
- Sweet & Sour Sauce

Louisiana Fish Fry ()
- Hot Sauce

Louisiana Hot Sauce
- Louisiana Hot Sauce

Meijer
- Chili Sauce
- Hot Dog Chili Sauce

Moore's 🍴 ✓
- Moore's Buffalo Wing Sauce
- Moore's Honey BBQ Wing Sauce

Nance's
- Chili Sauce
- Hot Wing Sauce
- Mild Wing Sauce

Original Louisiana Hot Sauce
- Original Louisiana Hot Sauce

Santa Barbara Salsa 🍴
- Santa Barbara Salsa (All)

Stop & Shop
- Chili Sauce

Tabasco ✓
- Chipotle Pepper Sauce
- Garlic Basting Sauce
- Garlic Pepper Sauce
- Habanero Pepper Sauce
- New Orleans Style Sauce
- Pepper Sauce

Taco Bell 🌀
- Hot Sauce
- Mild Hot Sauce

Taste of Thai, A
- Garlic Chili Pepper Sauce
- Sweet Red Chili Sauce

Texts Pete

Texas Pete
- Buffalo Chicken Wing Sauce - Extra Mild ☷
- Buffalo Chicken Wing Sauce - Hot ☷
- Buffalo Chicken Wing Sauce - Mild ☷
- Green Pepper Sauce ⓘ
- Hot Sauce - Garlic ☷
- Hot Sauce - Hotter ☷
- Hot Sauce - Original ☷

Thai Kitchen ⓘ
- Roasted Red Chili Paste
- Spicy Thai Chili Sauce
- Sweet Red Chili Sauce

Trappey ⓘ
- Hot Sauces

TryMe
- Cajun Sunshine
- Tennessee Sunshine
- Yucatan Sunshine Habanero Sauce

Winn-Dixie ⓘ
- Hot Sauce

Wizard's, The ✓
- Organic Hot Stuff

JAMS, JELLIES & PRESERVES

Bionaturae ☷
- Organic Fruit Spreads

Chugwater Chili
- Red Pepper Jelly

Crofter's
- Crofter's (All)

Crosse & Blackwell
- Crosse & Blackwell (All BUT Branston Pickle Relish, Fish & Chip Vinegar, and Plum Pudding)

Dickinson's
- Dickinson's (All)

Fischer & Wieser ⓘ
- Apricot Orange Marmalade
- Cinnamon-Orange Tomato Preserves
- Old Fashioned Peach Preserves
- Rhubarb Strawberry Preserves
- Texas Amaretto Peach Pecan Preserves
- Texas Hot Red Jalapeno Jelly
- Texas Jalapeach Preserves

- Texas Mild Green Jalapeno Jelly
- Whole Lemon Fig Marmalade

Giant
- Apple Jelly
- Apricot Preserves
- Apricot Spread
- Blueberry Preserves
- Cherry Preserves
- Concord Grape Jelly
- Currant Jelly
- Grape Preserves
- Mint Jelly
- Orange Marmalade
- Peach Preserves
- Pineapple Preserves
- Red Raspberry Preserves
- Red Raspberry Spread
- Seedless Blackberry Preserves
- Squeezable Grape Jelly
- Squeezable Strawberry Fruit Spread
- Strawberry Jam
- Strawberry Jelly
- Strawberry Preserves
- Strawberry Spread
- Sugar Free Preserves - Apricot
- Sugar Free Preserves - Blackberry
- Sugar Free Preserves - Red Raspberry
- Sugar Free Preserves - Strawberry

Goya
- Fruit Preserves (Jelly)

Hy-Vee
- Apple Jelly
- Apricot Preserves
- Blackberry Jelly
- Cherry Jelly
- Cherry Preserves
- Concord Grape Jelly
- Concord Grape Preserves
- Grape Jelly
- Orange Marmalade
- Peach Preserves
- Red Plum Jelly
- Red Raspberry Jelly
- Red Raspberry Preserves
- Strawberry Jelly
- Strawberry Preserves

Kroger ⓘ
Jams
Jellies
Preserves

Laura Lynn (Ingle's)
Grape Jelly/Peanut Butter
Jams (All)
Jellies (All)
Preserves (All)
Strawberry Jelly/Peanut Butter

Mediterranean Organics ⚱
Mediterranean Organics (All)

Meijer
Apple Jelly
Fruit Spread - Apricot
Fruit Spread - Blackberry Seedless
Fruit Spread - Red Raspberry
Fruit Spread - Strawberry
Grape Jam
Grape Jelly
Preserves - Apricot
Preserves - Blackberry Seedless
Preserves - Marmalade Orange
Preserves - Peach
Preserves - Red Raspberry
Preserves - Red Raspberry with Seeds
Preserves - Strawberry

Nature's Promise (Giant)
Organic Fruit Spread - Raspberry
Organic Fruit Spread - Strawberry
Organic Grape Jelly

Nature's Promise (Stop & Shop)
Organic Grape Jelly
Organic Raspberry Fruit Spread
Organic Strawberry Fruit Spread

Polaner ⓘ
All Fruit
Sugar Free Jams, Jellies & Preserves

Publix ()
Jams/Jellies/Preserves (All Flavors)

Robert Rothschild Farm
Caramelized Onion Balsamic Spread
Concord Grape Jelly
Golden Apricot Preserve
Hot Pepper Peach Preserves
Hot Pepper Raspberry Preserves
Marion Blackberry Preserves

Red Pepper Jelly
Red Raspberry Preserves
Rhubarb Strawberry Preserves
Seedless Raspberry Preserves
Sun-Ripened Strawberry Preserves
Tart Cherry Pomegranate Preserves
Wild Maine Blueberry Preserves

Safeway
Jams
Jellies
Select - Jams/Jellies

Simply Enjoy (Giant)
Balsamic Sweet Onion Preserves
Blueberry Preserves
Raspberry Champagne Peach Preserves
Red Pepper Jelly
Roasted Garlic and Onion Jam
Spiced Apple Preserves
Strawberry Preserves

Simply Enjoy (Stop & Shop)
Balsamic Sweet Onion Preserves
Blueberry Preserves
Raspberry Champagne Peach Preserves
Red Pepper Jelly
Roasted Garlic and Onion Jam
Spiced Apple Preserves
Strawberry Preserves

Smucker's
Jams, Jellies and Preserves (All)

St. Dalfour
Fruit Conserves ⚱

Stop & Shop
Apple Jelly
Apricot Preserves
Apricot Spread
Blueberry Spread
Concord Grape Jelly - Spreadable
Concord Grape Jelly - Squeezable
Currant Jelly
Grape Preserves
Mint Jelly
Orange Marmalade
Peach Preserves
Pineapple Preserves
Red Raspberry Preserves
Seedless Blackberry Preserves
Squeezable Grape Jelly

Strawberry Preserves
Strawberry Spread
Sugar Free Preserves - Apricot
Sugar Free Preserves - Blackberry
Sugar Free Preserves - Red Raspberry
Sugar Free Preserves - Strawberry

Walden Farms ☷
Walden Farms (All)

Welch's
Welch's (All)

KETCHUP

Annie's Naturals
Organic Ketchup

Del Monte ⓘ
Tomatoes & Tomato Products (All BUT
Spaghetti Sauce Flavored with Meat)

Gold's
Ketchup with Horseradish

Great Value (Wal-Mart)
Ketchup
Ketchup (Inverted Bottle)

Harvest Farms (Ingles)
Ketchup (All)

Heinz ⓘ
Hot & Spicy Ketchup Kick'rs
Ketchup
No Sodium Added Ketchup
One Carb Ketchup
Organic Ketchup
Reduced Sugar Ketchup

Hy-Vee
Ketchup
Squeezable Thick & Rich Tomato
Ketchup
Thick & Rich Tomato Ketchup

Laura Lynn (Ingle's)
Ketchup (All)

Meijer
Ketchup
Ketchup Squeeze
Tomato Ketchup - Organic

Midwest Country Fare (Hy-Vee)
Ketchup

Organicville
Organicville (All)

Publix GreenWise Market ⟨⟩
Organic Ketchup

Publix ⟨⟩
Ketchup

Red Gold
Tomato Products (All)

Safeway
Ketchup

Walden Farms ☷
Walden Farms (All)

Winn-Dixie ⓘ
Tomato Ketchup

MARASCHINO CHERRIES

Hy-Vee
Green Maraschino Cherries
Red Maraschino Cherries
Red Maraschino Cherries with Stems

Meijer
Maraschino Cherry Red
Maraschino Cherry Red with Stems

Midwest Country Fare (Hy-Vee)
Maraschino Cherries

Publix ⟨⟩
Maraschino Cherries

Safeway
Maraschino Cherries

MARINADES & COOKING SAUCES

Allegro
Gold Bucket Brisket Sauce
Hickory Smoke Marinade
Hot & Spicy Marinade
Original
Teriyaki Marinade

Annie's Naturals
Baja Lime Marinade
Roasted Garlic & Balsamic Marinade

Cains
Franklin Italian Marinade

Contadina ⓘ
Sweet & Sour Sauce

Fischer & Wieser ⓘ
Charred Pineapple Bourbon Sauce
Granny's Peach 'n' Pepper Pourin' Sauce
Sweet & Savory Onion Glaze

Follow Your Heart ⓘ ⅋
Unforgettable Balsamic Vinaigrette
Sauce
Unforgettable Balsamic Vinaigrette
Sauce - Lowfat

Giant
Lemon Pepper Marinade

Gold's
Saucy Chicken Sauce
Saucy Rib Sauce

Goya
Mojo Chipotle
Mojo Criollo

Hy-Vee
Citrus Grill Marinade
Herb & Garlic Marinade
Lemon Pepper Marinade
Mesquite Marinade

Jack Daniel's Sauces ⓘ
EZ Marinader - Garlic & Herb Variety

Johnny's Fine Foods ⓘ
Jamaica Me Sweet Hot & Crazy
Dressing/Marinade
Jamaica Mistake Dressing/Marinade
Salmon Sauce

Ken's ⓘ
Buffalo Wing Sauce Marinade

Mayacamas ✓
Béarnaise Sauce
Demi-Glace Sauce
Hollandaise Sauce

Meijer
Marinade - Garlic and Herb
Marinade - Lemon Pepper
Marinade - Mesquite

Moore's ⅋ ✓
Moore's Original Marinade

Mrs. Dash
Marinades (All)

Nellie & Joe's
Nellie & Joe's (All)

Newman's Own
Herb & Roasted Garlic Marinade
Lemon Pepper Marinade
Mesquite with Lime Marinade

Olde Cape Cod
Chipotle Grilling Sauce
Cranberry Grilling Sauce
Honey Orange Grilling Sauce
Lemon Ginger Grilling Sauce
Sweet & Bold Grilling Sauce

Regina ⓘ
Cooking Wines (All)

Robert Rothschild Farm
Anna Mae's Sweet Smoky Chipotle Oven
& Grill Sauce
Anna Mae's Sweet Smoky Oven & Grill
Sauce
Apricot Ginger Oven & Grill Sauce
Apricot Mango Wasabi Sauce
Asian Sesame Oven & Grill Sauce
Blackberry Chipotle Oven & Grill Sauce
Chop House Steak Sauce
Ginger Wasabi Sauce
Harissa Moroccan Sauce
Horseradish Tarter Sauce
Hot Pepper Peach Chipotle Sauce
Hot Pepper Raspberry Chipotle Sauce
Hot Raspberry Thunder Sauce
Lemon Dill & Capers
Lemon Dill Sauce
Lemon Wasabi Sauce
Pineapple Coconut Tequila Sauce
Plum Garlic Thai Sauce
Strawberry Balsamic Sauce
Tandoori Indian Sauce

Safeway
Select - Gourmet Dipping Sauces,
Cook'n Grill Plum

Soy Vay ✓
Toasted Sesame Dressing and Marinade

Stubb's ⓘ
Moppin' Sauce
Texas Steakhouse Marinade

TryMe
TryMe Tiger Sauce

MAYONNAISE

Best Foods
Dijonnaise
Mayonnaise Products - Canola
  Cholesterol Free
Mayonnaise Products - Light
Mayonnaise Products - Real
Mayonnaise Products - Real with Lime
Mayonnaise Products - Reduced Fat
Sandwich Spread

Blue Plate
Low Fat Mayonnaise
Mayonnaise
Sandwich Spread
Sugar Free Mayonnaise

Boar's Head
Condiments (All)

Cains
All-Natural Mayonnaise
Fat Free Mayonnaise
Kitchen Recipe Mayonnaise
Light Mayonnaise

French's
GourMayo - Caesar Ranch
GourMayo - Creamy Dijon
GourMayo - Smoke Chipotle
GourMayo - Sun Dried Tomato
GourMayo - Wasabi Horseradish

Hellmann's
see Best Foods

JFG Mayonnaise
Mayonnaise
Reduced Fat Mayonnaise
Sandwich Spread
Squeeze Mayonnaise

Kissle
Mayonnaise

Kraft Mayonnaise
All-Out Squeeze! Light Mayo
All-Out Squeeze! Real Mayo
Fat Free Dressing Mayo
Light
Light Mayo
Real Mayo Easy Squeeze
Real Mayonnaise

Real Mayonnaise Hot 'n Spicy Super
  Easy Squeeze
Real Mayonnaise Light Super Easy
  Squeeze
Real Mayonnaise Super Easy Squeeze
Reduced Fat with Olive Oil

Meijer
Mayonnaise
Mayonnaise Lite

Miracle Whip
All-Out Squeeze! Miracle Whip
  Dressing
Dressing
Easy Squeeze Dressing
Free Dressing
Free Nonfat Dressing
Light Dressing
Light Super Easy Squeeze Dressing
Super Easy Squeeze Dressing

Nasoya
Dijon Nayonaise
Fat Free Nayonaise
Nayonaise

Publix ()
Mayonnaise

Safeway
Enlighten - Mayonnaise
Select - Mayonnaise with Canola Oil
Select - Mayonnaise, Fat Free
Select - Mayonnaise, Reduced Fat
Select - Mayonnaise, Regular
Select - Salad Dressing

Smart Balance
Smart Balance (All)

Thummann's
Condiments (All)

Vegenaise ⓘ
Expeller
Grapeseed
Organic
Original

Walden Farms
Walden Farms (All)

Mexican, Misc.

Chi-Chi's
Taco Sauce

Great Value (Wal-Mart)
Mexican Hot Style Tomato Sauce,
   Bilingual
Red Taco Sauce

Hy-Vee
Hot Picante Sauce
Medium Picante Sauce
Medium Taco Sauce
Mild Enchilada Sauce
Mild Picante Sauce
Mild Taco Sauce

Kroger ⓘ
Picante Sauce Salsa - Hot
Picante Sauce Salsa - Medium
Picante Sauce Salsa - Mild

Las Palmas ⓘ
Crushed Tomatillos
Red Chile Sauce
Red Enchilada Sauce

Laura Lynn (Ingle's)
Picante Sauce (All)
Taco Sauce (All)

Ortega ⓘ
Picante - Hot
Picante - Medium
Picante - Mild
Taco Sauce - Hot
Taco Sauce - Medium
Taco Sauce - Mild

Para MiCasa (Giant)
Adobo - Pepper
Adobo - Regular

Para MiCasa (Stop & Shop)
Adobo - Pepper
Adobo - Regular

Safeway
Select - Enchilada Sauce (Mild)

Taco Bell ᗗ
Medium Taco Sauce
Mild Taco Sauce

Tostitos ⓘ
All Natural Medium Picante Sauce
All Natural Mild Picante Sauce

Mustard

Annie's Naturals
Organic Dijon Mustard
Organic Honey Mustard
Organic Horseradish Mustard
Organic Yellow Mustard

Best Foods
Mustard Products (All)

Boar's Head
Condiments (All)

Bone Suckin' Sauce ✔
Bone Suckin' Mustard

Bubbies ⚇
Bubbies (All)

Eden Foods ⓘ ✔
Brown Mustard - Organic
Yellow Mustard - Organic

Emeril's ⓘ
Dijon Mustard
Kicked Up Horseradish Mustard
NY Deli Style Mustard
Smooth Honey Mustard
Yellow Mustard

Fischer & Wieser ⓘ
Smokey Mesquite Mustard
Sweet, Sour & Smokey Mustard Sauce

French's
Honey Mustard
Prepared Mustards

Giant
Creamy Dijon Mustard
Dijon Mustard
Honey Mustard
Old Grainy Mustard
Raspberry Grainy Mustard
Tarragon Dijon Mustard
Yellow Mustard

Gold's
Deli Mustard
Dijon Mustard
Honey Mustard Sauce
Mustard with Horseradish
Squeeze Honey Mustard

Great Value (Wal-Mart)
Course Ground Mustard
Honey Mustard

Prepared Dijon Mustard
Prepared Mustard
Southwest Spicy Sweet, Hot Mustard
Spicy Brown Mustard
Squeeze Prepared Mustard

Grey Poupon 〰
Country Dijon Mustard
Deli Mustard
Dijon Mustard
Harvest Coarse Ground Mustard
Hearty Spicy Brown Mustard
Honey Mustard
Savory Honey Mustard
Spicy Brown Mustard

Heinz ⓘ
Mustard (All Varieties)

Hellmann's
see Best Foods

Hy-Vee
Dijon Mustard
Honey Mustard
Mustard
Spicy Brown Mustard

Laura Lynn (Ingle's)
Mustard (All)

Meijer
Mustard - Dijon Squeeze
Mustard - Honey Squeeze
Mustard - Horseradish Squeeze
Mustard - Hot & Spicy
Mustard - Salad
Mustard - Salad Squeeze
Mustard - Spicy Brown Squeeze

Midwest Country Fare (Hy-Vee)
Yellow Mustard

Nathan's
Deli Mustard

Olde Cape Cod
Mustards

Publix GreenWise Market ⟨⟩
Organic Creamy Yellow Mustard
Organic Spicy Brown Mustard
Organic Tangy Dijon Mustard

Publix ⟨⟩
Classic Yellow Mustard
Deli Style Mustard

Dijon Mustard
Honey Mustard
Spicy Brown Mustard

Raley's ⏱
Mustard

Robert Rothschild Farm
Anna Mae's Smoky Mustard
Champagne Garlic Mustard
Horseradish Mustard
Raspberry Honey Mustard
Raspberry Wasabi Mustard

Sabrett
Mustard

Safeway
Mustard (including Stone Ground
 Horseradish)
Select - Gourmet Dipping Sauces,
 Honey Mustard
Select - Mustard, Classic/Country Dijon
Select - Mustard, Spicy Brown
Select - Mustard, Stone Ground
 Horseradish

Sprecher Brewing Co. ✓
Beer Mustard
Rootbeer Mustard

Stop & Shop
Creamy Dijon Mustard
Deli Mustard
Dijon Mustard
Honey Mustard
Old Grainy Mustard
Raspberry Grainy Mustard
Spicy Brown Mustard
Tarragon Dijon Mustard
Yellow Mustard

Texas Pete
Honey Mustard Sauce (Ensure "Best By"
 11/2006 and Later) ⏱

Thummann's
Condiments (All)

Nut Butters

Adams Peanut Butter
Adams Peanut Butter

Arrowhead Mills ✓
Creamy Almond Butter

Creamy Cashew Butter
Creamy Peanut Butter
Crunchy Peanut Butter
Sesame Tahini

Fisher Nuts ()
Peanut Butter - Chunky
Peanut Butter - Creamy

Giant
Peanut Butter - All Natural
Peanut Butter - Creamy
Peanut Butter - Crunchy
Peanut Butter - No Added Salt
Peanut Butter - Reduced Fat
Peanut Butter - Regular

Great Value (Wal-Mart)
Creamy Peanut Butter
Crunchy Peanut Butter
Peanut Free Smooth Soy Butter

Hy-Vee
Creamy Peanut Butter
Crunchy Peanut Butter
Reduced Fat Creamy Peanut Butter

Ian's Natural Foods ⛎ ✓
Wheat and Gluten-Free Recipe
Soybutter 4 Me

Jif
Peanut Butters (All)

Kroger ⓘ
Creamy Peanut Butter
Crunchy Peanut Butter
Natural Creamy Peanut Butter
Natural Crunchy Peanut Butter
Reduced Fat Creamy Peanut Butter
Reduced Fat Crunchy Peanut Butter

Laura Scudder's Peanut Butter
Laura Scudder's Peanut Butter

Meijer
Peanut Butter - Creamy
Peanut Butter - Crunchy
Peanut Butter - Natural Creamy
Peanut Butter - Natural Crunchy

Midwest Country Fare (Hy-Vee)
Creamy Peanut Butter
Crunchy Peanut Butter

Nature's Promise (Giant)
Cashew Butter

Organic Almond Butter - Crunchy
Organic Almond Butter - Salted
Organic Almond Butter - Smooth
Organic Almond Butter - Unsalted
Organic Peanut Butter - Crunchy
Organic Peanut Butter - Salted
Organic Peanut Butter - Smooth
Organic Peanut Butter - Unsalted

Nature's Promise (Stop & Shop)
Cashew Butter
Organic Almond Butter - Smooth
Organic Almond Butter - Unsalted
Organic Peanut Butter (All Varieties)

Peanut Butter & Co
Peanut Butters (All)

Publix ()
Creamy Peanut Butter
Crunchy Peanut Butter
Fresh Ground Peanut Butter (Deli)
Old Fashioned Creamy Peanut Butter
Old Fashioned Crunchy Peanut Butter
Reduced Fat Spread Creamy Peanut
   Butter
Reduced Fat Spread Crunchy Peanut
   Butter

Safeway
Peanut Butter - Reduced Fat Creamy
Peanut Butter - Reduced Fat Crunchy
Peanut Butter - Regular

Santa Cruz Organic
Santa Cruz Organic (All)

Skippy
Reduced Fat Peanut Butter
Roasted Honey Nut
Skippy Peanut Butter (All Varieties)

Smart Balance
Smart Balance (All)

Stop & Shop
All Natural Smooth Peanut Butter -
   Regular, No Added Salt & Reduced Fat
Peanut Butter - Crunchy, Creamy &
   Smooth

Walden Farms ⛎
Walden Farms (All)

Olives

B&G Foods ⓘ
Black Olives
Green Olives

Bella Tavola (Ingles)
Olives (All)

DeLallo
Almond Stuffed Olives
Garlic & Jalapeno Stuffed Olives
Garlic Stuffed Olives
Green Olives Stuffed with Blue Cheese
in Oil
Jalapeno Stuffed Olives
Jumbo Pitted Olives
Small Pitted Olives
Stuffed Queen Olives
Super Colossal Black Greek Olives
Super Colossal Pitted Olives
X-Jumbo Calamata Olives
X-Large Pitted Calamata Olives

Di Lusso
Green Ionian Olives
Mediterranean Mixed Olives

Giant
Queen Olives - Plain
Queen Olives - Stuffed
Stuffed Manzanilla Olives
Stuffed Queen Olives

Goya
Olives

Great Value (Wal-Mart)
Chopped Ripe Olives
Jumbo Pitted Ripe Olives
Large Pitted Ripe Olives
Medium Pitted Ripe Olives
Minced Pimento Stuffed Manzanilla
Olives
Minced Pimento Stuffed Queen Olives
Sliced Ripe Olives
Sliced Salad Olives

Hy-Vee
Chopped Ripe Olives
Large Ripe Black Olives
Manzanilla Olives
Medium Ripe Black Olives
Queen Olives

Sliced Ripe Black Olives
Sliced Salad Olives

Kroger ⓘ
Black Olives - Not Stuffed
Green Olives - Not Stuffed
Green Olives - Pimento Stuffed

Laura Lynn (Ingle's)
Black Olives (All)
Green Olives (All)

Mediterranean Organics ⓨ
Mediterranean Organics (All)

Meijer
Olives - Manz Stuffed Placed
Olives - Manz Stuffed Thrown
Olives - Manz Stuffed Tree
Olives - Queen Stuffed Placed
Olives - Queen Whole Thrown
Olives - Ripe Large
Olives - Ripe Medium
Olives - Ripe Pitted Jumbo
Olives - Ripe Pitted Small
Olives - Ripe Sliced
Olives - Salad
Olives - Salad Sliced

Midwest Country Fare (Hy-Vee)
Large Ripe Black Olives
Sliced Ripe Black Olives

O Olive Oil ⓘ
O Olive Oil (All)

Peloponnese
Kalamata Olive Spread
Kalamata Olives

Publix ⟨⟩
Colossal Olives
Green Olives (All Sizes & Styles)
Large Olives
Ripe Olives
Small Olives

Raley's ⓨ
Canned Olives

Safeway
Black Olives
Manzanilla Olives

Santa Barbara Olive Co
Olives (All)

Stop & Shop
Manzanilla Olives - Stuffed & Sliced
Pitted Black Ripe Olives - Jumbo, Large, Medium & Small (Chopped, Whole & Sliced)
Stuffed Queen Olives

Winn-Dixie ⓘ
Small Pitted Olives

PASTA & PIZZA SAUCE

Amy's Kitchen ⓘ ✔
Family Marinara Pasta Sauce
Garlic Mushroom Pasta Sauce
Low Sodium Marinara Sauce
Puttanesca Pasta Sauce
Roasted Garlic Pasta Sauce
Tomato Basil Pasta Sauce

Barilla ()
Sauces (All)

Bertolli
Pasta Sauce (All)

Bove's of Vermont
Sauces (All)

Classico ⓘ
Alfredo Sauces (All Varieties)
Bruschetta (All Varieties)
Pesto Sauces (All Varieties)
Red Sauces   (All Varieties)

Colameco's
Beef Bolognese
Pomodoro Sauce
Turkey Bolognese

Colavita
Sauces (All)

Contadina ⓘ
Pasta Sauce (Glass Jar)
Pizza Sauces (All)
Pizza Squeeze

Dei Fratelli
Dei Fratelli (All BUT Tomato Soup)

Del Monte ⓘ
Tomatoes & Tomato Products (All BUT Spaghetti Sauce Flavored with Meat)

DeLallo
Fancy Pizza Sauce

Fat Free Marinara Sauce
Imported Arrabbiata Sauce
Imported Bruschetta Sauce
Imported Garlic, Oil, & Hot Pepper Sauce
Imported Italian Pizza Sauce
Imported Marinara Sauce
Imported Porcini Mushroom Sauce
Imported Primavera Sauce
Imported Puttanesca Sauce
Imported Roasted Garlic Sauce
Imported Sun Dried Tomato Sauce
Imported Tomato Basil Sauce
Organic Arrabbiata Sauce
Organic Marinara Sauce
Organic Tomato Basil Sauce
Pesto Sauce in Olive Oil
Pink Vodka Sauce
Red Clam Sauce
Roasted Garlic Marinara Sauce
Spaghetti Sauce with Meat
Spaghetti Sauce with Mushrooms
Sun Dried Tomato Pesto
Tomato Basil Sauce
Traditional Spaghetti Sauce
White Clam Sauce

Eden Foods ⓘ ✔
Pizza Pasta Sauce - Organic
Spaghetti Sauce - No Salt Added
Spaghetti Sauce - Organic

Emeril's ⓘ
Eggplant & Gaaahlic
Home Style Marinara Pasta Sauce
Italian Style Tomato and Basil
Kicked Up Tomato Pasta Sauce
Roasted Gaaahlic Pasta Sauce
Roasted Red Pepper Pasta Sauce
Sicilian Gravy Pasta Sauce
Three Cheeses
Vodka Pasta Sauce

Francesco Rinaldi ⓘ
Garden Style Sauces (All)
Hearty Sauces (All)
Organic Sauces (All)
Traditional Sauces (All)

Great Value (Wal-Mart)
Italian Garden Combination Chunky
   Pasta Sauce
Mushrooms & Green Peppers Spaghetti
   Sauce
Onions & Garlic Chunky Pasta Sauce
Pizza Sauce
Traditional Spaghetti Sauce

Harvest Farms (Ingles)
Organic Pasta Sauce (All)

HealthMarket (Hy-Vee)
Tomato Basil Sauce

Hy-Vee
3 Cheese Spaghetti Sauce
Garden Spaghetti Sauce
Mushroom Spaghetti Sauce
Pizza Sauce
Spaghetti Sauce with Meat
Traditional Spaghetti Sauce

Laura Lynn (Ingle's)
Spaghetti Sauce (All)

Lucini
Rustic Tomato Basil Sauce
Spicy Tuscan Tomato Sauce
Tuscan Marinara with Roasted Garlic
   Sauce

Manischewitz
Original Marinara Sauce
Tomato & Mushroom Sauce

Mayacamas ✔
Alfredo Sauce
Creamy Clam Sauce
Peppered Lemon Sauce

Meijer
Pasta Sauce Four Cheese-Select
Pasta Sauce Marinara-Select
Pasta Sauce Mushroom and Olive-Select
Pasta Sauce Onion and Garlic-Select
Pizza Sauce
Spaghetti Extra Chunk Garden Combo
Spaghetti Sauce Extra Chunk 3 Cheese
Spaghetti Sauce Extra Chunk Garlic and
   Cheese
Spaghetti Sauce Extra Chunk
   Mushroom/Green Pepper
Spaghetti Sauce Plain
Spaghetti Sauce with Meat

Spaghetti Sauce with Mushroom

Midwest Country Fare (Hy-Vee)
All Natural Garlic & Onion Spaghetti
Four Cheese Spaghetti Sauce
Garden Vegetable Spaghetti Sauce
Garlic & Herb Spaghetti Sauce
Meat Flavor Spaghetti Sauce
Mushroom Spaghetti Sauce
Traditional Spaghetti Sauce

Mom's ⓘ
Artichoke Heart & Asiago Cheese Pasta
   Sauce
Garlic & Basil Spaghetti Sauce
Martini Pasta Sauce
Organic Roasted Pepper Pasta Sauce
Organic Traditional Pasta Sauce
Puttanesca Spaghetti Sauce
Special Marinara Spaghetti Sauce
Spicy Arrabbiata

Nature's Promise (Giant)
Organic Pasta Sauce - Garden Vegetable
Organic Pasta Sauce - Original
Organic Pasta Sauce - Parmesan

Nature's Promise (Stop & Shop)
Organic Pasta Sauce - Garden Vegetable
Organic Pasta Sauce - Parmesan
Organic Pasta Sauce - Plain

Newman's Own
Bombolina (Basil)
Cabernet Marinara
Diavolo (Spicy Simmer Sauce)
Five Cheese
Italian Sausage & Peppers
Marinara (Venetian)
Marinara with Mushrooms
Organic Marinara Sauce
Organic Tomato Basil Sauce
Organic Traditional Herb Sauce
Pesto and Tomato
Roasted Garlic and Peppers
Sockarooni (Mushrooms, Onions,
   Peppers)
Sweet Onion and Roasted Garlic
Tomato and Roasted Garlic
Vodka Sauce

Prego ⓘ
Chunky Garden Combo

Chunky Garden Mushroom & Green
Pepper
Chunky Garden Mushroom Supreme
with Baby Portobello
Chunky Garden Tomato Onion & Garlic
Flavored with Meat
Fresh Mushroom
Heart Smart Mushroom
Heart Smart Onion & Garlic
Heart Smart Ricotta Parmesan
Heart Smart Roasted Red Pepper &
Garlic
Heart Smart Traditional
Italian Sausage & Garlic
Marinara
Mushroom & Garlic
Organic Mushroom
Organic Tomato & Basil
Roasted Garlic & Herb
Roasted Garlic Parmesan
Three Cheese
Tomato Basil Garlic
Traditional

Publix GreenWise Market ()
Organic Tomato Sauce

Rising Moon Organics ()
Pasta Sauces

Robert Rothschild Farm
Artichoke Pasta Sauce
Roasted Portabella & Roma Tomato
Pasta Sauce
Roma & Sun Dried Tomato Pasta Sauce
Vodka Pasta Sauce

Safeway
Meat Spaghetti Sauce
Mushroom Spaghetti Sauce
Select - Pasta Sauce, Classic Pesto
(Refrigerated)
Select - Pasta Sauce, Creamy Parmesan
Basil (Refrigerated)
Select - Pasta Sauce, Garden Vegetable &
Herb (Refrigerated)
Select - Pasta Sauce, Light Alfredo
(Refrigerated)
Select - Pasta Sauce, Mushroom/Onion
(Refrigerated)

Select - Pasta Sauce, Roasted Garlic &
Mushroom (Refrigerated)
Select - Pizza Sauce
Traditional Spaghetti Sauce

Santa Barbara Salsa 🍷
Santa Barbara Salsa (All)

Sauces 'n Love 🍷
Sauces 'n Love (All)

Simply Enjoy (Giant)
Fra Diavolo Sauce
Marinara Sauce
Roasted Garlic Sauce
Sicilian Eggplant Sauce
Tomato Basil Sauce
Vodka Sauce

Simply Enjoy (Stop & Shop)
Fra Diavolo Sauce
Marinara Sauce
Roasted Garlic Sauce
Sicilian Eggplant Sauce
Tomato Basil Sauce
Vodka Sauce

Ukrop's
Marinara Sauce (Deli)
Pizza Sauce (Deli)
Spaghetti Sauce with Meat (Deli)

Walden Farms 🍷
Walden Farms (All)

Winn-Dixie ⓘ
Classic Style Fine Pasta Sauce - Fat Free

PEPPERS

B&G Foods ⓘ
Peppers

Chi-Chi's
Green Chilies

DeLallo
Fried Peppers with Onions
Grilled Piquillo Peppers
Hot Banana Pepper Chunks
Hot Banana Pepper Rings
Hot Pepperoncini
Hot Peppers & Sauce
Hot Sliced Jalapeno Peppers
Medium Hot Peppers & Sauce
Mild Banana Pepper Chunks

Mild Banana Pepper Rings
Mild Pepperoncini
Red Hot Cherry Peppers
Roasted Piquillo Peppers
Roasted Red Peppers
Roasted Red Peppers with Garlic
Roasted Yellow & Red Peppers
Roasted Yellow & Red Peppers with
    Garlic
Roasted Yellow Peppers
Sliced Mild Pepperoncini
Sweet Peppers & Sauce
Whole Hot Banana Peppers
Whole Mild Banana Peppers
Whole Mild Pepperoncini

Di Lusso
Roasted Red Peppers

Goya
Red Pimientos

Great Value (Wal-Mart)
Fire Roasted Green Chiles, Bilingual
Nacho Sliced Jalapenos, Bilingual
Sliced Jalapenos
Whole Jalapenos, Bilingual

Heinz ⓘ
Peppers (All Varieties)

Hy-Vee
Green Salad Pepperoncini
Hot Banana Peppers
Mild Banana Peppers

Laura Lynn (Ingle's)
Jalapeno Peppers (All)
Pepperoncini (All)

Mediterranean Organics ⓾
Mediterranean Organics (All)

Meijer
Hot Pepper Rings
Mild Pepper Rings
Pepper Ring - Banana Hot
Pepper Rings - Banana Mild
Pepperoncini

Mount Olive Pickle Company ⓾
Mount Olive Pickle Company (All)

Ortega ⓘ
Chiles
Jalapenos

Peloponnese
Roasted Sweet Peppers

Strub's ⓞ
Strub's (All)

Thummann's
Condiments (All)

Trappey ⓘ
Peppers

Vlasic
Vlasic (All)

PICKLES

B&G Foods ⓘ
Pickles

Bubbies ⓾
Bubbies (All)

Claussen ⌒
Bread 'n Butter Chips Pickles
Burger Slices Pickles Kosher Dill
Deli Style Kosher Dill Halves Pickles
Deli Style Kosher Dill Spears Pickles
Hearty Garlic Deli Style Wholes Pickles
Kosher Dill Wholes Pickles
Kosher Dills Mini Pickles
Sweet Gherkins Pickles

DeLallo
Capote Capers
Hot Cauliflower
Hot Giardiniera
Mild Cauliflower
Non Pareil Capers

Gedney ⓾
Gedney (All)

Great Value (Wal-Mart)
Baby Dill Pickles
Bread & Butter Pickles
Dill Spears Pickles
Garlic Dill Slicers Pickles
Hamburger Dill Chips Pickles
Kosher Baby Dill Pickles
Kosher Dill Spears Pickles
Kosher Whole Dill Pickles
Sweet Gherkin Pickles
Sweet Whole Pickles
Whole Dill Pickles

Hans Jurgen
Pickles
Heinz ⓘ
Pickles (All Varieties)
Hermann Pickle ♨
Pickles (All)
Hy-Vee
Kosher Dill Halves (Refrigerated)
Kosher Dill Sandwich Slices
(Refrigerated)
Kosher Dill Spears (Refrigerated)
Kosher Dill Whole Pickles
(Refrigerated)
Special Recipe Baby Dills
Special Recipe Bread & Butter Slices
Special Recipe Hot & Spicy Zingers
Special Recipe Hot & Sweet Zinger
Chunks
Special Recipe Jalapeno Baby Dills
Special Recipe Sweet Garden Crunch
Laura Lynn (Ingle's)
Giardianiera (All)
Pickles (All)
Meijer
Bread & Butter Chips - Sugar Free
Bread & Butter Chips, FP
Dill Spears - Zesty, FP
Halves - Kosher Dill (Refrigerated)
Kosher Baby Dills, FP
Kosher Dills, FP
Pickle - Bread & Butter Chips - FP
Pickle - Dill Hamburger Slices-PROC
Pickle - Dill Kosher Baby, FP
Pickle - Dill Kosher Spears-FP
Pickle - Dill Kosher Whole - FP
Pickle - Dill Kosher Whole - PROC
Pickle - Dill Polish - FP
Pickle - Dill Polish Spears-FP
Pickle - Dill Whole-FP
Pickle - No Garlic Dill Spears
Pickle - Sweet Gherkin Whole - PROC
Pickle - Sweet Midgets Whole - PROC
Pickle - Sweet Whole - PROC
Pickles - Whole - Refrigerated
Sandwich Slice - Bread & Butter
Sandwich Slice - Kosher Dill
Sandwich Slice - Kosher Dill Zesty

Slickles Sandwich Slice - Kosher Dill
Slickles Sandwich Slice - Polish Dill
Sweet Pickles - Sugar Free
Wholes - Kosher Dill (Refrigerated)
Mount Olive Pickle Company ♨
Mount Olive Pickle Company (All)
Mrs. Renfro's
Mrs. Renfro's (All BUT Nacho Cheese
Sauce)
Publix ◖◗
Pickles (All Varieties)
Raley's ♨
Pickles
Safeway
Pickles (All)
Select - Capers
Strub's ◖◗
Strub's (All)
Thummann's
Pickles (All)
Vlasic
Vlasic (All)
Winn-Dixie ⓘ
Hamburger Chips

RELISH

B&G Foods ⓘ
Relishes
Bubbies ♨
Bubbies (All)
Cains
Relishes (All Retail Relishes)
Claussen ⌐
Sweet Squeeze Pickle Relish
Crosse & Blackwell
Crosse & Blackwell (All BUT Branston
Pickle Relish, Fish & Chip Vinegar,
and Plum Pudding)
Dickinson's
Dickinson's (All)
Giant
Relish - Dill
Relish - Sweet
Gold's
Squeeze Hot Dog Relish

Great Value (Wal-Mart)
Sweet Pickle Relish

Heinz ⓘ
Relish (All Varieties)

Meijer
Relish - Dill
Relish - Sweet
Sweet Relish - Sugar Free

Mount Olive Pickle Company ⌙
Mount Olive Pickle Company (All)

Mrs. Renfro's
Mrs. Renfro's (All BUT Nacho Cheese Sauce)

Nance's
Corn Relish

Raley's ⌙
Relish

Sabrett
Relish

Vlasic
Vlasic (All)

SALAD DRESSING & MIXES

Anchor Bar
Blue Cheese

Annie's Naturals
Artichoke Parmesan
Balsamic Dressing
Balsamic Vinaigrette
Caesar
Cowgirl Ranch
Lemon & Chive
Lite Italian Dressing
Low Fat Honey Mustard
Low Fat Raspberry
Mango Fat-Free Dressing
Organic Balsamic Dressing
Organic Buttermilk Dressing
Organic Cowgirl Ranch
Organic Creamy Asiago Dressing
Organic French Dressing
Organic Green Garlic
Organic Green Goddess
Organic Maple Ginger Dressing
Organic Oil & Vinegar with Balsamic Vinegar

Organic Papaya Poppyseed
Organic Pomegranate Vinaigrette
Organic Red Wine & Olive Oil
Organic Roasted Garlic Vinaigrette
Organic Sesame Ginger with Chamomile
Raspberry & Balsamic Fat Free Dressing
Roasted Red Pepper
Strawberry & Balsamic Fat-Free Dressing
Tuscany Italian

Big Y
Creamy French
French Lite
Italian
Lite Italian
Lite Ranch
Ranch
Thousand Island
Thousand Island Light Topco

Bragg
Bragg (All)

Briannas Fine Salad Dressings
Briannas Fine Salad Dressings (All BUT Asiago Caesar, Chipotle Cheddar, Ginger Mandarin, Lemon Tarragon, Monterey Ranch & Thousand Island)

Cains
Balsamic Vinaigrette Dressing
Bellisimo Italian Dressing
Blue Cheese Dressing
Blush Wine Vinaigrette Fat Free
Caesar Country Fat Free
Chipotle Ranch Dressing
Creamy Caesar
Creamy Italian Dressing
Deluxe Buttermilk Ranch
Fat Free Italian Dressing
Fat Free Raspberry Vinaigrette Country
French Dressing
Honey Dijon Fat Free
Italian Cheese Trio
Italian Country Dressing
Light Blush Wine Vinaigrette
Light Caesar Dressing
Light French Dressing
Light Italian

Light Ranch
Light Raspberry Vinaigrette Dressing
Peppercorn Parmesan Dressing
Peppercorn Ranch Fat Free
Ranch Dressing
Ranch with Bacon
Robust Italian Dressing
White Balsamic with Honey Dressing
Zesty Tomato & Onion French

Caroline's
Sweet Blue Onion Dressing
Sweet Celery Dressing
Sweet French Onion Dressing
Sweet Lemon Poppyseed
Sweet Orange Dressing
Sweet Razzmataz Dressing

Dave's
Coleslaw

DeLallo
Balsamic Vinaigrette Dressing
Classic Italian Dressing
Italian House Dressing

Drew's All Natural ⓘ
Buttermilk Ranch
Garlic Italian
Honey Dijon
Kalamata Olive & Caper
Poppy Seed
Raspberry
Roasted Garlic & Peppercorn
Romano Caesar
Rosemary Balsamic
Smoked Tomato

Durkee ⓘ
Buttermilk Ranch Dressing

Emeril's ⓘ
Balsamic Vinaigrette
Caesar Dressing
House Herb Vinaigrette Dressing
Italian Vinaigrette
Raspberry Balsamic Vinaigrette

Fischer & Wieser ⓘ
Citrus, Herb & Truffle Oil Vinaigrette
Creamy Garlic & Chile Dressing
Original Roasted Raspberry Chipotle
   Vinaigrette

Southwestern Herb & Tomato
   Vinaigrette
Spicy Lime & Coriander Dressing
Sweet Corn & Shallot Dressing

Follow Your Heart ⓘ ⛟
Caesar with Parmesan Dressing
Creamy Garlic Dressing
Honey Mustard Dressing
Lemon Herb Dressing
Low Fat Ranch Dressing
Organic Balsamic Vinaigrette Dressing
Organic Chipotle Lime Ranch Dressing
Organic Chunky Bleu Cheese Dressing
Organic Creamy Caesar Dressing
Organic Creamy Miso Ginger Dressing
Organic Creamy Ranch Dressing
Organic Italian Vinaigrette Dressing
Sesame Dijon Dressing
Sesame Miso Dressing
Spicy Southwest Ranch Dressing
Thousand Island Dressing
Vegan Caesar Dressing

Four Brothers
Greek House Dressing

Giant
Balsamic Vinaigrette
Blue Cheese
Caesar
French - Creamy
French - Regular
French - Spicy Sweet
Italian - Creamy
Italian - Fat Free
Italian - Lite
Italian - Regular
Ranch - Fat Free
Ranch - Lite
Ranch - Regular
Raspberry Vinaigrette - Reduced Fat
Raspberry Vinaigrette - Regular
Thousand Island

Good Seasons ⌒
Cheese Garlic Salad Dressing Mix
Classic Balsamic Vinaigrette with Extra
   Virgin Olive Dressing
Garlic & Herb Salad Dressing Mix
Italian Cruet Kit

Italian Salad Dressing & Recipe Mix
Italian Vinaigrette with Extra Virgin
  Olive Oil Dressing
Light Honey Dijon with Grey Poupon
  Mustard Dressing
Mild Italian Salad Dressing Mix
Red Raspberry Vinaigrette with
  Poppyseed Dressing
Sun Dried Tomato Vinaigrette with
  Roasted Red Pepper Dressing
Zesty Italian Salad Dressing Mix

HealthMarket (Hy-Vee)
Organic Creamy Caesar Dressing
Organic Honey Mustard Dressing
Organic Raspberry Vinaigrette

Henri's
Salad Dressings (All)

Hy-Vee
Chunky Blue Cheese Salad Dressing
French Dressing
Italian Dressing
Light French Salad Dressing
Light Italian Dressing
Light Ranch Dressing
Light Thousand Island Dressing
Ranch Dressing
Thousand Island Dressing
Zesty Italian Dressing

JFG Mayonnaise
Salad Dressing

Johnny's Fine Foods ⓘ
Great Caesar Dressing
Honey You're Terrific Dressing
Ranch Dressing & Dip

Ken's ⓘ
3 Cheese Italian
Balsamic & Basil
Balsamic Vinaigrette Lite Accent
  Dressing
Buttermilk Ranch
Caesar
Chef's Reserve Blue Cheese with
  Gorgonzola
Chef's Reserve Creamy Balsamic
Chef's Reserve Creamy Greek with
  Fresh Oregano

Chef's Reserve Farm House Ranch with
  Buttermilk
Chef's Reserve French with Applewood
  Smoked Bacon
Chef's Reserve Golden Vidalia Onion
Chef's Reserve Honey Dijon
Chef's Reserve Italian with Garlic and
  Asiago Cheese
Chef's Reserve Ranch
Chef's Reserve Russian
Christo's Yasou Greek
Chunky Blue Cheese
Country French with Vermont Honey
Creamy Caesar
Creamy French
Creamy Italian
Creamy Parmesan with Cracked
  Peppercorn
Fat Free Raspberry Pecan
Fat Free Sun Dried Tomato
Greek
Healthy Options Balsamic Vinaigrette
Healthy Options Honey Dijon
Healthy Options Honey French
Healthy Options Italian with Romano
  and Red Pepper
Healthy Options Olive Oil and Vinegar
Healthy Options Parmesan and
  Peppercorn
Healthy Options Ranch
Healthy Options Raspberry Walnut
Healthy Options Sweet Vidalia Onion
  Vinaigrette
Honey Mustard
Honey Mustard Vinaigette Lite Accent
  Dressing
Italian and Marinade
Italian Vinaigette Lite Accent Dressing
Italian with Aged Romano
Lite Balsamic & Basil
Lite Balsamic Vinaigrette
Lite Caesar
Lite Chunky Blue Cheese
Lite Country French with Vermont
  Honey
Lite Creamy Caesar
Lite Creamy Parmesan with Cracked
  Peppercorn

Lite Honey Mustard
Lite Italian
Lite Northern Italian
Lite Olive Oil Vinaigrette
Lite Ranch
Lite Raspberry Pomegranate
Lite Raspberry Walnut
Lite Red Wine Vinaigrette
Lite Sweet Vidalia Onion
New & Improved Ranch
Ranch
Raspberry Walnut Vinaigrette Lite
  Accent Dressing
Red Wine Vinegar & Olive Oil
Russian
Sweet Vidalia Onion
Thousand Island
Zesty Italian

Kissle
Italian Dressing
Salad Dressing

Kraft ↝
Coleslaw Maker
Tuna Salad Maker Super Easy Squeeze

Kraft Salad Dressing ↝
Balsamic Vinaigrette
Buttermilk Ranch
Caesar Vinaigrette with Parmesan
Caesar with Bacon
Catalina
Classic Caesar
Classic Italian Vinaigrette
Creamy French
Creamy Italian
Creamy Poppyseed
Free Caesar Italian
Free Catalina
Free Classic Caesar
Free French Style
Free Honey Dijon Fat Free
Free Italian
Free Zesty Italian
Garlic Ranch
Greek Vinaigrette
Honey Dijon
Honey Dijon Vinaigrette
Light Balsamic Vinaigrette

Light Balsamic Vinaigrette Parmesan
  Asiago
Light Balsamic Vinaigrette Sicilian
  Roasted Garlic
Light Creamy French Style
Light Done Right Red Wine Vinaigrette
Light Raspberry Vinaigrette with Extra
  Virgin Olive Oil
Light Thousand Island
Light Three Cheese Ranch
Peppercorn Ranch
Ranch
Ranch with Bacon
Roasted Red Pepper Italian with
  Parmesan
Roka Blue Cheese
Roka Brand Blue Cheese
Special Collection Parmesan Romano
Sun Dried Tomato Vinaigrette
Sweet Honey Catalina
Tangy Tomato Bacon
Thousand Island
Thousand Island with Bacon
Three Cheese Ranch
Tuscan House Italian
Vidalia Onion Vinaigrette with Roasted
  Red Pepper
Zesty Italian

La Martinique
Balsamic Vinaigrette
Blue Cheese Vinaigrette
Original Poppy Seed
True French Vinaigrette

Laura Lynn (Ingle's)
Bacon Ranch
Blue Cheese
CA French Style
French - Creamy
Honey Mustard
Italian - Fat Free
Italian - House
Poppyseed
Ranch
Ranch - Buttermilk
Ranch - Fat Free
Ranch Garden
Ranch Lite

Thousand Island
Vidalia Onion
Zesty Italian

Lily's Gourmet Dressings ⓘ

Balsamic Vinaigrette
Northern Italian
Poppyseed
Raspberry Walnut Vinaigrette

Litehouse

Bacon Bleu Cheese
Balsamic Vinaigrette
Barbecue Ranch
Big Bleu
Bleu Cheese Crumbles
Bleu Cheese Vinaigrette
Buttermilk Ranch
Caesar
Chunky Bleu Cheese
Chunky Garlic Caesar
Classic Feta
Coleslaw
Coleslaw with Pineapple
Creamy Cilantro
Garden Veggie Ranch Dressing
Garlic Vinaigrette
Greek Feta
Harvest Cranberry Vinaigrette
Homestyle Ranch
Honey Mustard
Huckleberry Vinaigrette
Jalapeno Ranch
Lite 1000 Island
Lite Bleu Cheese
Lite Caesar
Lite Coleslaw
Lite Greek
Lite Honey Dijon Vinaigrette
Lite Ranch
Organic Balsamic Vinaigrette
Organic Caesar
Organic Ranch
Organic Raspberry Lime Vinaigrette
Original Bleu Cheese
Pomegranate Blueberry Vinaigrette
Poppyseed Dressing
Ranch
Raspberry Walnut Vinaigrette

Red Wine Olive Oil Vinaigrette
Romano Caeser
Roquefort
Salsa Ranch
Spinach Salad
Sweet French
Thousand Island
Zesty Italian Vinaigrette

Lucini

Salad Dressing (All)

Marie's

Salad Dressings (All)

Mark's

Blue Cheese

Marukan

Lite Seasoned Gourmet Dressing
Organic Seasoned Dressing

Midwest Country Fare (Hy-Vee)

Ranch Dressing

Naturally Delicious

Balsamic
Barbeque Sauce
Blue Cheese
Chipotle Ranch
French
Honey Mustard
Italian
Light Blush Wine
Light Italian
Light Raspberry
Mayonnaise
Peppercorn Ranch

Newman's Own

Balsamic Spray Mist Dressing
Balsamic Vinaigrette
Caesar
Creamy Caesar
Creamy Italian (Parmesanio Italianio)
Italian Spray Mist Dressing
Light Balsamic Vinaigrette
Light Caesar Dressing
Light Cranberry and Walnut
Light Honey Mustard
Light Italian
Light Lime Vinaigrette
Light Raspberry and Walnut
Light Red Wine and Vinegar

Light Sun Dried Tomato
Olive Oil and Vinegar
Organic Creamy Caesar Dressing
Organic Light Balsamic Vinaigrette
   Dressing
Organic Tuscan Italian Dressing
Parmesan and Roasted Garlic
Ranch Dressing
Red Wine and Vinegar
Southwest
Three Cheese Balsamic Vinaigrette
Two Thousand Island

Olde Cape Cod
Blue Cheese & Chive
Chipotle Ranch
Garlic & Herb
Honey Dijon
Honey French Lite
Lemon Poppyseed
Lite Blush Wine Vinaigrette
Lite Caesar
Lite Raspberry Vinaigrette
Lite Sweet & Sour Poppyseed
Orange Poppyseed
Parmesan & Peppercorn
Sundried Tomato Lite

Organicville
Organicville (All)

Oxford
Italian
Ranch

Publix ()
Balsamic Vinaigrette
Caesar
California French
Chunky Blue Cheese
Creamy Parmesan
Fat Free Italian
Fat Free Thousand Island
Italian
Lite Caesar
Lite Honey Dijon
Lite Ranch
Lite Raspberry Walnut
Ranch
Thousand Island
Zesty Italian

Robert Rothschild Farm
Buffalo Bleu Cheese Dressing
Chipotle Ranch Dressing
Fat Free Raspberry Dressing
Maple Balsamic Dressing
Raspberry Dressing
Raspberry Wasabi Dressing

Rooties
Blue Cheese

Safeway
1000 Island Dressing
Creamy Italian Dressing
Enlighten - Balsamic & Red Wine
   Vinaigrette
Enlighten - Garden Italian Dressing
Enlighten - Honey Mustard Dressing
Enlighten - Roasted Sweet Pepper &
   Garlic Vinaigrette
Fat Free 1000 Island Dressing
Italian Dressing Mix
Light Ranch Dressing
Light Zesty Italian Salad Dressing
Ranch Dressing
Ranch Dressing Mix
Ranch with Bacon Dressing
Select - Italian Salad Dressing Mix
Select - Salad Dressing, Basil Ranch
Select - Salad Dressing, Blue Cheese
Select - Salad Dressing, Cranberry/
   Orange
Select - Salad Dressing, Creamy Goat
   Cheese/Dried Tomato
Select - Salad Dressing, Harvest
   Vegetable
Select - Salad Dressing, Ranch
Select - Salad Dressing, Raspberry
   Cranberry Vinaigrette
Select - Salad Dressing, Raspberry
   Vinaigrette
Select - Salad Dressing, Red Wine
   Balsamic
Select - Salad Dressing, Roasted Red
   Pepper & Garlic Vinaigrette
Select - Salad Dressing, Tuscan Basil
   Herb
Select - Salad Dresssing, Balsamic &
   Olive Oil Vinaigrette

Zesty Italian Dressing

Seven Seas Salad Dressing ⌇
Green Goddess Dressing
Red Wine Vinaigrette Dressing

South Beach Living ⌇
Balsamic with Extra Virgin Olive Oil
Italian with Extra Virgin Olive Oil
Ranch

Stop & Shop
Balsamic Vinaigrette
Blue Cheese
Caesar
French - Creamy
French - Regular
Italian - Creamy
Italian - Fat Free
Italian - Lite
Ranch - Fat Free
Ranch - Regular
Raspberry Vinaigrette
Thousand Island

Taste of Thai, A
Peanut Salad Dressing

Walden Farms ☒
Walden Farms (All)

Winn-Dixie ⓘ
Creamy French Dressing

Salsa

Amy's Kitchen ⓘ ✓
Black Bean & Corn Salsa
Fire Roasted Vegetable Salsa
Medium Salsa
Mild Salsa
Spicy Chipotle Salsa

Arriba!
Arriba! (All)

Bone Suckin' Sauce ✓
Bone Suckin' Salsa - Hot
Bone Suckin' Salsa - Regular

Dei Fratelli
Dei Fratelli (All BUT Tomato Soup)

Drew's All Natural ⓘ
Salsa (All)

EatSmart
Fire-Roasted Salsa
Salsa Con Queso

Emerald Valley Kitchen
Emerald Valley Kitchen (All)

Emeril's ⓘ
Gaaahlic Lovers Medium Salsa
Kicked Up Chunky Hot Salsa
Original Recipe Medium Salsa
Southwest Style Medium Salsa

Fischer & Wieser ⓘ
Das Peach Haus Peach Salsa
Salsa A La Charra
Salsa Verde Ranchera
Timpone's Organic Salsa Muy Rica

Garden Fresh Gourmet ☒
Salsas (All)

Giant
Salsa - Hot
Salsa - Medium
Salsa - Mild

Gold's
Extra Chunky Salsa - Hot
Extra Chunky Salsa - Mild

Goya
Salsas - Pico De Gallo
Salsas - Taquera
Salsas - Verde

Grande ⓘ
Fire Roasted Salsa Dip
Sweet Garden Salsa Dip

Great Value (Wal-Mart)
Salsa Con Queso
White Salsa Con Queso

Green Mountain Gringo
Salsa - Hot ☒
Salsa - Medium ☒
Salsa - Mild ☒
Salsa - Roasted Chile ☒
Salsa - Roasted Garlic ☒

Guiltless Gourmet
Salsas (All) ☒

Harvest Farms (Ingles)
Organic Salsa (All)

HealthMarket (Hy-Vee)
Organic Medium Salsa

Organic Mild Salsa
Organic Pineapple Salsa

Herr's ()
Medium Chunky Salsa
Mild Chunky Salsa

Hy-Vee
Thick & Chunky Hot Salsa
Thick & Chunky Medium Salsa
Thick & Chunky Mild Salsa

Kroger ⓘ
Thick & Chunky Salsa - Hot
Thick & Chunky Salsa - Medium
Thick & Chunky Salsa - Mild
Traditional Salsa - Hot
Traditional Salsa - Medium
Traditional Salsa - Mild

Laura Lynn (Ingle's)
Salsa (All)

Litehouse
Medium Salsa

Meijer
Salsa - Hot
Salsa - Medium
Salsa - Mild
Salsa - Restaurant Style Hot
Salsa - Restaurant Style Medium
Salsa - Restaurant Style Mild
Salsa - Santa Fe Style Medium
Salsa - Santa Fe Style Mild
Salsa - Thick & Chunky Hot
Salsa - Thick & Chunky Medium
Salsa - Thick & Chunky Mild

Mrs. Renfro's
Mrs. Renfro's (All BUT Nacho Cheese
Sauce)

Nathan's
Salsa - Hot
Salsa - Mild

Nature's Promise (Giant)
Chipotle Organic Salsa - Medium
Chipotle Organic Salsa - Mild

Nature's Promise (Stop & Shop)
Chipotle Organic Salsa
Organic Salsa - Medium
Organic Salsa - Mild

Newman's Own
Black Bean & Corn Salsa
Farmer's Garden Salsa
Hot Salsa
Mango Salsa
Medium Salsa
Mild Salsa
Organic Chunky Medium Salsa
Organic Cilantro Medium Salsa
Peach Salsa
Pineapple Salsa
Roasted Garlic Salsa
Tequila Lime Salsa

Organicville
Organicville (All)

Ortega ⓘ
Black Bean & Corn (Mexican)
Garden - Medium
Garden - Mild
Original - Medium
Original - Mild
Roasted Garlic
Thick & Chunky - Medium
Thick & Chunky - Mild

Publix GreenWise Market ()
Organic Salsa - Medium
Organic Salsa - Mild

Publix ()
All Natural - Hot Salsa
All Natural - Medium Salsa
All Natural - Mild Salsa
Southwestern Black Bean and Corn
Salsa
Thick & Chunky - Hot Salsa
Thick & Chunky - Medium Salsa
Thick & Chunky - Mild Salsa

Red Gold
Tomato Products (All)

Rising Moon Organics ()
Salsas

Robert Rothschild Farm
Cilantro Lime Salsa
Mango Salsa
Raspberry Chipotle Salsa
Raspberry Salsa "Original"

Safeway
Salsa Con Queso

Select - Fiesta Fajita Salsa
Select - Salsa (All Varieties)

Santa Barbara Salsa ⚕
Santa Barbara Salsa (All)

Simply Enjoy (Giant)
Black Bean and Corn Salsa
Peach Mango Salsa
Pineapple Chipotle Salsa
Raspberry Chipotle
Tequila Lime Salsa

Simply Enjoy (Stop & Shop)
Black Bean and Corn Salsa
Peach Mango Salsa
Pineapple Chipotle Salsa
Raspberry Chipotle
Tequila Lime Salsa

Snyder's of Hanover ⓘ
Fire Roasted Salsa Dip
Sweet Salsa Dip

Stop & Shop
Salsa - Hot
Salsa - Medium
Salsa - Mild

Taco Bell Ꮹ
Home Originals Medium Salsa Con Queso
Home Originals Mild Salsa Con Queso
Thick 'n Chunky Medium Salsa
Thick 'n Chunky Mild Salsa

TGI Friday's (Heinz) ⓘ
Salsa (All Varieties)

Timpone's ⓘ
Salsa Muy Rica

Tostitos ⓘ
All Natural Hot Chunky Salsa
All Natural Medium Black Bean & Corn Salsa
All Natural Medium Chunky Salsa
All Natural Medium Pineapple & Peach Salsa
All Natural Mild Chunky Salsa
Creamy Salsa
Salsa Con Queso

Ukrop's
Pico De Gallo (Deli)
Salsa (Deli)

Utz ⚕ ✓
Mt. Misery Mike's Salsa Dip
Sweet Salsa Dip

SAUERKRAUT

B&G Foods ⓘ
Sauerkraut

Bubbies ⚕
Bubbies (All)

Claussen Ꮹ
Premium Crisp Sauerkraut

Dei Fratelli
Dei Fratelli (All BUT Tomato Soup)

Eden Foods ⓘ ✓
Sauerkraut - Organic

Giant
Sauerkraut (Canned)

Great Value (Wal-Mart)
Sauerkraut

Hy-Vee
Shredded Kraut

Meijer
Sauerkraut

Sabrett
Sauerkraut

Safeway
Sauerkraut

Stop & Shop
Sauerkraut

Strub's ()
Strub's (All)

Thummann's
Condiments (All)

SLOPPY JOE SAUCE

Heinz ⓘ
Sloppy Joe Sauce

Hy-Vee
Sloppy Joe Sauce

Laura Lynn (Ingle's)
Sloppy Joes

Meijer
Sloppy Joe Sauce

Safeway
Sloppy Joe

Steak Sauce

A.1. ↺
Carb Well Steak Sauce
New York Steakhouse
Roasted Garlic
Smoky Mesquite
Steak House Chicago
Steak House Cracked Peppercorn
Steak House New Orleans Cajun
Steak House Sweet Hickory with Bull's
Eye BBQ Sauce
Steak Sauce
Steakhouse Jamaican Jerk
Thick & Hearty
Crosse & Blackwell
Crosse & Blackwell (All BUT Branston
Pickle Relish, Fish & Chip Vinegar,
and Plum Pudding)
Fischer & Wieser ⓘ
Jethro's Heapin' Helping Steak Sauce
Steak & Grilling Sauce
Gold's
Steak Sauce with Horseradish
Great Value (Wal-Mart)
Steak Sauce
Heinz ⓘ
Traditional Steak Sauce
Hy-Vee
Classic Steak Sauce
Jack Daniel's Sauces ⓘ
Steak Sauce (Both Varieties)
Lea & Perrins ⓘ
Traditional Steak Sauce
Meijer
Steak Sauce
Safeway
Select - Steak Sauce
Tabasco ✓
Caribbean Style Steak Sauce
TryMe
Bullfighter Steak & Burger Sauce

Syrup, Pancake & Maple

Aunt Jemima ()
Syrups (All)
Cary's
Cary's (All)
Eggo 🍴
Kellogg's Eggo Syrup
Hungry Jack
Syrups (All)
Hy-Vee
Artificial Butter Flavored Syrup
Lite Syrup
Pancake & Waffle Syrup
Karo 🍴
Golden Griddle
Old Tyme
Log Cabin
Log Cabin
MacDonald's
MacDonald's (All)
Meijer
Syrup - Butter Flavored
Syrup - Lite
Syrup - Lite Butter
Syrup - Regular
Midwest Country Fare (Hy-Vee)
Pancake & Waffle Syrup
Mrs. Butterworth's
Mrs. Butterworth's (All)
Mrs. Renfro's
Mrs. Renfro's (All BUT Nacho Cheese
Sauce)
Publix ()
Butter Flavor Pancake Syrup
Lite Butter Flavor Pancake Syrup
Lite Maple Flavor Pancake Syrup
Maple Flavor Pancake Syrup
Robert Rothschild Farm
Maple Praline Gourmet Syrup
Roasted Pecan Gourmet Syrup
Safeway
Select - Pure Maple Syrup
Select - Syrup Blueberry
Syrup - Butter Light
Syrup - Light

Syrup - Old Fashioned
Syrup - Original
Syrup - Pure Maple

Spring Tree
Spring Tree (All)

Vermont Maid ⓘ
Vermont Maid Syrup (All Varieties)

Walden Farms ⊌
Walden Farms (All)

Wholesome Sweeteners ⊌
Organic Pancake & Waffle Syrup

TARTAR SAUCE

Best Foods
Tartar Sauce

Cains
Tartar Sauce

Crosse & Blackwell
Crosse & Blackwell (All BUT Branston
Pickle Relish, Fish & Chip Vinegar,
and Plum Pudding)

Gold's
Squeeze Tartar Sauce

Heinz ⓘ
Tartar Sauce

Hellmann's
see Best Foods

Kraft ⌇
Fat Free Tartar Sauce
Hot & Spicy Tartar Sauce
Lemon & Herb Tartar Sauce
Tartar Sauce

Legal
Tartar Sauce

Louisiana Fish Fry ◌
Remoulade Sauce
Tartar Sauce

VINEGAR

Bionaturae ⊌
Organic Balsamic Vinegar

Bragg
Bragg (All)

Colavita
Vinegars/Glaces (All)

DeLallo
Balsamic Vinegar
Balsamic Vinegar Spray
Garlic Wine Vinegar
Private Stock Balsamic Vinegar
Red Wine Vinegar

Di Lusso
Red Wine Vinegar

Eden Foods ⓘ ✓
Apple Cider Vinegar - Organic
Brown Rice Vinegar - Organic
Red Wine Vinegar - Organic

Giant
Cider Vinegar
Red Wine Vinegar
White Distilled Vinegar

Goya
Cider Vinegar

Grand Selections (Hy-Vee)
Balsamic Vinegar of Modena
Red Wine Vinegar
White Wine Vinegar

Great Value (Wal-Mart)
Apple Cider Vinegar
Balsamic Vinegar
Distilled White Vinegar
Premium Garlic Flavored Red Wine
Vinegar
Premium Red Wine Vinegar

Heinz ⓘ
Apple Cider Flavored Vinegar
Apple Cider Vinegar
Distilled White Vinegar
Garlic Wine Vinegar
Red Wine Vinegar

Holland House ◌
Premium Vinegars (All BUT Malt
Vinegar)

Hy-Vee
Apple Cider Flavored Distilled Vinegar
White Distilled Vinegar

Knouse Foods ⊌
Apple Cider Vinegar
White Distilled Vinegar

Lorenzi ()
Balsamic Vinegar

Lucini
Balsamic Vinegar (All)

Marukan
Genuine Brewed Rice Vinegar
Organic Rice Vinegar
Seasoned Gourmet Rice Vinegar
Dressing

Meijer
Vinegar
Vinegar - Balsamic 12 Year Aged
Vinegar - Balsamic 4 Year Aged
Vinegar - Cider
Vinegar - Red Wine
Vinegar - White
Vinegar - White Wine

Nakano ()
Nakano (All)

Newman's Own Organics ⓘ
Balsamic Vinegar

O Olive Oil ⓘ
O Olive Oil (All)

Ortalli
Ortalli (All)

Publix ()
Red Wine Vinegar
White Distilled Vinegar

Raley's ⍲
Vinegar

Rapunzel
Balsamic Vinegar ()
White Balsamic Vinegar ()

Regina ⓘ
Vinegar (All)

Safeway
Select - Vinegar (All BUT Malt Vinegar)

Simply Enjoy (Giant)
Balsamic Vinegar of Modena
White Balsamic Vinegar

Simply Enjoy (Stop & Shop)
Balsamic Vinegar of Modena
White Balsamic Vinegar

Stop & Shop
Cider Vinegar
White Vinegar

Wine Vinegar

WORCESTERSHIRE SAUCE

French's
Worcestershire Sauce

Great Value (Wal-Mart)
Worcestershire Sauce

Hy-Vee
Worcestershire Sauce

Lea & Perrins ⓘ
Worcestershire Sauce

Meijer
Worcestershire Sauce

Safeway
Worcestershire Sauce

TryMe
Wine & Pepper Worcestershire

Wizard's, The ✓
Organic Wheat-Free Vegan
Worcestershire

MISCELLANEOUS

B&G Foods ⓘ
Capers

Boar's Head
Condiments (All)

Crosse & Blackwell
Crosse & Blackwell (All BUT Branston
Pickle Relish, Fish & Chip Vinegar,
and Plum Pudding)

Rising Moon Organics ()
Pesto Sauces

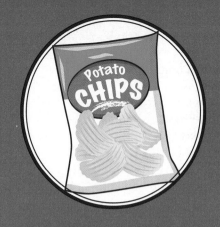
©iStockphoto.com/Alison Hess

SNACKS & CONVENIENCE FOODS

APPLESAUCE

Applesnax ()
Applesnax Products (All)

Eden Foods (i) ✔
Apple Cherry Sauce - Organic
Apple Cinnamon Sauce - Organic
Apple Sauce - Organic
Apple Strawberry Sauce - Organic

Giant
Applesauce - Chunky
Applesauce - Cinnamon
Applesauce - Mixed Berry
Applesauce - Natural
Applesauce - Strawberry

Great Value (Wal-Mart)
Apple Sauce
Cinnamon Apple Sauce
Natural Apple Sauce
No Salt Added Apple Sauce Sweetened
w/Splenda
Unsweetened Apple Sauce

Hy-Vee
Applesauce
Cinnamon Applesauce
Natural Applesauce
Natural Style Applesauce

Knouse Foods ⚕
Apple-Cherry Sauce
Apple-Grape Sauce
Apple-Orange-Mango Sauce
Apple-Peach Sauce
Apple-Raspberry Sauce
Apple-Strawberry Sauce
Golden Delicious Apple Sauce

Granny Smith Apple Sauce
Healthy Picks Sauce - Blueberry
Pomegranate
Healthy Picks Sauce - Cupucacu Key
Lime
Healthy Picks Sauce - Raspberry Acai
McIntosh Apple Sauce
Red Delicious Apple Sauce
Sweetened Apple Sauce
Totally Fruit Sauce - Apple
Totally Fruit Sauce - Chunky Apple
Sauce
Totally Fruit Sauce - Cinnamon Apple
Sauce
Totally Fruit Sauce - Peach
Unsweetened Apple Sauce

Kroger (i)
Applesauce - Flavored
Applesauce - Plain

Meijer
Applesauce
Applesauce Chunky
Applesauce Cinnamon
Applesauce Mixed Berry Single Serve
Applesauce Natural
Applesauce Organic Cinnamon
Applesauce Organic Sweetened
Applesauce Organic Unsweetened
Applesauce Original
Applesauce Strawberry Single Serve

Midwest Country Fare (Hy-Vee)
Applesauce with Cinnamon
Applesauce with Peaches
Applesauce with Raspberries
Applesauce with Strawberries

Home Style Applesauce
Natural Applesauce

Mott's
Sauces (All)

Publix GreenWise Market ()
Organic Unsweetened Apple Sauce

Publix ()
Applesauce - Chunky
Applesauce - Cinnamon
Applesauce - Old Fashioned
Applesauce - Unsweetened

Safeway
Applesauce - Cups, Natural & Sweetened

Stop & Shop
Applesauce - Chunky
Applesauce - Cinnamon
Applesauce - Mixed Berry
Applesauce - Natural
Applesauce - Regular
Applesauce - Strawberry

Tree Top
Apple Sauce (All)

Baked Goods

Ener-G ☘
Brownies
Cinnamon Rolls
Doughnut Holes - Plain
Doughnuts - Plain
Poundcake

Foods by George ☘
Blueberry Muffins
Brownies
Corn Muffins
Crumb Cake
Pound Cake

Frankly Natural Bakers ⓘ ✔
Gluten-Free Carob Almondine Brownie
Gluten-Free Cherry Berry Brownie
Gluten-Free Java Jive Brownie
Gluten-Free Misty Mint Brownie
Gluten-Free Wacky Walnut Brownie

French Meadow Bakery
Gluten-Free Fudge Brownie Bites
Gluten-Free Fudge Brownies

Gillian's Foods ☘
Gillian's Foods (All)
Gillian's Foods (All)

Gluten-Free & Fabulous ☘ ✔
Brownie Bites

Mariposa Baking Company ☘
Biscotti (All)
Brownies (All)
Cakes (All)
Lemon Poppyseed Tea Loaf
Morning Glory Tea Loaf
Squares (All)

Publix ()
New York Style Cheesecake, Plain 6 Inch
  Round (Bakery)

Bars

ALPSNACK ✔
Alpsnack (All)

Attune ()
Dark Chocolate Probiotic Bar (All)
Milk Chocolate Probiotic Bar (All)

Bakery on Main
Cranberry Maple Nut Gluten-Free
  Granola Bar
Extreme Trail Mix Gluten-Free Granola
  Bar
Peanut Butter Chocolate Chip Gluten-
  Free Granola Bar

Balance
BalancePure-Cherry Pecan
BalancePure-Chocolate Cashew

Betty Lou's ✔
Krispy Bites

BoomiBar ☘ ✔
Almond Protein Plus
Apricot Cashew
Apricot Goji
Apricot Pumpkin
Cashew Almond
Cashew Protein Plus
Cinnamon Apple
Coconut Acai
Cranberry Apple
Fruit and Nut
Health Hazel

Macadamia Paradise
Maple Pecan
Pear Ginseng
Perfect Pumpkin
Pineapple Ginger
Pistachio Pineapple
Walnut Date

BumbleBar ✓
BumbleBar (All)

Cascade Fresh
Cascade Fresh (All)

Clif
Clif Nectar ()

Ener-G ⚇
Chocolate Chip Snack Bars

Enjoy Life Foods ⚇
Caramel Apple Snack Bars
Cocoa Loco Snack Bars
Sunbutter Crunch Snack Bars
Very Berry Snack Bars

EnviroKidz ⓘ ✓
Crispy Rice Bars - Cheetah Berry
Crispy Rice Bars - Koala Chocolate
Crispy Rice Bars - Lemur Choco Drizzle
Crispy Rice Bars - Panda Peanut Butter
Crispy Rice Bars - Penguin Fruity Burst

Frankly Natural Bakers ⓘ ✓
Gluten-Free Apricot Energy Bar
Gluten-Free Date Nut Energy Bar
Gluten-Free Raisin Energy Bar
Gluten-Free Tropical Energy Bar

Glucerna
Caramel Nut Glucerna Snack Bar ⓘ

Gluten Free Café ✓
Chocolate Sesame Bar
Cinnamon Sesame Bar
Lemon Sesame Bar

Glutino ⚇ ✓
Breakfast Bars Apple
Breakfast Bars Blueberry
Breakfast Bars Chocolate
Breakfast Bars Cranberry
Organic Bar - Chocolate & Peanuts
Organic Bar - Chocolate Banana
Organic Bar - Wildberry

GoMacro ✓
Banana Almond
Cashew Butter Bar
Cashew Mesquite
Peanut Protein Bar
Tahini Date Bar

Ian's Natural Foods ⚇ ✓
Wheat and Gluten-Free Apple Pie Go
Bar
Wheat and Gluten-Free Cinnamon Bun
Go Bar

Jamfrakas
Jamfrakas (All)

Jŏcalat
Jŏcalat (All)

KIND ✓
Almond & Apricot
Almond & Apricots in Yogurt
Almond & Coconut
Fruit & Nut Delight
Fruit & Nuts in Yogurt
Macadamia & Apricot
Nut Delight
PLUS: Almond Cashew + OMEGA-3
PLUS: Almond Walnut Macadamia +
PROTEIN
PLUS: Cranberry Almond +
ANTIOXIDANTS
PLUS: Mango Macadamia + CALCIUM
PLUS: Passion Fruit Macadamia +
B-COMPLEX
PLUS: Strawberry Nut Delight +
CALCIUM
Sesame & Peanuts with Chocolate
Walnut & Date

Lärabar
Lärabar (All)

Luna ()
Luna Sports Products (All)

Manischewitz
Raspberry Jell Bars

Meijer
Xtreme Snack Bars

Orgran ⚇
Orgran (All)

Planters Carb Well ⌇
  Crunchy Nut Bar - Caramel Chocolate Crunch
  Crunchy Nut Bar - Peanut Butter Crunch

Planters ⌇
  Original Peanut Bar

PranaBar
  PranaBar (All)

Publix ()
  Peanut Butter Bars

PureFit ✓
  PureFit (All 4 Flavors)

Raw Revolution
  Raw Revolution Bars (All)

Schar ☷ ✓
  Chocolate Hazelnut Bars

Sharkies
  Sharkies (All)

South Beach Living ⌇
  Caramel Peanut Crisp Meal Replacement Bar
  Chocolate Caramel Meal Replacement Bar
  Chocolate Crisp Meal Replacement Bar
  Chocolate Peanut Butter Meal Replacement Bar
  Chocolate Raspberry Snack Bars
  Cinnamon & Creme Meal Replacement Bar
  High Protein Cereal Bar - Chocolate
  High Protein Cereal Bar - Cinnamon Raisin
  Peanut Butter Snack Bars
  Vanilla Creme Meal Replacement Bar

SoyJoy ()
  SoyJoy

thinkProducts
  thinkProducts (All)

Tiger's Milk ()
  Peanut Butter
  Peanut Butter & Honey
  Protein Rich

ZonePerfect ()
  Banana Nut
  Chocolate Almond Raisin

  Chocolate Caramel Cluster
  Chocolate Coconut Crunch
  Chocolate Peanut Butter
  Chocolate Raspberry
  Dark Chocolate Caramel Pecan
  Dark Chocolate Mocha
  Double Dark Chocolate
  Fudge Graham
  Peanut Toffee

BEEF JERKY & OTHER MEAT SNACKS

Bridgford
  Hickory Beef Jerky
  Original Beef Jerky
  Peppered Beef Jerky
  Sweet & Hot Beef Jerky
  Turkey Summer Sausage

Garrett County Farms
  Turkey Tom Tom Snack Sticks

Golden Valley Natural ⓘ
  Organic Beef Jerky

Hy-Vee
  Original Beef Jerky
  Summer Sausage

Old Wisconsin ⓘ
  Old Wisconsin (All BUT Beef Jerky Products)

Safeway
  Original Beef Jerky
  Peppered Beef Jerky

Shelton's
  Beef Jerky
  Turkey Jerky
  Turkey Jerky Hot
  Turkey Pepperoni Sticks
  Turkey Sticks Regular

CANDY & CHOCOLATE

3 Musketeers
  3 Musketeers (All)

Alse Tois ✓
  Chocolate Raspberry Pecan Brittle

Alter Eco Fair Trade
  Dark Black Out Chocolates
  Dark Cacao Chocolates

Dark Mint Chocolates
Dark Twist Chocolates
Milk Hazelnut Chocolates

Altoids
Altoids (All BUT Dark Chocolate
Dipped Mints)

Andes
Andes (All)

Atomic FireBall 🍵
Atomic Fireball (All)

Baby Ruth
Baby Ruth

Before & After Candy
Before & After Candy (All)

Betty Lou's ✔
Chocolate Walnut Balls
Coconut Macadamia Balls
Peanut Butter Balls

Big Hunk
Big Hunk (2 oz size)

Bit-O-Honey
Bit-O-Honey

Black Forest Gummies 🍵
Black Forest Gummies

Boston Baked Beans 🍵
Boston Baked Beans

BottleCaps
BottleCaps

Butterfinger
Butterfinger (But NOT Butterfinger
Crisp & Butterfinger Stixx)

Canada Mints 🍵
Mint Lozenges
Wintergreen Lozenges

Candy Carnival
Candy Carnival (All)

Caramel Apple Pops
Caramel Apple Pops (All)

Cella Cherries
Cella Cherries (All)

Certs
Certs

Charleston Chew
Charleston Chew (All)

Charms Blow Pops
Charms Blow Pops (All)

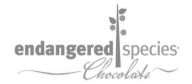

Savor chocolate.
Save our planet.

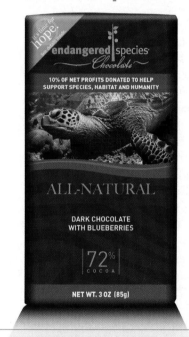

10% OF NET PROFITS DONATED TO HELP
SUPPORT SPECIES, HABITAT AND HUMANITY

ALL-NATURAL

DARK CHOCOLATE
WITH BLUEBERRIES

72% COCOA

NET WT. 3 OZ (85g)

Have your
chocolate...
and eat it too.

Charms Flat Pops
  Charms Flat Pops (All)
Child's Play
  Child's Play (All)
Chuao ()
  Chuao (All BUT BonBon Pan Con
    Chocolate and Panko Chocolate Bar)
Clark Bar ☉
  Clark Bar
Clorets
  Clorets
Crispy Cat Candy Bars ✓
  Chocolate Sundae
  Mint Coconut
  Toasted Almond
Crows
  Crows
Cry Baby
  Cry Baby (All)
Dagoba ✓
  Dagoba (All)
Dots
  Dots (All)
Dove
  Dove Chocolate Products
Endangered Species Chocolate ☉ ✓
  70% Cran/Almonds Bag Wolf
  70% Mint Bag Rainforest
  Assorted 70% Bag Sea Turtle/Grizzly
  Assorted 72% & 88% Bag Chimpanzee/
    Panther
  Bat Bar
  Black Panther Bar
  Black Rhino Bar
  Bug Bites Dark Treats
  Bug Bites Milk Treats
  Butterfly Bar
  Cheetah Bar
  Chimp Mints Treats
  Chimpanzee Bar
  Chocolate Covered Peanut Brittle - All-
    Natural Dark Chocolate Covered
    Peanut Butter Brittle
  Crane Bar
  Dolphin Bar
  Giraffe Bar

Grizzly Bar
Halloween Dark Treats
Halloween Milk Treats
Hoppy Dark Treats
Hoppy Milk Treats
Koala Bar
Lion Bar
Love Dark Treats
Love Milk Treats
Organic 70% Bag Butterfly
Organic Double Dipped Truffles (Dark/
  Dark) 9) Dark/Milk Peanut Butter
  Cup Truffles
Organic Double Dipped Truffles (Dark/
  Milk) 9) Dark/Milk Peanut Butter Cup
  Truffles
Organic Double Dipped Truffles (Milk/
  Milk) 9) Milk/Milk Peanut Butter Cup
  Truffles
Otter Bar
Rainforest Bar
Sea Turtle Bar
Spider Monkey Bar
Tiger Bar
Toucan Bar
Tree Frog Bar
Winter Holiday Dark Treats
Winter Holiday Milk Treats
Wolf Bar
Zebra Bar
Enjoy Life Foods ☉
  boom CHOCO boom Crispy Rice Bar
  boom CHOCO boom Dark Chocolate
    Bar
  boom CHOCO boom Rice Milk Bar
Fannie May
  Almond Clusters (All)
  Apricot Bon Bon & Creams (All)
  Candy Bars (All)
  Chocolate Toffee
  Chocolate Wafers
  Citrus Peel
  English Toffee
  Irish Toffee
  Ivory and Dark Bark
  Milk Chocolate Peanut Butter Crunch
  Mint Meltaways

Solid Chocolate Novelties (All)
Walnut Clusters (All)

Ferrara Pan Candy Company 🏅
Ferrara Pan Candy (All)

Fluffy Stuff Cotton Candy
Fluffy Stuff (All)

Frooties
Frooties (All)

Giant
Assorted Fruit Filled Candy
Assorted Star Drops
Assorted Starlights
Blue Gummi Sharks
Butter Toffee
Butterscotch Disks
Canada Wintergreen
Candy Corn
Candy Necklaces
Cinnamon Starlights
Circus Peanuts
Gum Drops
Gummi Bears
Jelly Beans
Kiddie Mix
Lemon Drops
Neon Sour Crawlers
Orange Slices
Pastel Mints
Peach Rings
Red Ju Ju Coins
Red Ju Ju Fish
Root Beer Barrels
Royal Mix
Silver Mints
Smarties
Soft Peppermints
Sour Balls
Sour Gummi Worms
Spearmint Leaves
Spearmint Starlights
Spice Drops
Starlight Mints
Strawberry Buds
Watermelon Hard Candy

Ginger People, The
Crystallized Ginger 🏅
Gin-Gins BOOST

Gin-Gins Hard Candy
Hot Coffee Ginger Chews
Original Ginger Chews
Peanut Ginger Chews
Spicy Apple Ginger Chews

Glutino 🏅 ✓
Chocolate Peanut Butter Candy Bar
Dark Chocolate Candy Bar
Milk Chocolate Candy Bar

Go Lightly
Go Lightly (All)

Go Naturally
Go Naturally (All)

Gobstoppers
Chewy
Original

Goobers
Goobers

Great Value (Wal-Mart)
Butterscotch Discs
Candy Corn
Cinnamon Disc
Fruit Smiles (Sour Apple, Watermelon, Blue Raspberry, Tropical Punch)
Fruit Smiles Bag (Strawberry, Grape, Orange, Lemon)
Gummy Bears
Gummy Worms
Jelly Beans
Spearmint Starlight Mint
Spice Drops
Starlight Mints

Guittard
Guittard (All)

Haviland 🏅
Candy Stix (All)
Peppermint Patties
Thin Mints (All)
Wintergreen Patties

Hershey's
Milk Chocolate Bar (Plain)
Milk Chocolate Bar with Almonds
Plain Milk Chocolate Kisses

Hillside Sweets
Hillside Sweets (All)

Honees Candies
Honees Bars
Honees Cough Drops
Milk-N-Honees Bars

Hot Tamales
Hot Tamales

Hy-Vee
Caramels
Chocolate Caramel Clusters
Chocolate Covered Raisins
Chocolate Peanut Clusters
Chocolate Stars
Circus Peanuts
Double Dipped Chocolate Covered
   Peanuts
Gum Drops
Gummi Bears
Gummi Sour Squiggles
Gummi Squiggles
Lemon Drops
Milk Chocolate Caramel Cups
Milk Chocolate Peanut Butter Cups
Orange Slices
Smarties
Spice Drops
Tootsie Pops
Wax Bottles

JawBusters
JawBusters

Jelly Belly
Jelly Beans (All)

Jolly Rancher
Hard Candies
Lollipops

Junior Mints
Junior Mints (All)

Kroger ⓘ
Hard Candy

Laffy Taffy
Laffy Taffy Fruitarts Chews
Laffy Taffy Rope

Laura Lynn (Ingle's)
Orange Slice Candy

Lemonhead & Friends
Lemonhead & Friends

Let's Do...Organic ✓
Organic Classic Gummi Bears
Organic Jelly Gummi Bears
Organic Super Sour Gummi Bears

LifeSavers
LifeSavers

Lik-M-Aid Fun Dip
Lik-M-Aid Fun Dip

M&M'S
M&M's (All Including Mint Crisp)

Manischewitz
Caramel Cashew Patties
Chocolate Frolic Bears
Fruit Slices
Hazelnut Truffles
Mallo Cups
Max's Magic Lollycones
Mini Sour Fruit Slices
Peppermint Patties
Swiss Chocolate Mints
Viennese Crunch

Mary Janes
Mary Janes
Peanut Butter Kisses

Meijer
Peanuts - Butter Toffee

Mentos
Mentos

Mike and Ike
Mike and Ike

Milka Chocolate ᕲ
Alpine Milk Chocolate Confection

Milky Way
Milky Way Products (All BUT Milky
   Way Bar)

Munch Bar
Munch Bar

Necco
Banana Split Chews
Candy Buttons
Candy Eggs (Easter)
Marshmallow Eggs
Mint Julep Chews
Peach Blossoms
Sky Bars
Squirrel Nut Caramels

Squirrel Nut Zippers
Talking Pumpkins (Halloween)
Wafers

Nerds
Nerds Gumballs
Nerds Rope

Nestlé Milk Chocolate
Nestlé Milk Chocolate

Newman's Own Organics ⓘ
Chocolate Bars (All BUT Crisp Rice)
Chocolate Cups (All)
Mint Rolls
Mints in Tins

Nik-L-Nip
Nik-L-Nip (All)

Nips
Regular
Sugar Free

Now and Later
Now and Later Candies

Oh Henry!
Oh Henry!

Old Dominion Peanut Company
Old Dominion Peanut Company (All)

Orgran ⛾
Orgran (All)

Pangburn's ()
Pangburn's (All BUT S'mores and
Cookies & Cream Rabbits [Seasonal,
Easter])

Peanut Chews
Peanut Chews

Pearson Candy Company
Candies (All)

Peeps
Marshmallow Peeps

PEZ
PEZ

Pixy Stix
Pixy Stix

Planters 〰
Cashews - Chocolate Covered
Cashews - Chocolate Lovers Milk
Chocolate
Mixed Nuts - Almonds, Cashews &
Mixed Nuts In Milk Chocolate

Peanuts - Rich Roasted Whole In Milk
Chocolate

Pop Rocks
Pop Rocks

Publix ()
Butterscotch Discs
Chocolate Covered Peanut Brittle
Double Dipped Chocolate Covered
Peanuts
Gummi Worms
Lollipops
Pixy Stick Candy
Smarties Candy
Sour Worms
Spearmint Starlight Mints
Starlight Mints Candy
Strawberry Bon Bons

Queen Anne
Queen Anne (All)

Rain-Blo
Rain-Blo Gum

Raisinets
Raisinets

Rapunzel
Chocolate Hazelnut Butter ()
Dark Chocolate 55% ()
Dark Chocolate 70% ()
Dark Chocolate with Almonds 55% ()
Dark Chocolate with Hazelnuts 55% ()
Dark Espresso Chocolate 55% ()
Lady Truffles with NutTruffle Crème ()
Milk Chocolate ()
Milk Chocolate with Hazelnuts ()
Milk Chocolate with Nut Truffle Crème ()

Razzles
Razzles (All)

Red Bird ⛾
Red Bird Brand (All)

Red Hots ⛾
Red Hots

Reed's
Crystallized Ginger
Ginger Chews

Reese's
Reese's Peanut Butter Cups
Reese's Pieces

Riesen ()
Riesen

Runts
Chewy
Original

Russell Stover ()
Russell Stover (All BUT S'Mores and
Cookies + Cream Bunny (Easter))

Safeway
Candy Corn
Cinnamon Imperials
Dessert Mints
Gummi Bears
Gummi Worms - Regular
Gummi Worms - Sour
Jelly Eggs - Classic Jelly Beans
Lemon Drops
Orange Slices with Vitamin C Fat Free
Candies
Select - Soft Caramel Cups
Select - Truffles, Butterscotch
Select - Truffles, Chocolate/Raspberry
Select - Truffles, Milk Chocolate
Select - Truffles, Mocha
Spice Drops
Star Light Mints

Scharffen Berger
Bars (1 & 3 oz.) ()
Chocolate Covered Products ()
Panned Products ()

Shockers
Shockers

Simply Enjoy (Giant)
Dark Chocolate Amaretto Coated
Cranberries
Dark Chocolate Cappuccino Crunch
Bits
Dark Chocolate Caramel Squares
Dark Chocolate Covered Cherries
Dark Chocolate Covered Coffee Beans
Dark Chocolate Covered Cranberries
Dark Chocolate Covered Kona Almond
Coffee Beans
Dark Chocolate Covered Strawberries
Dark Chocolate Raspberry Sticks
Milk Chocolate Butter Toffee Squares
Milk Chocolate Coated Cashews

Milk Chocolate Cocoa Almonds
Milk Chocolate Covered Cashews
Milk Chocolate Covered Cherries
Milk Chocolate Covered Peanuts
Milk Chocolate Covered Raisins
Milk Chocolate Pecan Caramel Patties
White Chocolate Coated Coffee Nuggets
Whole Chocolate Covered Raspberries
Yogurt Coated Cranberries

Simply Enjoy (Stop & Shop)
Dark Chocolate Amaretto Coated
Cranberries
Dark Chocolate Cappuccino Crunch
Bits
Dark Chocolate Caramel Squares
Dark Chocolate Covered Cherries
Dark Chocolate Covered Coffee Beans
Dark Chocolate Covered Cranberries
Dark Chocolate Covered Kona Almond
Coffee Beans
Dark Chocolate Covered Strawberries
Dark Chocolate Raspberry Sticks
Milk Chocolate Butter Toffee Squares
Milk Chocolate Coated Cashews
Milk Chocolate Cocoa Almonds
Milk Chocolate Covered Cashews
Milk Chocolate Covered Cherries
Milk Chocolate Covered Peanuts
Milk Chocolate Covered Raisins
Milk Chocolate Pecan Caramel Patties
White Chocolate Coated Coffee Nuggets
Whole Chocolate Covered Raspberries
Yogurt Coated Cranberries

Skittles
Skittles

Skybar ♨
Skybars

Smarties
Smarties (All with UPC starting with
0 11206)

Snickers
Snickers Bars
Snickers Dark Bars

Sno-Caps
Sno-Caps

Sour Patch Kids
Sour Patch Kids

South Beach Living ᨠ
  Snack Pack Delights - Dark Chocolate
    Covered Soynuts

Spangler Candy Company
  Candy Canes
  Chocolately Chewy Candy Canes
  Circus Marshmallow Peanuts
  Dum Dum Chewy Pops
  Dum Dums
  Jelly Belly Candy Canes
  Marshmallow Treats
  Saf-T-Pops
  Sour Punch Candy Canes

Spree
  Spree

Starburst
  Starburst

Stop & Shop
  Assorted Fruit Filled Candy
  Assorted Star Drops
  Assorted Starlights
  Blue Gummi Sharks
  Butter Toffee
  Butterscotch Disks
  Canada Wintergreen
  Candy Corn
  Candy Necklaces
  Cinnamon Starlights
  Circus Peanuts
  Gum Balls
  Gum Drops
  Gummi Bears
  Jelly Beans
  Kiddie Mix
  Lemon Drops
  Neon Sour Crawlers
  Orange Slices
  Pastel Mints
  Peach Rings
  Pina Colada Coated Cashews
  Red Ju Ju Coins
  Red Ju Ju Fish
  Root Beer Barrels
  Royal Mix
  Silver Mints
  Smarties
  Soft Peppermints

  Sour Balls
  Sour Gummi Worms
  Spearmint Leaves
  Spearmint Starlights
  Spice Drops
  Starlight Mints
  Strawberry Buds
  Watermelon Hard Candy

Sugar Babies
  Sugar Babies (All)

Sugar Daddy
  Sugar Daddy (All)

Surf Sweets ♻
  Surf Sweets (All)

Swedish Fish
  Swedish Fish

SweeTARTS
  SweeTARTS

Sweethearts ♻
  Sweethearts Conversation Hearts
    (Valentines Only)

Teenee Beanee
  Jelly Beans

Terrys ᨠ
  Orange Dark Chocolate
  Orange Milk Chocolate
  Pure Milk Chocolate

Toblerone ᨠ
  Minis Swiss Chocolate with Honey &
    Almond Nougat
  Minis White Confection with Honey &
    Almond Nougat
  Swiss Bittersweet with Honey & Almond
    Nougat
  Swiss Milk Chocolate with Honey &
    Almond Nougat
  Swiss White Confection with Honey &
    Almond Nougat
  Truffle Peaks

Too Tarts ()
  Too Tarts (All)

Tootsie Pops
  Tootsie Pops (All)

Tootsie Rolls
  Tootsie Rolls (All)

Trolli ()
Trolli (All)

VerMints ⛛
VerMints (All)

Wack-O-Wax
Wack-O-Wax (All)

Werther's Original ()
Werther's Original

Wonka Mix-Ups
Mix-Ups

Zip-A-Dee Mini Pop
Zip-A-Dee-Mini Pop (All)

Zotz
Bulk Straight Flavors
Cherry Apple Watermelon
Lemon Orange Grape

CHEESE PUFFS & CURLS

Baked! Cheetos ⓘ
Crunchy Cheese Flavored Snacks
Flamin' Hot Cheese Flavored Snacks

Cheetos ⓘ
Cheddar Jalapeno Cheese Flavored
Snacks
Chile Limon Flavored Snacks
Crunchy Cheese Flavored Snacks
Crunchy Salsa Roja Cheese Flavored
Snacks
Crunchy Wild White Cheddar Cheese
Flavored Snacks
Fantastix! Chili Cheese Flavored Baked
Corn/Potato Snack
Fantastix! Flamin' Hot Flavored Baked
Corn/Potato Snacks
Flamin' Hot Cheese Flavored Snacks
Flamin' Hot Limon Cheese Flavored
Snacks
Giant Puffs Cheese Flavored Snacks
Giant Puffs Flamin' Hot Cheese Flavored
Snacks
Jumbo Puffs Cheese Flavored Snacks
Jumbo Puffs Flamin' Hot Cheese
Flavored Snacks
Natural White Cheddar Puffs Cheese
Flavored Snacks
Puffs Cheese Flavored Snacks

Twisted Cheese Flavored Snacks
Xxtra Flamin' Hot Cheese Flavored
Snacks

Chester's ⓘ
Cheddar Cheese Flavored Popcorn
Cheese Flavored Puffcorn Snacks

EatSmart
CheddAirs

Giant
Crunchy Cheese Corn Snacks
Puff Cheese Corn Snacks

Golden Flake ⓘ
Cheese Curls
Cheese Puff Corn
Cheese Puffs
Puff Corn

Great Value (Wal-Mart)
Cheddar Cheese Crunch
Cheddar Cheese Puffs
Cheddar Flavor Cheese Sensations

Herr's ()
Cheese Curls
Honey Cheese Curls
Hot Cheese Curls

Jay's ⓘ
Hot Stuff Crunchy Cheezlets

Meijer
Cheese Pops
Cheese Puffs
Cheezy Treats
White Cheddar Puffs

Michael Season's
Baked Cheddar Cheese Curl
Baked Cheddar Cheese Puff
Baked Hot Chili Pepper Curl
Baked White Cheddar Pops
Ultimate Cheddar Cheese Curls
Ultimate Cheddar Cheese Puffs
Ultimate White Cheddar Cheese Puffs

Mike-Sell's
Cheese Curls

O-Ke-Doke ⓘ
Baked Cheese Puffs

Pirate's Booty ⓘ ⛛
Pirate's Booty

Publix ()
- Crunchy Cheese Curls
- Crunchy Cheese Curls (Deli)
- Crunchy Cheese Puffs
- Jumbo Cheese Puffs (Deli)

Safeway
- Cheese Curls
- Puffed Cheese Snacks

Snyder's of Hanover ⓘ
- Apple Cinnamon CheddAirs
- CheddAirs
- Cheese Twists
- Multigrain Aged Cheddar Puffs
- Multigrain White Cheddar Puffs
- Zesty Cheddar CheddAirs

Stop & Shop
- Crunchy Cheese Corn Snacks
- Puff Cheese Corn Snacks

Utz ⚇ ✓
- Baked Cheese Balls
- Baked Cheese Curls
- Cheese Puff'n Corn
- Crunchy Cheese Curls
- White Cheddar Cheese Curls

CHIPS & CRISPS, OTHER

Arico Natural Foods Company
- Cassava Chips (All)

BHUJA ⚇ ✓
- Original Mix

Chester's ⓘ
- Flamin' Hot Flavored Fries

Corn Nuts ⌇
- Barbecue Crunchy Corn Snacks
- Chile Picante Con Limon Crunchy Corn Snacks
- Chile Picante Crunchy Corn Snacks
- Limon Crunchy Corn Snacks
- Nacho Cheese Crunchy Corn Snacks
- Original Crunchy Corn Snacks
- Ranch Crunchy Corn Snacks
- Salsa Jalisco Crunchy Corn Snacks

EatSmart
- Soy Crisps (All Flavors)
- Veggie Crisps (All Flavors)

Eden Foods ⓘ ✓
- Brown Rice Chips

Fritos ⓘ
- Flavor Twists Honey BBQ Flavored Corn Chips
- Original Corn Chips
- Scoops! Corn Chips
- Spicy Jalapeño Flavored Corn Chips

Funyuns ⓘ
- Flamin' Hot Onion Flavored Rings
- Onion Flavored Rings

Golden Flake ⓘ
- Chili Cheese Corn Chips
- Corn Chips

Good Health Natural Products ()
- Apple Chips
- Avocado Chips
- Barbeque Polenta Chips
- Guacamole Polenta Chips
- Mediterranean Lime Polenta Chips
- Sea Salt Polenta Chips
- Veggie Chips

Goya
- Garlic Plantain Chips
- No Salt Plantain Chips
- Plantain Chips
- Plantain Chips - Loose
- Plantain Strips

Great Value (Wal-Mart)
- Bigger Corn Chips
- Corn Chips

Herr's ()
- BBQ Corn Chips
- Cheddar Friez
- Hot Friez
- Regular Corn Chips

Jay's ⓘ
- Hot Stuff Corn Chips

Kitchen Table Bakers ⓘ ✓
- Wafer Crisps (All)

LesserEvil ⓘ ✓
- Classic Sea Salt Krinkle Sticks
- Old School Bar-B-Que Krinkle Sticks
- Sour Cream & Onion Krinkle Sticks
- Zesty Pizza Krinkle Sticks

Lundberg Family Farms
- Rice Chips - Fiesta Lime ⓘ ✓
- Rice Chips - Honey Dijon ⓘ ✓
- Rice Chips - Nacho Cheese ⓘ ✓
- Rice Chips - Pico De Gallo ⓘ ✓
- Rice Chips - Santa Fe Barbecue ⓘ ✓
- Rice Chips - Sea Salt ⓘ ✓
- Rice Chips - Sesame & Seaweed ⓘ ✓
- Rice Chips - Wasabi ⓘ ✓

Michael Season's
- Cheddar Baked Multigrain Chips
- Honey Chipotle Baked Multigrain Chips
- Original Baked Multigrain Chips

Mike-Sell's
- Puffcorn Delights (All)

Mr. Krispers ✓
- Almond Nut Chip
- Barbeque
- Multiseed Chip
- Nacho
- Sea Salt & Pepper
- Sour Cream & Onion
- Sun Dried Tomato & Basil
- White Cheddar & Herb

Nature's Promise (Giant)
- Soy Crisps - BBQ
- Soy Crisps - Ranch

Nature's Promise (Stop & Shop)
- Soy Crisps - BBQ
- Soy Crisps - Ranch

Newman's Own Organics ⓘ
- Barbeque Soy Crisps
- Cinnamon Sugar Soy Crisps
- Lightly Salted Soy Crisps
- White Cheddar Soy Crisps

Pirate's Booty ⓘ ♟
- Pirate's Booty
- Tings

Publix ()
- Corn Chips - King Size

Snyder's of Hanover ⓘ
- Cheddar Jalapeno Veggie Crisps
- Parmesan Garlic & Olive Oil Soy Crisps
- Sundried Tomato & Pesto Veggie Crisps
- Tomato Romano & Olive Oil Soy Crisps
- Veggie Crisps, Unseasoned

Stacy's ♟
- Soy Crisps

Stop & Shop
- BBQ Rice Crisps
- Cheddar Rice Crisps
- Ranch Rice Crisps

Utz ♟ ✓
- Barbeque Corn Chips
- Plain Corn Chips

CHIPS & CRISPS, POTATO

Baked! Lay's ⓘ
- Cheddar & Sour Cream Flavored Potato Crisps
- Original Potato Crisps
- Sour Cream & Onion Artificially Flavored Potato Crisps
- Southwestern Ranch Flavored Potato Crisps

Baked! Ruffles ⓘ
- Cheddar & Sour Cream Flavored Potato Crisps
- Original Potato Crisps

Cape Cod
- Cape Cod Products (All)

French's
- Potato Sticks - Barbecue Flavor
- Potato Sticks - Cheezy Cheddar
- Potato Sticks - Original Flavor

Giant
- Plain Potato Chips
- Salt and Vinegar Potato Chips
- Sour Cream and Onion Chips
- Wavy Cut Potato Chips

Golden Flake ⓘ
- BBQ Potato Chips
- Cheddar & Sour Cream Dip Style Chips
- Dill Pickle Potato Chips
- Dip Style Potato Chips
- Hot Potato Chips
- Mesquite Dip Style Potato Chips
- Mrs. B's Cajun Hot Potato Chips
- Mrs. B's Regular Potato Chips
- Regular Potato Chips
- Sweet Heat Potato Chips
- Vinegar & Salt Potato Chips

Good Health Natural Products ()
Au Gratin Bistro Chips
Blue Cheese Bistro Chips
Cracked Pepper Olive Oil Chips
Crème Fraishe Bistro Chips
Garlic Olive Oil Chips
Rosemary Olive Oil Chips
Sea Salt Bistro Chips
Sea Salt Olive Oil Chips

Herr's ()
Baked Cheddar & Sour Cream Crisps
Baked Crisps
Cheddar & Sour Cream Potato Chips
Honey BBQ Potato Chips
Jalapeno Kettle Potato Chips
Jalapeno Ripple Potato Chips
Ketchup Potato Chips
Kettle Blue Potato Chips
Kettle Potato Chips
Kettle Reduced Fat Potato Chips
Lightly Salted Potato Chips
Natural Kettle Cooked with Sea Salt Potato Chips
No Salt Added Potato Chips
Old Bay Potato Chips
Old Fashioned Potato Chips
Potato Stix - Regular
Red Hot Potato Chips
Regular Potato Chips
Ripple Potato Chips
Salt & Pepper Potato Chips
Salt & Vinegar Potato Chips

Jay's ⓘ
BBQ Potato Chips
Crispy Ridged Potato Chips, Unseasoned
Crispy Ridged Sour Cream & Cheddar Potato Chips
Curly Dippettes Potato Chips
Extra Hot Stuff Ridged Potato Chips
Hot Stuff Potato Chips
Kettle Cooked Old Fashioned Potato Chips
No Salt Potato Chips
Original Potato Chips, Unseasoned
Salt & Sour Potato Chips
Shoe String Potatoes

Sour & Dill Potato Chips
Sour Cream & Onion Potato Chips

Kettle Brand
Potato Chips (All)

Kroger ⓘ
Plain Potato Chips

Krunchers! ⓘ
Baked Bar-B-Que Potato Crisps
Baked Cheddar & Sour Cream Potato Crisps
Baked Original Potato Crisps
Cheddar & Sour Cream Kettle Chips
Hot Buffalo Wing Kettle Chips
Jalapeno Kettle Chips
Kosher Dill Kettle Chips
Original Kettle Chips, Unseasoned
Sea Salt & Cracked Pepper Kettle Chips
Sweet Hawaiian Onion Kettle Chips

Lay's ⓘ
Cheddar & Sour Cream Artificially Flavored Potato Chips
Chile Limon Potato Chips
Classic Potato Chips
Deli Style Original Potato Chips
Dill Pickle Flavored Potato Chips
Hot & Spicy Barbecue Flavored Potato Chips
Kettle Cooked Jalapeno Flavored Extra Crunchy Potato Chips
Kettle Cooked Mesquite BBQ Flavored Extra Crunchy Potato Chips
Kettle Cooked Original Potato Chips
Kettle Cooked Reduced Fat Original Flavored Potato Chips
Kettle Cooked Sweet Chili & Sour Cream Flavored Potato Chips
Light Original Potato Chips
Lightly Salted Potato Chips
Limon Tangy Lime Flavored Potato Chips
Natural Country BBQ Thick Cut Potato Chips
Natural Sea Salt Thick Cut Potato Chips
Salt & Vinegar Artificially Flavored Potato Chips
Sour Cream & Onion Artificially Flavored Potato Chips

Wavy Au Gratin Flavored Potato Chips
Wavy Hickory BBQ Flavored Potato Chips
Wavy Ranch Flavored Potato Chips
Wavy Regular Potato Chips

Lay's Stax ⓘ ⚋

Cheddar Flavored Potato Crisps
Hot'n Spicy Barbecue Flavored Potato Crisps
Jalapeno Cheddar Flavored Potato Crisps
Mesquite Barbecue Flavored Potato Crisps
Original Flavored Potato Crisps
Ranch Flavored Potato Crisps
Salt & Vinegar Flavored Potato Crisps
Sour Cream & Onion Flavored Potato Crisps

Manischewitz

Potato Chips (All Varieties)

Maui Style ⓘ

Regular Potato Chips
Salt & Vinegar Flavored Potato Chips

Meijer

Potato Sticks

Michael Season's

Baked Thin Potato Crisps - Cheddar & Sour Cream
Baked Thin Potato Crisps - Original
Baked Thin Potato Crisps - Sweet Barbeque
Thin & Crispy Potato Chips - Honey Barbeque
Thin & Crispy Potato Chips - Lightly Salted
Thin & Crispy Potato Chips - Ripple
Thin & Crispy Potato Chips - Salt & Pepper
Thin & Crispy Potato Chips - Unsalted
Thin & Crispy Potato Chips - Yogurt & Green Onion

Mike-Sell's

Bold Bahama Kettle Chips
Good 'n Hot Potato Chips
Green Onion Potato Chips
Jalapeno Kettle Chips
Mesquite Smoked Bacon Potato Chips

Regular Potato Chips
Salt 'n Pepper Potato Chips
Sea Salt and Vinegar Potato Chips
Sour Cream and Sweet Onion Kettle Chips
Zesty Barbeque Potato Chips

Miss Vickie's ⓘ

Country Onion with 3 Cheeses Kettle Cooked Potato Chips
Creamy Buttermilk Ranch Kettle Cooked Flavored Potato Chips
Hand Picked Jalapeno Kettle Cooked Flavored Potato Chips
Sea Salt & Vinegar Kettle Cooked Flavored Potato Chips
Simply Sea Salt Kettle Cooked Potato Chips
Smokehouse BBQ Kettle Cooked Flavored Potato Chips

Munchos ⓘ

Regular Potato Crisps

Old Dutch Foods ⟨⟩

Original Dutch Crunch Potato Chips
Original Regular Potato Chips
Original Rip-L Potato Chips
Original Ripples Potato Chips

Pringles ⓘ

Fat Free Original Pringles
Fat Free Sour Cream & Onion Pringles

Publix ⟨⟩

Potato Chips - Dip Style
Potato Chips - Original Thins
Potato Chips - Salt & Vinegar

Ruffles ⓘ

Authentic Barbecue Flavored Potato Chips
Cheddar & Sour Cream Flavored Potato Chips
Light Cheddar & Sour Cream Flavored Potato Chips
Light Original Potato Chips
Natural Reduced Fat Regular Sea Salted Potato Chips
Reduced Fat Potato Chips
Regular Potato Chips
Sour Cream & Onion Flavored Potato Chips

Thick Cut Cheddar Baked Potato
Flavored Potato Chips

Sabritas ⓘ

Chile Piquin Flavored Potato Chips

Snyder's of Hanover ⓘ

French Onion Potato Chips
Hot Buffalo Wing Potato Chips
Jalapeno Potato Chips
Kosher Dill Potato Chips
Original Potato Chips, Unseasoned
Ripple Potato Chips, Unseasoned
Salt and Vinegar Potato Chips
Sour Cream and Onion Potato Chips
Sweet BBQ Potato Chips

Stop & Shop

Kettle Cooked Potato Chips
Plain Potato Chips
Rippled Potato Chips
Salt & Vinegar Potato Chips
Sour Cream & Onion Chips
Wavy Cut Potato Chips

Utz ⚕ ✓

All Natural Dark Russet Kettle Cooked
Potato Chips
All Natural Gourmet Medley Kettle
Cooked Potato Chips
All Natural Lightly Salted Kettle Cooked
Potato Chips
All Natural Sea Salt & Vinegar Kettle
Cooked Potato Chips
Barbeque Potato Chips
Carolina BBQ Potato Chips
Cheddar & Sour Cream Potato Chips
Crab Potato Chips
Grandma Utz BBQ Kettle Cooked
Potato Chips
Grandma Utz Plain Kettle Cooked
Potato Chips
Homestyle Kettle Cooked Potato Chips
- Plain
Honey BBQ Potato Chips
Kettle Classic Dark Russet Potato Chips
Kettle Classic Jalapeno Potato Chips
Kettle Classic Plain Potato Chips
Kettle Classic Smokin' Sweet BBQ
Potato Chips

Kettle Classic Sour Cream & Chive
Potato Chips
Kettle Classic Sweet Potato Chips
Mystic Dark Russet Kettle Potato Chips
Mystic Kettle Potato Chips - Plain
Mystic Sea Salt & Vinegar Kettle Cooked
Potato Chips
No Salt BBQ Potato Chips
No Salt Potato Chips
Red Hot Potato Chips
Reduced Fat Potato Chips
Ripple Potato Chips - Regular, Plain
Salt & Pepper Potato Chips
Salt & Vinegar Potato Chips
Sour Cream & Onion Potato Chips
Wavy Cut Potato Chips - Regular, Plain

Winn-Dixie ⓘ

Salt & Vinegar Potato Chips

CHIPS, TORTILLA

Baked! Tostitos ⓘ

Scoops! Tortilla Chips

Chi-Chi's

Chips (All Varieties)

Doritos ⓘ

Blazin' Buffalo & Ranch Flavored
Tortilla Chips
Collisions Hot Wings and Blue Cheese
Flavored Tortilla Chips
Collisions Pizza Cravers and Ranch
Flavored Tortilla Chips
Collisions Zesty Taco and Chipotle
Ranch Flavored Tortilla Chips
Cool Ranch Flavored Tortilla Chips
Diablo Flavored Tortilla Chips
Fiery Habanero Flavored Tortilla Chips
Last Call Jalapeño Pepper Flavored
Tortilla Chips
Reduced Fat Cool Ranch Flavored
Tortilla Chips
Salsa Verde Flavored Tortilla Chips
Spicy Nacho Flavored Tortilla Chips
Taco Flavored Tortilla Chips
Toasted Corn Tortilla Chips
Toro Habañero Flavored Tortilla Chips

Food Should Taste Good ⛐ ✓
  Chips (All)
Garden Fresh Gourmet ⛐
  Tortilla Chips (All)
Giant
  Nacho Tortilla Chips
  White Restaurant Tortilla Chips -
    Regular
  White Restaurant Tortilla Chips -
    Rounds
Golden Flake ⓘ
  Nacho Tortilla Chips
Grande ⓘ
  Original Tortilla Chips
  Reduced Fat Tortilla Chips
  Restaurant Style Tortilla Chips
  Salsa Limon Tortilla Chips
Green Mountain Gringo
  Tortilla Strips - Organic Blue Corn ⓘ
  Tortilla Strips - Organic White Corn ⓘ
  Tortilla Strips - Original ⓘ
Guiltless Gourmet
  Tortilla Chips (All) ()

HealthMarket (Hy-Vee)
  Organic Blue Corn Tortilla Chips
  Organic White Corn Tortilla Chips
  Organic Yellow Corn Tortilla Chips
Herr's ()
  Bite Size Dipper Tortilla Chips
  Nacho Tortilla Chips
  Restaurant Style Tortilla Chips
Kroger ⓘ
  Plain Tortilla Chips
Mission Foods
  Corn Products (All)
Padrino's ⓘ
  Lightly Salted Tortilla Strips
  No Salt Tortilla Chips
  Reduced Fat Tortilla Chips
  Restaurant Style Tortilla Chips
Publix GreenWise Market ()
  Blue Tortilla Chips
  Yellow Tortilla Chips
Publix ()
  White Corn Tortilla Chips - Restaurant
    Style

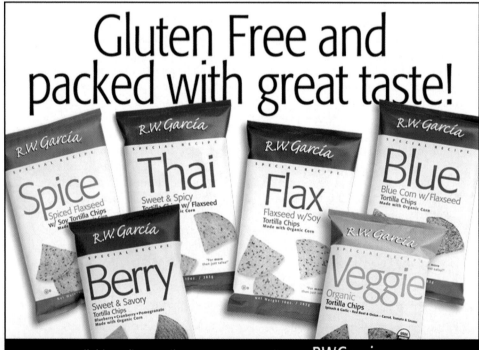

Yellow Corn Tortilla Chips - Round
Style

R.W. Garcia
Berry Tortilla Chips
Blue Corn Tortilla Chips
Blue Corn with Flaxseed Tortilla Chips
Extra Thin Tortilla Chips
Flaxseed with Soy Tortilla Chips
MixtBag Yellow & Blue Corn Tortillla
Chips
MixtBag Yellow and White Corn Tortilla
Chips
Organic Veggie Tortilla Chips
Salsa Fresca Tortilla Chips
Spice Flaxseed with Soy Tortilla Chips
Stone Ground Yellow Corn Tortilla
Chips
Thai Sweet and Spicy Tortilla Chips

Ricos ✔
Chips (All)

Robert Rothschild Farm
Tortilla Chips

Safeway
White Corn Tortilla Chips

Santitas ⓘ
White Corn Restaurant Style Tortilla
Chips
Yellow Corn Tortilla Chips

Snyder's of Hanover ⓘ
Restaurant Style Tortilla Chips
White Triangle Tortilla Chips
Yellow Round Tortilla Chips

Stop & Shop
Nacho Tortilla Chips
White Restaurant Tortilla Chips -
Regular & Round
Yellow Round Tortilla Chips

Tostitos ⓘ
100% White Corn Restaurant Style
Tortilla Chips
Bite Size Gold Tortilla Chips
Bite Size Rounds Tortilla Chips
Crispy Rounds Tortilla Chips
Light Restaurant Style Tortilla Chips
Natural Blue Corn Restaurant Style
Tortilla Chips

Natural Yellow Corn Restaurant Style
Tortilla Chips
Restaurant Style with A Hint of Lime
Flavor Tortilla Chips
Scoops! Hint of Jalapeno Tortilla Chips
Scoops! Tortilla Chips

Utz ♟ ✔
Baked Tortilla Chips
Cheesier Nacho Tortilla Chips
Restaurant Style Tortilla Chips
White Corn Tortilla Chips

Winn-Dixie ⓘ
Ground White Tortilla Chips

COOKIES

Andean Dream ♟
Quinoa Cookies - Chocolate Chip
Quinoa Cookies - Cocoa-Orange
Quinoa Cookies - Coconut
Quinoa Cookies - Orange Essence
Quinoa Cookies - Raisins & Spice

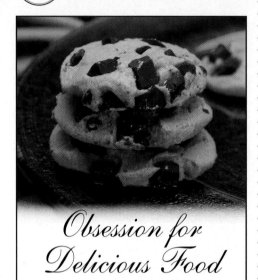

Obsession for Delicious Food

For over 21 years, our passion has been creating amazing cookies and baking mixes ... Wheat-free & Gluten-free.

www.**PamelasProducts**.com

Arico Natural Foods Company
Cookie Pouches (All)

Cherrybrook Kitchen ⓘ ✓
Gluten-Free Dreams Mini-Chocolate Chip Cookie
Gluten-Free Dreams Mini-Vanilla Graham Cookies

Ener-G ☷
Chocolate Chip Biscotti Cookies
Chocolate Chip Potato Cookies
Chocolate Cookies
Cinnamon Cookies
Ginger Cookies
Sunflower Cookies
Vanilla Cookies
White Chocolate Chip Cookies

Enjoy Life Foods ☷
Chewy Chocolate Chip Cookie Pack
Chewy Chocolate Chip Cookies
Double Chocolate Brownie Cookies
Gingerbread Spice Cookies
Happy Apple Cookies
Lively Lemon Cookies
No-oats "Oatmeal" Cookies

Snickerdoodle Cookie Pack
Snickerdoodle Cookies

EnviroKidz ⓘ ✓
Vanilla Animal Cookies

French Meadow Bakery
Gluten-Free Chocolate Chip Cookie
Gluten-Free Coconutty Macaroons

Gillian's Foods ☷
Gillian's Foods (All)

Gluten-Free & Fabulous ☷ ✓
Butterscotch Cookie Bites
Chocolate Chip Cookie Bites
Shortbread Cookie Bites

Glutino ☷ ✓
Chocolate Wafers - Chocolate Coated
Gluten-Free Dream Cookies Chocolate and Vanilla Crème
Gluten-Free Dream Cookies Chocolate Chip
Gluten-Free Dream Cookies Vanilla Crème
Lemon Wafers
Strawberry Wafers
Vanilla Wafers - Chocolate Coated

Ian's Natural Foods ☷ ✓
Wheat and Gluten-Free Chocolate Chip Cookie Buttons
Wheat and Gluten-Free Crunchy Cinnamon Cookie Buttons

Manischewitz
Banana Split Macaroons
Cappuccino Chip Macaroons
Chocolate Chip Macaroons
Chocolate Chunk Cherry Macaroons
Chocolate Macaroons
Coconut Macaroons
Fudgey Nut Brownie Macaroons
Honey Nut Macaroons
Rocky Road Macaroons
Tender Coconut Patties
Toffee Crunch Macaroons
Ultimate Triple Chocolate Macaroons

Mi-Del ✓
Chocolate Caramel Bite-Size Cookies
Gluten-Free Arrowroot Cookies
Gluten-Free Chocolate Chip Cookies

Gluten-Free Chocolate Sandwich Cookies
Gluten-Free Cinnamon Snaps
Gluten-Free Ginger Snaps
Gluten-Free Pecan Cookies
Gluten-Free Royal Vanilla Sandwich Cookies

Nana's

No Gluten Cookie - Chocolate
No Gluten Cookie - Chocolate Crunch
No Gluten Cookie - Ginger
No Gluten Cookie - Lemon
No Gluten Cookie Bars - Berry Vanilla
No Gluten Cookie Bars - Chocolate Munch
No Gluten Cookie Bars - Nana Banana
No Gluten Cookie Bites - Fudge
No Gluten Cookie Bites - Ginger Spice
No Gluten Cookie Bites - Lemon Dreams

Orgran 🍼

Orgran (All)

Pamela's Products 🍼 ✓

Almond Anise Biscotti
Butter Shortbread
Chocolate Chip Mini Cookies
Chocolate Chip Walnut
Chocolate Chunk Pecan Shortbread
Chocolate Walnut Biscotti
Chunky Chocolate Chip Cookies
Dark Chocolate-Chocolate Chunk
Espresso Chocolate Chunk
Extreme Chocolate Mini Cookies
Ginger Mini Snapz
Ginger with Sliced Almonds
Lemon Almond Biscotti
Lemon Shortbread
Old Fashioned Raisin Walnut
Peanut Butter
Peanut Butter Chocolate Chip
Pecan Shortbread
Shortbread Swirl
Spicy Ginger with Crystallized Ginger

Schar 🍼 ✓

Chocolate Sandwich Creams
Chocolate-Dipped Cookies
Cocoa Wafers

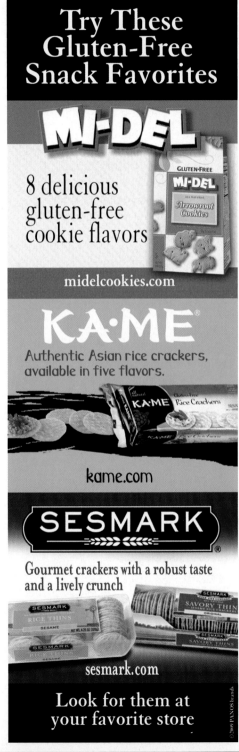

Hazelnut Wafers
Ladyfingers
Shortbread Cookies
Vanilla Sandwhich Creams
Vanilla Wafers

CORN CAKES

Giant
Corn Cakes - Butter
Corn Cakes - Caramel
Corn Cakes - White Cheddar
Safeway
Popcorn Cakes (All BUT White
   Cheddar and Mini Caramel Corn) ()
Stop & Shop
Corn Cakes - Caramel
Corn Cakes - Multigrain Unsalted

CRACKERS

BHUJA ☷ ✓
Cracker Mix
Blue Diamond Growers ⓘ
Nut-Thins Crackers (All) ☷ ✓
Brown Rice Snaps
Black Sesame
Cheddar
Onion Garlic
Salsa
Tamari Seaweed
Tamari Sesame
Toasted Onion
Unsalted Plain
Unsalted Sesame
Vegetable
Corn Thins ☷
Cracked Pepper & Lemon Corn Thins ☷
Flax & Soy Corn Thins (Organic) ☷ ✓
Multigrain Corn Thins ☷ ✓
Original Corn Thins (Organic) ☷ ✓
Rice Thins ☷ ✓
Sesame Corn Thins (Organic) ☷ ✓
Crunchmaster ✓
Artisan Four Cheese
Multigrain
Multiseed - Original

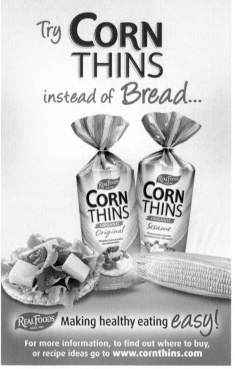

Multiseed - Roasted Garlic
Multiseed - Rosemary & Olive Oil
Multiseed - Sweet Onion
Toasted Sesame
Eden Foods ⓘ ✓
Brown Rice Crackers
Nori Maki Rice Crackers
Ener-G ☷
Cinnamon Crackers
Ener-G Gourmet Crackers
Gourmet Onion Crackers
Seattle Crackers
Exotic Rice Toast ✓
Brown Rice & Spring Onion
Purple Rice & Black Sesame
Thai Red Rice & Flaxseeds
Gluten-Free & Fabulous ☷ ✓
Sweet Savory Bites
Glutino ☷ ✓
Breadsticks Pizza
Breadsticks Sesame
Crackers - Cheddar
Crackers - Multigrain

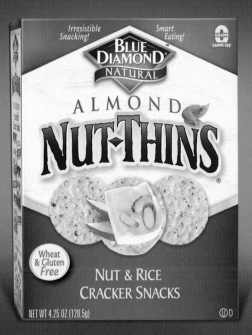

WHAT MORE COULD YOU WANT FROM A DELICIOUS TASTING CRACKER? OK THEY'RE GLUTEN FREE.

12 CRACKERS = 100 CALORIES

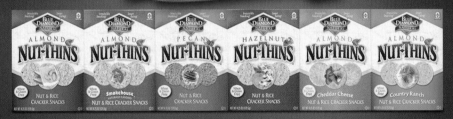

Indulge in a scrumptious line of crackers that are sure to satisfy. In fact, the only things missing are wheat, gluten,* trans fat and artificial ingredients. Try all 6 irresistible flavors with your favorite topping or all by themselves.

 Strong supporter of the Celiac Foundation

Crackers - Original
Crackers - Vegetable

Hol-Grain
Brown Rice Crackers - Lightly Salted
Brown Rice Crackers - No Salt
Brown Rice Crackers - Onion & Garlic
Flavor
Brown Rice Crackers - Organic Lightly
Salted
Brown Rice Crackers - Sesame Lightly
Salted

KA-ME ✓
Gluten-Free Mini Rice Crackers (90
Calorie Packs)
Gluten-Free Rice Crackers
Original Brown Rice Crisps
Szechuan Brown Rice Crisps
Teriyaki Brown Rice Crisps

Mariposa Baking Company ☺
Crostini - Garlic

Mary's Gone Crackers ☺ ✓
Black Pepper Crackers
Caraway Crackers

Herb Crackers
Onion Crackers
Original Crackers

Mr. Krispers ✓
Tasty Snack Cracker

Orgran ☺
Orgran (All)

R.W. Garcia
5-Seed Onion and Chive Crackers
5-Seed Rosemary and Garlic Crackers
5-Seed Tellicherry Cracked Pepper
Crackers

Schar ☺ ✓
Crispbread
Snack Crackers
Table Crackers

SESMARK ✓
Garlic Hummus Ancient Grains
Crackers
Mini Rice Crackers – Lightly Salted
Mini Rice Crackers – Sesame Garlic
Parmesan Herb Ancient Grains
Crackers

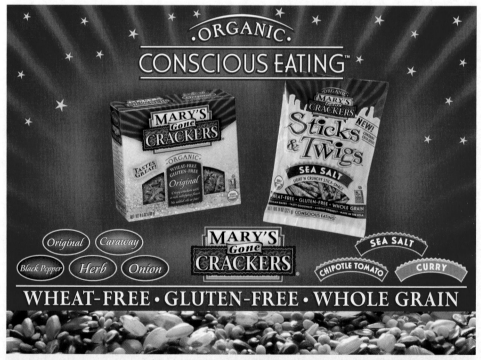

Rice Thins – Brown Rice
Rice Thins – Cheddar
Rice Thins – Sesame
Rice Thins – Teriyaki
Savory Thins – Black Sesame & Garlic
Savory Thins – Original
Savory Thins – Teriyaki
Savory Thins – Three Cheese & Tomato
Savory Thins – Toasted Onion & Garlic
Sea Salt Ancient Grains Crackers

DRIED FRUIT

BHUJA ♼ ✔
Fruit Mix
Craisins
Cherry
Orange
Original
Crunchies
Crunchies (All)
Dole ()
Dried Fruits (All)
Eden Foods ⓘ ✔
Dried Cranberries - Organic
Dried Wild Blueberries - Organic
Montmorency Dried Tart Cherries
Wild Berry Mix - Organic
Great Value (Wal-Mart)
California Pitted Prunes
California Sun-Dried Raisins
Harvest Farms (Ingles)
Raisins (All)
Hy-Vee
California Sun Dried Raisins
Just Tomatoes
Just Tomatoes (All)
Laura Lynn (Ingle's)
Raisins (All)
Mariani ()
Mariani (All BUT Vanilla and Chocolate
Yogurt Raisins)
Meijer
Prunes - Pitted Canister
Raisins - Seedless

Newman's Own Organics ⓘ
Apples
Apricots
Berry Blend
Cranberries
Pitted Prunes
Raisins
Publix ()
Raisins
Safeway
Dried Fruit - Apples
Dried Fruit - Apricots
Dried Fruit - Cherries
Dried Fruit - Peaches
Dried Fruit - Prunes
Raisins
Sensible Foods ♼
Sensible Foods (All)
St. Dalfour
Dried Fruits ♼
Sun-Maid
Sun-Maid Natural Sun-Dried Raisins
Zante Currants
Sunsweet ♼
Sunsweet (All BUT Chocolate Plum
Sweets)
Welch's
Welch's (All)

FRUIT CUPS

Del Monte ⓘ
Fruit Snack Cups (Metal & Plastic)
Hy-Vee
Diced Peaches Fruit Cups
Mandarin Orange Fruit Cups
Mixed Fruit in Light Syrup Fruit Cups
Pineapple Tidbit Fruit Cup
Tropical Fruit Cups
Kroger ⓘ
Fruit - Cups

FRUIT SNACKS

Annie's Homegrown
Fruit Snacks

Clif
Twisted Fruit

Fruit by the Foot
Fruit by the Foot (All)

Fruit Gushers
Fruit Gushers (All)

Fruit Roll-Ups
Fruit Roll-Ups (All)
Fruit Stickerz (All)

Fruit Shapes
Fruit Shapes (All)

Giant
Build A Bear Fruit Snacks
Curious George Fruit Snacks
Dinosaur Fruit Snacks
Justice League Fruit Snacks
Peanuts Fruit Flavored Snacks
Sharks Fruit Snacks
Underwater World Fruit Snacks
Veggie Tales Fruit Snacks

Great Value (Wal-Mart)
Berry Medley

Hy-Vee
Dinosaurs Fruit Snacks
Fruit Snacks (Variety Pack)
Sharks Fruit Snacks
Snoopy Fruit Snacks
Veggie Tales Fruit Snacks

Kellogg's ⛹
Fruit Flavored Snacks

Kroger ⓘ
Fruit Snacks

Laura Lynn (Ingle's)
Fruit Snacks (All)

Meijer
Fruit Roll - Justice League Berry
Fruit Roll - Rescue Heroes
Fruit Roll - Strawberry
Fruit Roll - Strawberry Garfield
Fruit Roll - Wildberry Rush
Fruit Snack - Dinosaurs
Fruit Snack - Sharks
Fruit Snack - Veggie Tales
Fruit Snacks - African Safari
Fruit Snacks - Curious George
Fruit Snacks - Jungle Adventure

Fruit Snacks - Justice League
Fruit Snacks - Peanuts
Fruit Snacks - Rescue Heroes Big Box
Fruit Snacks - Underwater World

Paas ⛹
Painted Fruit Snack Eggs

Publix ⟨⟩
Dinosaurs Dry Fruit
Rescue Heroes Dry Fruit
Sharks Dry Fruit
Snoopy Dry Fruit
Veggie Tales Dry Fruit

Safeway
Fruit Snacks (All)

Stop & Shop
Build A Bear Fruit Snacks
Curious George Fruit Snacks
Dinosaur Fruit Snacks
Justice League Fruit Snacks
Peanuts Fruit Flavored Snacks
Sharks Fruit Snacks
Tom & Jerry Fruit Snacks
Underwater World Fruit Snacks
Variety Pack Fruit Snacks
Veggie Tales Fruit Snacks

Welch's
Welch's (All)

Yogos ⛹
Yogos

GELATIN SNACKS & MIXES

Giant
Cherry Gelatin Mix
Orange Gelatin Mix
Raspberry Gelatin Mix
Refrigerated Gelatin Fun Pack
Refrigerated Rainbow Fruit Gelatin
Refrigerated Rainbow Parfait
Refrigerated Sugar Free Gelatin - Black
Cherry
Refrigerated Sugar Free Gelatin - Cherry
Refrigerated Sugar Free Gelatin -
Strawberry
Refrigerated Sugar Free Gelatin Fun
Pack

Great Value (Wal-Mart)

Cherry Gelatin Dessert
Lemon Gelatin Dessert
Lime Gelatin Dessert
Orange Gelatin Dessert
Peach Gelatin Dessert
Strawberry Banana Gelatin Dessert
Strawberry Gelatin Dessert
Sugar Free Cherry Gelatin Dessert
Sugar Free Lime Gelatin Dessert
Sugar Free Orange Gelatin Dessert
Sugar Free Peach Gelatin Dessert
Sugar Free Raspberry Gelatin Dessert
Sugar Free Strawberry Banana Gelatin Dessert
Sugar Free Strawberry Gelatin Dessert

Hy-Vee

Cherry Gelatin
Cranberry Gelatin
Lemon Gelatin
Lime Gelatin
Orange Gelatin
Raspberry Gelatin
Strawberry Gelatin
Sugar Free Cherry Gelatin
Sugar Free Cranberry Gelatin
Sugar Free Lime Gelatin
Sugar Free Orange Gelatin
Sugar Free Raspberry Gelatin
Sugar Free Strawberry Gelatin

Jell-O

Apricot Artificial Flavor Gelatin Dessert
Berry Blue Gelatin Dessert
Black Cherry Gelatin Dessert
Blackberry Fusion Gelatin Dessert
Cherry & Black Cherry Sugar Free Gelatin Snacks
Cherry Gelatin Dessert
Cranberry Gelatin Dessert
Grape Gelatin Dessert
Island Pineapple Gelatin Dessert
Lemon Gelatin Dessert
Lime & Orange Variety Pack Sugar Free Gelatin Snacks
Lime Gelatin Dessert
Margarita Limited Edition Gelatin Dessert
Melon Fusion Gelatin Dessert
Orange Gelatin Dessert
Peach & Watermelon Sugar Free Gelatin Snacks
Peach Gelatin Dessert
Pear Chunks In Cherry Pomegranate Gelatin Snacks
Pina Colada Limited Edition Gelatin Dessert
Raspberry & Orange Sugar Free Gelatin Snacks
Raspberry Gelatin Dessert
Real Chunks Of Pineapple In Tropical Fusion Sugar Free Gelatin Snacks
Strawberry & Orange Variety Pack Sugar Free Gelatin Snacks
Strawberry & Raspberry Gelatin Snacks
Strawberry Banana Gelatin Dessert
Strawberry Daiquiri Limited Edition Gelatin Dessert
Strawberry Gelatin Dessert
Strawberry Gelatin Snacks
Strawberry Kiwi Gelatin Dessert
Strawberry Sugar Free Gelatin Snacks
Sugar Free Black Cherry Low Calorie Gelatin Dessert
Sugar Free Cherry Low Calorie Gelatin Dessert
Sugar Free Cranberry Low Calorie Gelatin Dessert
Sugar Free Lemon Low Calorie Gelatin Dessert
Sugar Free Lime Low Calorie Gelatin Dessert
Sugar Free Mixed Fruit Low Calorie Gelatin Dessert
Sugar Free Orange Low Calorie Gelatin Dessert
Sugar Free Peach Low Calorie Gelatin Dessert
Sugar Free Raspberry Low Calorie Gelatin Dessert
Sugar Free Strawberry Banana Low Calorie Gelatin Dessert
Sugar Free Strawberry Kiwi Low Calorie Gelatin Dessert
Sugar Free Strawberry Low Calorie Gelatin Dessert

Sugar Free Tropical Blends Strawberry
Kiwi Low Calorie Gelatin Dessert
Tropical Fusion Gelatin Dessert
Watermelon Gelatin Dessert
Wild Strawberry Gelatin Dessert
X-Treme Cherry & Blue Raspberry Gel
Cups
X-Treme Watermelon & Green Apple
Gel Cups

Kool-Aid Gels ✍

Cherry Tropical Punch Gel Snacks
Groovalicious Grape Gel Snacks
Ice Blue Raspberry Gel Snacks
Oh Yeah Orange Gel Snacks
Soarin' Strawberry Gel Snacks

Kroger ⓘ

Gelatin - Flavored
Gelatin - Plain
Gelatin - Snack Cups

Laura Lynn (Ingle's)

Boxed Gelatins (All)

Meijer

Gelatin Dessert - Berry Blue
Gelatin Dessert - Cherry
Gelatin Dessert - Cherry Sugar Free
Gelatin Dessert - Cranberry
Gelatin Dessert - Cranberry Sugar Free
Gelatin Dessert - Grape
Gelatin Dessert - Lime
Gelatin Dessert - Lime Sugar Free
Gelatin Dessert - Orange
Gelatin Dessert - Orange Sugar Free
Gelatin Dessert - Raspberry
Gelatin Dessert - Raspberry Sugar Free
Gelatin Dessert - Strawberry
Gelatin Dessert - Strawberry Sugar Free
Gelatin Dessert - Strawberry Wild
Gelatin Dessert - Unflavored

Publix ()

Mandarin Oranges in Gel
Sugar Free Black Cherry & Cherry
Gelatin
Sugar Free Raspberry & Orange Gelatin
Sugar Free Strawberry Gelatin

Safeway

Gelatin Mix (All Flavors)
Instant Gelatins - Regular

Instant Gelatins - Sugar Free
Pineapple Lime Gel Cups

Stop & Shop

Cherry Gelatin Mix
Cranberry Gelatin Mix
Orange Gelatin Mix
Raspberry Gelatin Mix
Refrigerated Gelatin Fun Pack
Refrigerated Rainbow Fruit Gelatin
Refrigerated Rainbow Parfait
Refrigerated Sugar Free Gelatin Fun
Pack

GUM

5

5 Products

Beechies

Beechies Gum

Big Red

Big Red Gum

Bubblicious

Bubblicious

Chiclets

Chiclets

Clorets

Clorets

Dentyne

Dentyne (All)

Doublemint

Doublemint Gum

Dubble Bubble

Dubble Bubble (All)

Eclipse

Eclipse Gum

Extra

Extra Gum

Freedent

Freedent Gum

Giant

Gum Balls

Hy-Vee

Dubble Bubble Gum

Juicy Fruit

Juicy Fruit Gum

Orbit
Orbit Gum
Orbit White Gum

Publix ()
Super Bubble Bubble Gum

Stride
Stride

Trident
Trident

Winterfresh
Winterfresh Gum

Wrigley
Wrigley's Spearmint Gum

Nuts, Seeds & Mixes

Arrowhead Mills ✓
Sesame Seeds
Sesame Seeds (Whole)

BHUJA ⚇ ✓
Nut Mix

Blue Diamond Growers
Cinnamon-Brown Sugar Oven Roasted Almonds ⓘ
No Salt Oven Roasted Almonds ⓘ
Sea Salt Oven Roasted Almonds ⓘ
Vanilla Bean Oven Roasted Almonds ⓘ

Carole's Soycrunch ⚇
Cinnamon Raisin
Coconut
Original
Sesame
Toffee

Chugwater Chili
Chili Nuts

DeLallo
Pignoli Nuts

Earth Family ✓
Organic Peanuts with Sea Salt

Eden Foods ⓘ ✓
All Mixed Up
All Mixed Up Too
Tamari Almonds - Dry Roasted - Organic
Tamari Roasted Spicy Pumpkin Seeds

Fannie May
Assorted Nuts
Cashews

Fire Dancer ✓
Jalapeno Seasoned Peanuts

Fisher Nuts ()
Almonds
Butter Toffee Peanuts
Cashews
Chef's Naturals (All)
Dry Roasted Sunflower Kernels
Fusions Country Honey Snack Mix
Fusions Martini Mix
Honey Roasted Peanuts
Macadamia Nuts
Mixed Nuts
Nature's Nut Mix
Party Peanuts
Pecans
Pine Nuts
Pistachios
Salad Buddies Sunflower Kernels - No Salt
Salted In-Shell Sunflower Seeds
Spanish Peanuts
Unsalted Golden Roast Peanuts
Walnuts

Frito Lay ⓘ
Cashews
Deluxe Mixed Nuts
Flamin' Hot Flavored Sunflower Seeds
Honey Roasted Cashews
Honey Roasted Peanuts
Hot Peanuts
Praline Pecans
Ranch Sunflower Seeds
Salted Almonds
Salted Peanuts
Smoked Almonds
Sunflower Seed Kernels
Sunflower Seeds

Giant
Pina Colada Coated Cashews
Pistachios

Hy-Vee
Black Walnuts
English Walnut Pieces

English Walnuts
Natural Almonds
Natural Sliced Almonds
Pecan Pieces
Pecans
Raw Spanish Peanuts
Salted Blanched Peanuts
Salted Spanish Peanuts
Slivered Almonds

Meijer

Almonds - Blanched Sliced
Almonds - Blanched Slivered
Almonds - Natural Sliced
Almonds - Slivered
Almonds - Whole
Cashew Halves with Pieces
Cashew Halves with Pieces Lightly
  Salted
Cashews Whole
Nut Topping
Nuts - Blanched Peanuts
Nuts - Blanched Peanuts Slightly Salted
Nuts - Deluxe Mixed
Nuts - Mixed
Nuts - Mixed Lightly Salted
Peanuts - Dry Roasted
Peanuts - Dry Roasted Lightly Salted
Peanuts - Dry Roasted Unsalted
Peanuts - Honey Roasted
Peanuts - Hot and Spicy
Peanuts - Spanish
Pecan Chips
Pecan Halves
Pine Nuts
Sunflower Seeds
Sunflower Seeds Salted in Shell
Walnut Chips
Walnuts Black
Walnuts Halves and Pieces

Nut Harvest ⓘ

Natural Honey Roasted Peanuts
Natural Lightly Roasted Almonds
Natural Sea Salted Peanuts
Natural Sea Salted Whole Cashews

Planters ⌒

Almonds- Recipe Ready
Almonds- Sliced

- Almonds- Slivered
- Almonds- Smoked
- Cashew Sesame Mix Made with Pure
  Sea Salt
- Cashews - Dry Roasted
- Cashews - Halves & Pieces
- Cashews - Halves & Pieces Lightly
  Salted
- Cashews - Halves & Pieces Made with
  Pure Sea Salt
- Cashews - Halves & Pieces Salted
- Cashews - Halves And Pieces
- Cashews - Honey Roasted
- Cashews - Jumbo
- Cashews - Salted
- Cashews - Whole
- Cashews - Whole Honey Roasted
- Cashews - Whole Lightly Salted
- Cashews with Almonds & Pecans Select
- Cocktail Peanuts
- Cocktail Peanuts - Lightly Salted
- Cocktail Peanuts - Lightly Salted Made
  with Pure Sea Salt
- Cocktail Peanuts - Unsalted
- Go Nuts Lightly Salted Almonds
- Go Nuts Lightly Salted Heart Healthy
  Mix.
- Hazelnuts - Chopped
- Macadamia Cashew Mix & Almonds
  Select
- Macadamias
- Macadamias - Chopped
- Mixed Nuts
- Mixed Nuts - Deluxe Cashews,
  Almonds, Brazils, Hazelnuts & Pecans
- Mixed Nuts - Deluxe Lightly Salted
- Mixed Nuts - Honey Roasted
- Mixed Nuts - Lightly Salted
- Mixed Nuts - Unsalted
- Nut-Rition Almonds- Lightly Salted
- Nut-Rition Heart Healthy Mix
- Nut-Rition Mix - Almonds
- Nut-Rition Mix - Cashews, Almonds &
  Macadamia Lightly Salted
- Nut-Rition Mix - Lightly Salted
- Nut-Rition Smoked Almonds - Lightly
  Salted
- Peanuts - Cocktail

Peanuts - Dry Roasted
Peanuts - Dry Roasted Honey Roasted
Peanuts - Dry Roasted Lightly Salted
Peanuts - Dry Roasted Unsalted
Peanuts - Heat
Peanuts - Honey & Dry Roasted
Peanuts - Honey Roasted
Peanuts - Salted
Peanuts - Sweet N' Crunchy
Peanuts - Wicked Hot Chipotle
Pecan Chips - Recipe Ready
Pecan Halves
Pecan Halves - Recipe Ready
Pecan Lovers Mix with Cashews &
    Pistachios
Pecan Pieces
Pecan Pieces - Recipe Ready
Pepitas - Made with Pistachios Peanuts
    & Almonds
Pepitas - Roasted Salted
Pepitas - Wicked Hot Chipotle
Pine Nuts
Pistachio Lovers Mix with Cashews &
    Almonds
Pistachios - Dry Roasted
Spanish Peanuts - Redskin
Sunflower Kernels
Sunflower Kernels - Dry Roasted
Sunflower Seeds - Roasted & Salted
Sweet Roasts - Honey Peanuts &
    Cashews
Walnut Pieces - Recipe Ready
Walnuts
Walnuts Black - Recipe Ready

Publix ()

Almonds - Natural Whole
Almonds - Salted
Almonds - Sliced
Cashews - Dry Roasted
Cashews - Halves & Pieces
Cashews - Halves & Pieces, Lightly
    Salted
Cashews - Whole
Mixed Nuts
Mixed Nuts- Deluxe
Mixed Nuts- Dry Roasted
Mixed Nuts- Lightly Salted

Peanuts - Dry Roasted, Lightly Salted
Peanuts - Dry Roasted, Salted
Peanuts - Dry Roasted, Unsalted
Peanuts - Oil Roasted, Honey Roasted
Peanuts - Salted Party
Pecans
Pistachios
Sunflower Seeds
Sunflower Seeds - Raw-Shelled, All
    Natural
Walnuts

Raley's ♟

In-shell Peanuts

Sabritas ⓘ

Picante Peanuts
Salt & Lime Peanuts

Safeway

Butter Toffee Peanuts (All varieties with
    S3012)
Cashews - Halves & Pieces
Cashews - Whole
Dry Roasted Peanuts
Roasted/Salted Spanish Peanuts
Sunflower Seeds - Kernels

Sensible Foods ♟

Sensible Foods (All)

True North ⓘ

Almond Clusters
Almond Cranberry Vanilla Clusters
Almonds Pistachios Walnuts Pecans
Peanut Clusters
Pecan Almond Peanut Clusters

Wine Nuts ✓

Chardonnay
Choco~Late
Lemoncella
Margarita Mix
Merlot

POPCORN

Arrowhead Mills ✓

Whole Yellow Popcorn

Chester's ⓘ

Butter Flavored Puffcorn Snacks

Cracker Jack ⓘ
Original Caramel Coated Popcorn &
Peanuts

Eden Foods ⓘ ✓
Popcorn - Yellow - Organic

Giant
Microwave Popcorn - 94% Fat Free
Butter
Microwave Popcorn - Butter Flavored -
Light
Microwave Popcorn - Butter Flavored -
Regular
Microwave Popcorn - Kettle Corn
Microwave Popcorn - Movie Theatre
Butter Flavored
Microwave Popcorn - Natural Light
Microwave Popcorn - Sweet & Buttery
White Cheddar Popcorn
Yellow Popcorn

Good Health Natural Products ⟨⟩
Half-Naked Popcorn
Organic Popcorn

Herr's ⟨⟩
Hulless Popcorn
Light Popcorn
Original Popcorn

Hy-Vee
94% Fat Free Butter Microwave Popcorn
Butter Microwave Popcorn
Extra Butter Lite Microwave Popcorn
Extra Butter Microwave Popcorn
Kettle Microwave Popcorn
Light Butter Microwave Popcorn
Natural Flavor Microwave Popcorn
White Popcorn
Yellow Popcorn

Jay's ⓘ
Caramel Corn
Fat Free Caramel Corn

Jolly Time ⓘ
American's Best 94% Fat Free Butter
Flavor
Better Butter
Blast O Butter
Blast O Butter Light
Butter-Licious
Butter-Licious Light

Crispy'n White
Crispy'n White Light
Healthy Pop 94% Fat Free Butter Flavor
Healthy Pop 94% Fat Free Caramel
Apple
Healthy Pop 94% Fat Free Kettle Corn
Healthy Pop Butter Flavor Low Sodium
Kernel Corn - American's Best White
Kernel Corn - American's Best Yellow
Kernel Corn - White Pop Corn
Kernel Corn - Yellow Pop Corn
KettleMania
Mallow Magic
Sassy Salsa
Sea Salt & Cracked Pepper
The Big Cheez
White & Buttery

Kroger ⓘ
Plain Popcorn Kernels

LesserEvil ⓘ ✓
Black & White Kettle Corn
Classic Kettle Kettle Corn
Cocoa Coal Kettle Corn
Gingerbread Kettle Corn
MaplePecan Kettle Corn
Peanut Butter & Choco Kettle Corn
Peppermint Kettle Corn

Meijer
Caramel Corn
Cheese Popcorn
Chicago Style Popcorn
Popcorn
Popcorn - Micro Kettle Sweet & Salty
Popcorn - Microwave 94% Fat Free
Popcorn - Microwave Butter
Popcorn - Microwave Butter 75% Fat
Free
Popcorn - Microwave Butter GP
Popcorn - Microwave Extra Butter
Popcorn - Microwave Extra Butter GP
Popcorn - Microwave Extra Butter Lite
Popcorn - Microwave Hot n' Spicy
Popcorn - Microwave Natural Lite
Popcorn - White
Popcorn - Yellow
Purple Cow Butter Popcorn
White Cheddar Popcorn

Miss Vickie's ⓘ
Salty Sweet Kettle Corn

Newman's Own
Microwave Popcorn - 94% Fat Free
Microwave Popcorn - Butter
Microwave Popcorn - Butter Boom
Microwave Popcorn - Light Butter
Microwave Popcorn - Natural
Microwave Popcorn - Natural 100
Calorie Mini Bags
Microwave Popcorn - Tender White
Kernel
Microwave Popcorn - White Cheddar
Cheese
Regular Pop (Jar)

Newman's Own Organics ⓘ
Pop's Corn - Butter Flavored
Pop's Corn - Light Butter
Pop's Corn - No Butter/No Salt

O-Ke-Doke ⓘ
Buttery Popcorn
Cheese Flavored Popcorn
Hot Cheese Popcorn
White Cheddar Popcorn
White Popcorn

Oogie's
Oogie's (All)

Pirate's Booty ⓘ ⓤ
Smart Puffs

Publix ◌
Popcorn (Deli)

Ricos ✔
Popcorn (All)

Safeway
Microwave Popcorn (All Varieties)
Popcorn - Kettle
Popcorn - Light Butter Microwave
Popcorn - Yellow

Smart Balance
Smart Balance (All)

Smartfood ⓘ
Cranberry Almond Popcorn Clusters
Reduced Fat White Cheddar Cheese
Flavored Popcorn
White Cheddar Cheese Flavored
Popcorn

Snyder's of Hanover ⓘ
Butter Popcorn

Stop & Shop
Microwave Popcorn - 94% Fat Free
Butter
Microwave Popcorn - Butter Flavored
Microwave Popcorn - Butter Light
Microwave Popcorn - Kettle Corn
Microwave Popcorn - Movie Theatre
Butter Flavored
Microwave Popcorn - Natural Light
Microwave Popcorn - Sweet & Buttery
Yellow Popcorn

Utz ⓤ ✔
Butter Popcorn
Caramel Puff'n Corn
Cheese Popcorn
Plain Puff'n Corn
White Cheddar Popcorn

Winn-Dixie ⓘ
Microwavable Natural Popcorn

PORK SKINS & RINDS

Baken-Ets ⓘ
BBQ Flavored Fried Pork Skins
Fried Pork Skins
Hot 'N Spicy Flavored Pork Skins
Hot 'n Spicy Flavored Cracklins

Golden Flake ⓘ
Hot Pork Skins
Pork Cracklins
Pork Skins
Sweet Heat Pork Skins
Vinegar & Salt Pork Cracklins
Vinegar & Salt Pork Skins

Herr's ◌
Pork Rinds - Original

Jay's ⓘ
Cracklins
Pork Skins
Pork Skins Hot
Pork Skins with Hot Sauce

PRETZELS

Ener-G ♀
- Crisp Pretzels
- Sesame Pretzel Rings
- Wylde Poppyseed Pretzels
- Wylde Pretzels
- Wylde Sesame Pretzels

Glutino ♀ ✓
- Pretzel Sticks
- Pretzel Twists
- Pretzel Twists - Family Bag
- Pretzels - Sesame Rings
- Pretzels - Snack Pack
- Unsalted Pretzel Twists

Mary's Gone Crackers ♀ ✓
- Sticks & Twigs - Chipotle Tomato
- Sticks & Twigs - Curry
- Sticks & Twigs - Sea Salt

PUDDING & PUDDING MIXES

Dr. Oetker ()
- Organic Pudding Mix - Chocolate
- Organic Pudding Mix - Coconut
- Organic Pudding Mix - Mocha
- Organic Pudding Mix - Vanilla

Giant
- Butterscotch Pudding Mix
- Chocolate Fudge Pudding Snack Cups
- Chocolate Instant Pudding and Pie Filling
- Chocolate Pudding Snack Cups - Fat Free
- Chocolate Pudding Snack Cups - Regular
- Refrigerated Chocolate Pudding - Fat Free
- Refrigerated Chocolate Pudding - Regular

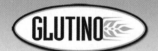
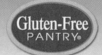
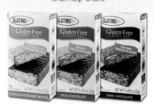
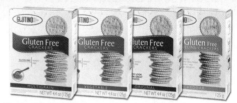
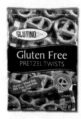
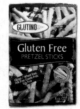
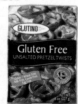
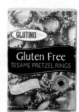

Refrigerated Chocolate/Vanilla Pudding - Fat Free
Refrigerated Chocolate/Vanilla Pudding - Regular
Rice Pudding
Tapioca Pudding Mix
Vanilla Pudding Snack Cups

Great Value (Wal-Mart)
Banana Cream Instant Pudding
Chocolate Family Size Instant Pudding
Chocolate Instant Pudding
French Vanilla Instant Pudding
Pistachio Instant Pudding
Sugar Free Chocolate Instant Pudding
Sugar Free French Vanilla Instant Pudding
Vanilla Family Size Instant Pudding
Vanilla Instant Pudding

Handi-Snacks Pudding ✍
Banana
Butterscotch
Chocolate
Pudding Doubles - Banana Split
Pudding Doubles - Chocolate Chip Cookie Doubles
Pudding Doubles - Chocolate Vanilla
Pudding Doubles - Fudge Rocky Road
Rice Pudding
Sugar Free Chocolate Reduced Calorie
Sugar Free Creamy Caramel Reduced Calorie
Sugar Free Vanilla Reduced Calorie
Vanilla

Hy-Vee
Butterscotch Pudding Cups
Chocolate Fudge Pudding Cups
Chocolate Pudding Cups
Cooked Chocolate Pudding
Cooked Vanilla Pudding
Fat Free Chocolate Pudding Cups
Instant Butterscotch Pudding
Instant Chocolate Pudding
Instant Fat Free/Sugar Free Chocolate Pudding
Instant Fat Free/Sugar Free Vanilla Pudding
Instant Lemon Pudding

Instant Pistachio Pudding
Instant Vanilla Pudding
Tapioca Pudding Cups
Vanilla Pudding Cups

Jell-O ✍
Americana Fat Free Rice Pudding
Cheesecake Snacks Strawberry
Chocolate Fat Free Pudding Snacks
Chocolate Fudge Sundaes Pudding Snacks
Chocolate Pudding Snacks
Chocolate Sugar Free Pudding Snacks
Chocolate Vanilla Swirls Fat Free Pudding Snacks
Chocolate Vanilla Swirls Pudding Snacks
Chocolate Vanilla Swirls Sugar Free Pudding Snacks
Cook & Serve Banana Cream Pudding & Pie Filling
Cook & Serve Butterscotch Pudding & Pie Filling
Cook & Serve Chocolate Fudge Pudding & Pie Filling
Cook & Serve Chocolate Pudding & Pie Filling
Cook & Serve Chocolate Sugar Free Pudding & Pie Filling
Cook & Serve Coconut Cream Pudding & Pie Filling
Cook & Serve Lemon Pudding & Pie Filling
Cook & Serve Tapioca Fat Free Pudding
Cook & Serve Vanilla Pudding & Pie Filling
Cook & Serve Vanilla Sugar Free Pudding & Pie Filling
Creamy Caramel Sugar Free Pudding Snacks
Devil's Food & Chocolate Fat Free Pudding Snacks
Double Chocolate Sugar Free Pudding Snacks
Instant Banana Cream Pudding & Pie Filling
Instant Banana Cream Sugar Free & Fat Free Pudding & Pie Filling

Instant Butterscotch Pudding & Pie Filling

Instant Butterscotch Sugar Free & Fat Free Pudding & Pie Filling

Instant Cheesecake Pudding & Pie Filling

Instant Cheesecake Sugar Free & Fat Free Pudding & Pie Filling

Instant Chocolate Caramel Chip Pudding & Pie Filling

Instant Chocolate Fudge Pudding & Pie Filling

Instant Chocolate Fudge Sugar Free & Fat Free Pudding & Pie Filling

Instant Chocolate Mint Chip Pudding & Pie Filling

Instant Chocolate Pudding & Pie Filling

Instant Chocolate Sugar Free & Fat Free Pudding & Pie Filling

Instant Coconut Cream Pudding & Pie Filling

Instant Devil's Food Fat Free Pudding & Pie Filling

Instant French Vanilla Pudding & Pie Filling

Instant Lemon Pudding & Pie Filling

Instant Lemon Sugar Free & Fat Free Pudding & Pie Filling

Instant Pistachio Pudding & Pie Filling

Instant Pistachio Sugar Free & Fat Free Pudding & Pie Filling

Instant Pumpkin Spice Pudding & Pie Filling

Instant Vanilla Chocolate Chip Pudding & Pie Filling

Instant Vanilla Pudding & Pie Filling

Instant Vanilla Sugar Free & Fat Free Pudding & Pie Filling

Instant White Chocolate Fat Free Pudding & Pie Filling

Instant White Chocolate Sugar Free & Fat Free Pudding & Pie Filling

Mixed Berry Smoothie Snacks

Oreo Pudding Snacks

Rice Creme Brulee Sugar Free Pudding

Strawberries & Creme Swirled Pudding Snacks Creme Savers

Strawberry Banana Smoothie Snacks

Sundae Toppers Chocolate with Chocolate Topping Pudding

Sundae Toppers Vanilla with Caramel Topping Pudding Snacks

Sundae Toppers Vanilla with Chocolate Topping Pudding

Tapioca Fat Free Pudding Snacks

Tapioca Pudding Snacks

Vanilla & Chocolate 100 Calorie Packs Fat Free Pudding Snacks

Vanilla Caramel Sundaes 100 Calorie Packs Fat Free Pudding Snacks

Vanilla Pudding Snacks

Vanilla Sugar Free Pudding Snacks

X-Treme Chocolate Pudding Sticks

Kroger ⓘ

Pudding - Boxed

Pudding - Snack Cups

Laura Lynn (Ingle's)

Boxed Puddings (All)

Lifeway ⚕

Lifeway Products (All BUT Probiotic Wellness Bars)

Meijer

Pudding - Cook & Serve Butterscotch

Pudding - Cook and Serve Chocolate

Pudding - Cook and Serve Vanilla

Pudding and Pie Filling Instant - Chocolate

Pudding and Pie Filling Instant - Coconut Cream

Pudding and Pie Filling Instant - French Vanilla

Pudding and Pie Filling Instant - Pistachio

Pudding and Pie Filling Instant - Vanilla

Pudding Instant - Banana Cream

Pudding Instant - Butterscotch Fat Free & Sugar Free

Pudding Instant - Chocolate Fat Free and Sugar Free

Pudding Instant - Vanilla Fat Free and Sugar Free

Pudding Premium - Chocolate Peanut Butter

Pudding Premium - French Vanilla

Pudding Premium - Orange Dream

Pudding Snack - Banana
Pudding Snack - Butterscotch
Pudding Snack - Chocolate
Pudding Snack - Chocolate Fat Free
Pudding Snack - Chocolate Fudge
Pudding Snack - Multi-Pack Chocolate
and Vanilla
Pudding Snack - Tapioca
Pudding Snack - Vanilla

Mori-Nu
Mates Chocolate Pudding Mix
Mates Lemon Crème Pudding Mix
Mates Vanilla Pudding Mix

Publix ()
Chocolate Pudding
Fat Free Chocolate Pudding
Fat Free Chocolate-Vanilla Swirl
Pudding
Rice Pudding
Sugar Free Chocolate-Vanilla Swirl
Pudding
Tapioca Pudding

Safeway
Instant Pudding (All Flavors)
Pudding Snack Cups (All Flavors)
Ready-to-Eat Pudding (All Flavors)

Stop & Shop
Butterscotch Pudding Mix
Chocolate Fudge Pudding Snack Cups
Chocolate Instant Pudding & Pie Filling
Chocolate Pudding Snack Cups
Instant Low Calorie Vanilla Pudding &
Pie Mix
Refrigerated Chocolate Pudding
Refrigerated Chocolate/Vanilla Pudding
Refrigerated Fat Free Chocolate
Pudding
Refrigerated Fat Free Chocolate/Vanilla
Pudding
Rice Pudding
Sugar Free Chocolate Instant Pudding
Mix
Tapioca Pudding Mix
Vanilla Pudding Snack Cups

ZenSoy
ZenSoy Products (All)

Rice Cakes

Giant
Rice Cakes - Multigrain Unsalted
Rice Cakes - Plain Unsalted
Rice Cakes - Sour Cream & Onion

Koyo Foods ☦
Rice Cakes (All)

Lundberg Family Farms
Eco-Farmed Rice Cakes - Apple
Cinnamon
Eco-Farmed Rice Cakes - Brown Rice
Eco-Farmed Rice Cakes - Brown Rice
(Salt Free)
Eco-Farmed Rice Cakes - Buttery
Caramel
Eco-Farmed Rice Cakes - Honey Nut
Eco-Farmed Rice Cakes - Sesame
Tamari
Eco-Farmed Rice Cakes - Toasted
Sesame
Organic Rice Cakes - Brown Rice
Organic Rice Cakes - Brown Rice (Salt
Free)
Organic Rice Cakes - Caramel Corn
Organic Rice Cakes - Cinnamon Toast
Organic Rice Cakes - Koku Seaweed
Organic Rice Cakes - Mochi Sweet
Organic Rice Cakes - Popcorn
Organic Rice Cakes - Sesame Tamari
Organic Rice Cakes - Sweet Green Tea
with Lemon
Organic Rice Cakes - Tamari with
Seaweed
Organic Rice Cakes - Wild Rice

Publix ()
Lightly Salted Rice Cakes
Mini Caramel Rice
Mini Cheddar Rice
Mini Ranch Rice
Unsalted Rice Cakes
White Cheddar Rice Cakes

Stop & Shop
Apple Cinnamon Rice Cakes
Rice Cakes - Caramel
Rice Cakes - Plain Salted & Unsalted
Rice Cakes - Sesame Unsalted

Rice Cakes - Sour Cream & Onion
Rice Cakes - White Cheddar

Trail Mix

BHUJA ☷ ✓
Cracker Mix
Original Mix
Enjoy Life Foods ☷
Not Nuts! Beach Bash Trail Mix
Not Nuts! Mountain Mambo Trail Mix
Fisher Nuts ()
Fusions Trail Blazer Snack Mix
Frito Lay ⓘ
Original Trail Mix
Nut Harvest ⓘ
Natural Nut & Fruit Mix
Planters ⌇
Trail Mix - Fruit & Nut
Trail Mix - Mixed Nuts & Raisins
Trail Mix - Nut & Chocolate Mix
Publix ()
Party Time Mix
Safeway
Trail Mix with Candy Pieces

Miscellaneous

Clif
Shot Bloks ()
Shot Gels ()
Crunchies
Crunchies (All)
Great Value (Wal-Mart)
Naturally Smoked Kipper Snacks
Let's Do... ✓
Gluten-Free Ice Cream Cones

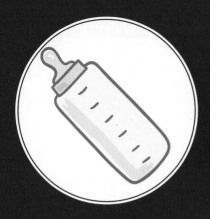

BABY FOOD & FORMULA

BABY FOOD

Beech-Nut

DHA Plus Rice Cereal
Good Evening Whole Grain Brown Rice Cereal
Good Evening Whole Grain Brown Rice with Bananas & Raspberries
Let's Grow! - Mini Meals Apple Cinnamon Oatmeal
Let's Grow! - Mini Meals Mixed Fruit Oatmeal
Let's Grow! Tummy Tray Savory Beef Potato
Let's Grow! Tummy Tray Turkey Vegetable
Let's Grow! Tummy Tray Vegetable Beef Rice Cereal
Stage 1 - Applesauce
Stage 1 - Beef & Beef Broth
Stage 1 - Butternut Squash
Stage 1 - Chicken & Chicken Broth
Stage 1 - Chiquita Bananas
Stage 1 - Peaches
Stage 1 - Pears
Stage 1 - Tender Golden Sweet Potatoes
Stage 1 - Tender Sweet Carrots
Stage 1 - Tender Sweet Peas
Stage 1 - Tender Young Green Beans
Stage 1 - Turkey & Turkey Broth
Stage 2 - Apples & Bananas
Stage 2 - Apples & Blueberries
Stage 2 - Apples & Cherries
Stage 2 - Apples & Chicken
Stage 2 - Apples, Mango & Kiwi
Stage 2 - Apples, Pears & Bananas

Stage 2 - Applesauce
Stage 2 - Apricots with Pears & Apples
Stage 2 - Banana Apple Yogurt
Stage 2 - Butternut Squash
Stage 2 - Carrots & Peas
Stage 2 - Chicken & Rice Dinner
Stage 2 - Chicken Noodle Dinner
Stage 2 - Chiquita Bananas
Stage 2 - Chiquita Bananas & Strawberries
Stage 2 - Corn & Sweet Potatoes
Stage 2 - Country Garden Vegetables
Stage 2 - DHA Plus Apple Delight
Stage 2 - DHA Plus Banana Supreme
Stage 2 - DHA Plus Butternut Squash with Corn
Stage 2 - DHA Plus Sweet Potatoes
Stage 2 - Good Evening - Creamy Chicken Noodle Dinner
Stage 2 - Good Evening - Ham, Pineapple & Rice
Stage 2 - Good Evening - Hearty Vegetable Stew
Stage 2 - Good Evening - Sweet Potato & Turkey
Stage 2 - Good Evening - Turkey Tetrazzini
Stage 2 - Good Morning Cinnamon Raisin Granola
Stage 2 - Good Morning Country Breakfast
Stage 2 - Good Morning Mixed Fruit Yogurt
Stage 2 - Good Morning Peaches, Oatmeal & Bananas
Stage 2 - Guava

Stage 2 - Homestyle Chicken Soup
Stage 2 - Macaroni & Beef with
  Vegetables
Stage 2 - Mango
Stage 2 - Mixed Cereal & Apple
Stage 2 - Mixed Vegetables
Stage 2 - Oatmeal & Apples
Stage 2 - Papaya
Stage 2 - Peaches
Stage 2 - Peaches & Bananas
Stage 2 - Pears
Stage 2 - Pears & Pineapple
Stage 2 - Pears & Raspberries
Stage 2 - Pineapple Glazed Ham
Stage 2 - Plums with Apples & Pears
Stage 2 - Rice Cereal & Apples with
  Cinnamon
Stage 2 - Sweet Corn Casserole
Stage 2 - Sweet Potatoes & Apples
Stage 2 - Sweet Potatoes & Chicken
Stage 2 - Tender Golden Sweet Potatoes
Stage 2 - Tender Sweet Carrots
Stage 2 - Tender Sweet Peas
Stage 2 - Tender Young Green Beans
Stage 2 - Turkey Rice Dinner
Stage 2 - Vegetables & Beef
Stage 2 - Vegetables & Chicken
Stage 3 - Apples & Bananas
Stage 3 - Banana Pudding
Stage 3 - Chiquita Bananas
Stage 3 - Country Vegetables & Chicken
Stage 3 - Good Evening Country
  Vegetables with Beef
Stage 3 - Good Evening Vegetable
  Turkey Dinner
Stage 3 - Green Beans, Corn & Rice
Stage 3 - Oatmeal & Pears with
  Cinnamon
Stage 3 - Pears
Stage 3 - Rice Cereal & Pears
Stage 3 - Sweet Potatoes
Stage 3 - Turkey Rice Dinner

Ella's Kitchen

Apples + Bananas
Broccoli, Pear, + Peas
Carrot, Apple, + Parsnip
Peaches + Bananas

Strawberries + Apples
Sweet Potato, Pumpkin, Apple, +
  Blueberries
The Red One
The Yellow One

Meijer

Little Fruit - Apple
Little Fruit - Strawberry/Banana
Little Veggies - Corn

PBM Products

Stage II Fruit Tubs
Toddler Freeze Dried Little Fruits

BABY JUICE & OTHER DRINKS

Beech-Nut

Apple Juice from Concentrate
DHA Plus Yogurt Blends with Juice-
  Mixed Berry
DHA Plus Yogurt Blends with Juice-
  Tropical Fruit
Good Evening Veggie Delight Juice
Good Morning Chiquita Banana Juice
  with Yogurt
Let's Grow! - Smoothie Surprise Berry
  Medley
Let's Grow! - Smoothie Surprise
  Chiquita Banana Orange
Let's Grow! - Smoothie Surprise Vanilla
  Apple
Stage 2 - DHA Plus Apples with
  Pomegranate Juice
White Grape Juice from Concentrate

Hy-Vee

Mother's Choice Infant Water
Mother's Choice Infant Water with
  Fluoride
Mother's Choice Pediatric Vanilla Drink
Mother's Choice Pediatric Vanilla with
  Fiber Drink

Meijer

Bright Beginnings Soy Vanilla Pediatric
  Nutritional Drink
Chocolate Pediatric Nutritional Drink
Gluco-Burst - Arctic Cherry
Strawberry Pediatric Nutritional Drink
Vanilla Pediatric Nutritional Drink

Vanilla Soy Pediatric Nutritional Drink
Vanilla with Fiber Pediatric Nutritional
Drink

Pedialyte
Pedialyte (All)

PediaSure
Pediasure (All)

FORMULA

Bright Beginnings
Infant Formulas (All)

EleCare
Unflavored
Vanilla

Enfamil
Mead Johnson Infant Formula &
Pediatric Products (All)

Meijer
Gentle Protein with DHA
Lactose Free with DHA
Milk with DHA
Regular Term Formula
Soy Term Formula
Soy with DHA

PBM Products
Infant Formula (All)

Pregestimil
Mead Johnson Infant Formula &
Pediatric Products

Similac
Infant Formulas (All)

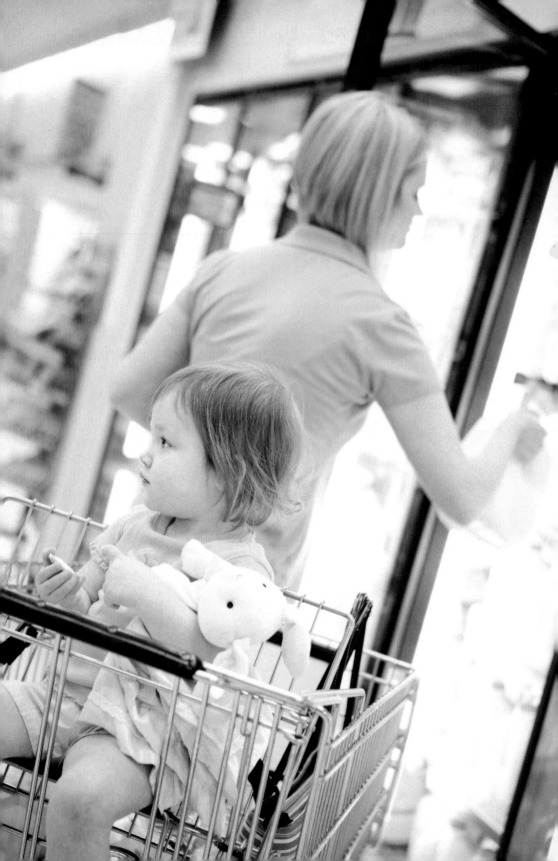

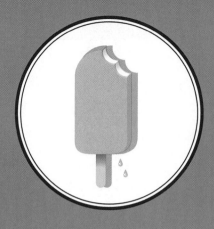

FROZEN FOODS

Beans

Giant
Baby Lima Beans
Fordhook Lima Beans

Great Value (Wal-Mart)
Microwavable Cut Green Beans

Hy-Vee
Frozen Baby Lima Beans

Meijer
Frozen Beans - Baby Lima
Frozen Beans - Lima Fordhook

Nature's Promise (Stop & Shop)
Organic Edamame in Pod

Publix ()
Limas - Baby
Limas - Fordhook
Spec. Butter Beans

Stop & Shop
Baby Lima Beans
Fordhook Lima Beans

Cookie Dough

French Meadow Bakery
Gluten-Free Chocolate Chip Cookie
Dough

Glutenfreeda Real Cookies! ♨ ✓
Chip Chip Hooray!
Chocolate Minty Python
Peanut Envy
Peanut, Paul & Mary
Snicker Poodles
Sugar Kookies

Dough

Chebe ♨ ✓
Bread Sticks
Rolls
Sandwich Buns
Tomato-Basil Breadsticks

Frozen Yogurt

Dreyer's
Fat Free Vanilla Yogurt
Slow Churned Yogurt Blend Black
Cherry Vanilla Swirl
Slow Churned Yogurt Blend Cappuccino
Chip
Slow Churned Yogurt Blend Caramel
Praline Crunch
Slow Churned Yogurt Blend Chocolate
Vanilla Swirl
Slow Churned Yogurt Blend Peach
Slow Churned Yogurt Blend Strawberry
Slow Churned Yogurt Blend Tart Honey
Slow Churned Yogurt Blend Tart Mango
Slow Churned Yogurt Blend Vanilla

Edy's
see Dreyer's

Lucerne (Safeway)
Fat Free Vanilla Frozen Yogurt

Publix ()
Black Cherry Premium Low Fat Frozen
Yogurt
Butter Pecan Premium Low Fat Frozen
Yogurt

Chocolate Premium Low Fat Frozen
Yogurt
Neapolitan Premium Low Fat Frozen
Yogurt
Peach Premium Low Fat Frozen Yogurt
Peanut Butter Cup Premium Low Fat
Frozen Yogurt
Strawberry Premium Low Fat Frozen
Yogurt
Vanilla Orange Premium Low Fat
Frozen Yogurt
Vanilla Premium Low Fat Frozen Yogurt

Turkey Hill ⓘ
Frozen Yogurt - Banana Split
Frozen Yogurt - Chocolate Cherry
Cordial
Frozen Yogurt - Chocolate
Marshmallow
Frozen Yogurt - Fudge Ripple
Frozen Yogurt - Neapolitan
Frozen Yogurt - Nutty Caramel Caribou
(Limited Edition)
Frozen Yogurt - Orange Cream Swirl
Frozen Yogurt - Peach Mango
Frozen Yogurt - Vanilla Bean

WholeSoy & Co. ⓘ ✔
Black Cherry
Chocolate Hazelnut
Crème Caramel
French Vanilla
Mocha Fudge
Swiss Dark Chocolate
Vanilla Bean

FRUIT

Birds Eye Foods
Fruit Berry Medley
Fruit Blueberries
Fruit Mango Chunks
Fruit Mixed Fruit
Fruit Red Raspberries
Fruit Sliced Peaches
Fruit Strawberries, Lite Syrup
Fruit Strawberries, Regular Syrup
Fruit Strawberries, Sliced
Fruit Strawberries, Whole

Dole ()
Frozen Fruits (All)

Giant
Berry Medley
Blackberries
Blueberries
Dark Sweet Cherries
Mango
Mixed Fruit
Peaches
Pineapple
Raspberries - In Syrup
Raspberries - Plain
Sliced Strawberries - Plain
Sliced Strawberries with Artificial
Sweetener
Sliced Strawberries with Sugar
Strawberries

Goya
Guava Paste

Great Value (Wal-Mart)
Sliced Strawberries

Hy-Vee
Frozen Blueberries
Frozen Cherry Berry Blend
Frozen Red Raspberries
Frozen Sliced Strawberries
Frozen Whole Strawberries

Kroger ⓘ
Plain Frozen Fruit

Meijer
Frozen Berry Medley
Frozen Blackberries
Frozen Blueberries
Frozen Dark Sweet Cherries
Frozen Mango Chunks
Frozen Mango Sliced
Frozen Mixed Fruit
Frozen Organic Blueberries
Frozen Organic Peaches
Frozen Organic Raspberries
Frozen Organic Strawberries
Frozen Pineapple Chunks
Frozen Raspberries
Frozen Raspberries - Individually Quick
Frozen
Frozen Sliced Peaches

Frozen Strawberries - Individually
Quick Frozen
Frozen Strawberries - Sliced
Frozen Tart Cherries
Frozen Triple Berry Blend
Frozen Tropical Fruit Blend

Publix ()

Blackberries
Blueberries
Cherries - Dark Sweet
Cranberries
Mixed Berries
Mixed Fruit
Peaches - Sliced
Raspberries
Strawberries - Sliced, Sweetened
Strawberries - Whole

Stahlbush Island Farms (i)

Stahlbush Island Farms (All)

Stop & Shop

Berry Medley
Blackberries
Blueberries
Dark Sweet Cherries
Mango
Mixed Fruit
Peaches
Pineapple
Raspberries
Raspberries in Syrup
Sliced Strawberries
Sliced Strawberries in Sugar
Sliced Strawberries with Artificial
Sweetener
Strawberries

Tropic Isle Coconut

Coconut

Wyman's

Wyman's (All)

ICE CREAM

Dreyer's

Banana Split
Butter Pecan Grand Ice Cream Pints
Chocolate Grand Ice Cream Pints

Chocolate Peanut Butter Chunk Maxx
Pints
Eggnog
Fat Free No Sugar Added Chocolate
Fudge
Fat Free No Sugar Added Vanilla
Chocolate
Fun Flavors - Butter Pecan
Fun Flavors - Cherry Chocolate Chip
Fun Flavors - Dulce de Leche
Fun Flavors - Mango
Fun Flavors - Mocha Almond Fudge
Fun Flavors - Peanut Butter Cup
Fun Flavors - Spumoni
Grand Ice Cream - Chocolate
Grand Ice Cream - Chocolate Chip
Grand Ice Cream - Coffee
Grand Ice Cream - Double Vanilla
Grand Ice Cream - French Vanilla
Grand Ice Cream - Fudge Swirl
Grand Ice Cream - Mint Chocolate Chip
Grand Ice Cream - Neapolitan
Grand Ice Cream - Real Strawberry
Grand Ice Cream - Rocky Road
Grand Ice Cream - Vanilla
Grand Ice Cream - Vanilla Bean
Grand Ice Cream - Vanilla Chocolate
Java MashUp Maxx Pints
Loaded - Chocolate Peanut Butter Cup
Loaded - Nestle Butterfinger
Mint Chocolate Chip Grand Ice Cream
Pints
Nestlé Butterfinger Maxx Pints
Peppermint
Pumpkin
Slow Churned Light Butter Pecan
Slow Churned Light Caramel Delight
Slow Churned Light Chocolate
Slow Churned Light Chocolate Chip
Slow Churned Light Chocolate Fudge
Chunk
Slow Churned Light Coffee
Slow Churned Light French Vanilla
Slow Churned Light Fudge Tracks
Slow Churned Light Mint Chocolate
Chip
Slow Churned Light Neapolitan
Slow Churned Light Peanut Butter Cup

Slow Churned Light Rocky Road
Slow Churned Light Strawberry
Slow Churned Light Take the Cake
Slow Churned Light Vanilla
Slow Churned Light Vanilla Bean
Slow Churned Limited Edition Eggnog
Slow Churned Limited Edition Hot
  Cocoa
Slow Churned Limited Edition
  Peppermint
Slow Churned Limited Edition Pumpkin
Slow Churned No Sugar Added Butter
  Pecan
Slow Churned No Sugar Added Coffee
Slow Churned No Sugar Added French
  Vanilla
Slow Churned No Sugar Added Fudge
  Tracks
Slow Churned No Sugar Added Mint
  Chocolate Chip
Slow Churned No Sugar Added
  Neapolitan
Slow Churned No Sugar Added Triple
  Chocolate
Slow Churned No Sugar Added Vanilla
Slow Churned No Sugar Added Vanilla
  Bean
Strawberry Grand Ice Cream Pints
Vanilla Grand Ice Cream Pints

Edy's
Fun Flavors - Espresso Chip (Edy's
  Only)
see Dreyer's

Giant
Andes Crème De Menthe Ice Cream
Black Cherry Ice Cream
Black Raspberry Ice Cream
Butter Pecan Ice Cream
Butterscotch Ripple Ice Cream
Cherry Vanilla Ice Cream
Chocolate Ice Cream
Chocolate Marshmallow Ice Cream
Coffee Ice Cream
Light Butter Pecan Ice Cream
Light Vanilla Ice Cream
Mint Chocolate Chip Ice Cream
Moose Tracks Ice Cream

Natural Butter Pecan Ice Cream
Natural Chocolate Chip Ice Cream
Natural Chocolate Ice Cream
Natural Coffee Ice Cream
Natural French Vanilla Ice Cream
Natural Mint Chocolate Chip Ice Cream
Natural Mocha Almond Ice Cream
Natural Strawberry Ice Cream
Natural Vanilla Bean Ice Cream
Natural Vanilla Fudge Ripple Ice Cream
Peanut Butter Jumble Ice Cream
Strawberry Ice Cream
Toffee Crunch Ice Cream
Vanilla Fudge Ice Cream
Vanilla Ice Cream

Guaranteed Value (Stop & Shop)
Chocolate Ice Cream
Chocolate Marshmallow
Fudge Royal Ice Cream
Neapolitan Ice Cream
Vanilla Ice Cream
Vanilla Orange Ice Cream

Hood
Chippedy Chocolaty
Chocolate
Classic Trio
Creamy Coffee
Fudge Twister
Golden Vanilla
Holiday Eggnog (Seasonal)
Maple Walnut
Natural Vanilla Bean
New England Creamery - Bear Creek
  Caramel
New England Creamery - Boston
  Vanilla Bean
New England Creamery - Cape Cod
  Fudge Shop
New England Creamery - Light Butter
  Pecan
New England Creamery - Light
  Chocolate Chip
New England Creamery - Light Coffee
New England Creamery - Light French
  Silk
New England Creamery - Light Maine
  Blueberry & Sweet Cream

New England Creamery - Light Martha's Vineyard Black Raspberry

New England Creamery - Light Mint Chocolate Chip

New England Creamery - Light Under The Stars

New England Creamery - Light Vanilla

New England Creamery - Maine Blueberry & Sweet Cream

New England Creamery - Martha's Vineyard Black Raspberry

New England Creamery - Moosehead Lake Fudge

New England Creamery - Mystic Lighthouse Mint

New England Creamery - New England Homemade Vanilla

New England Creamery - New England Lighthouse Coffee

New England Creamery - Vermont Maple Nut

Patchwork

Peppermint Stick (Seasonal)

Red Sox Ice Cream (All Flavors)

Strawberry

Hy-Vee

Butter Crunch Ice Cream

Cherry Nut Ice Cream

Cherry Nut Light Ice Cream

Chocolate Chip Ice Cream

Chocolate Chip Light Ice Cream

Chocolate Ice Cream

Chocolate Marshmallow Ice Cream

Chocolate/Vanilla Flavored Ice Cream

Dutch Chocolate Light Ice Cream

Fudge Marble Ice Cream

Mint Chip Ice Cream

Neapolitan Ice Cream

Neapolitan Light Ice Cream

New York Vanilla Ice Cream

Peppermint Stick Ice Cream

Strawberry Ice Cream

Vanilla Flavored Ice Cream

Vanilla Light Ice Cream

It's Soy Delicious ✓

Almond Pecan

Awesome Chocolate

Black Leopard

Carob Peppermint

Chocolate Almond

Chocolate Peanut Butter

Espresso

Green Tea

Mango Raspberry

Pistachio Almond

Raspberry

Tiger Chai

Vanilla

Vanilla Fudge

Lucerne (Safeway)

Egg Nog Ice Cream

Meijer

Awesome Strawberry Ice Cream

Black Cherry Ice Cream

Bordeaux Cherry Chocolate Ice Cream

Butter Pecan Ice Cream

Candy Bar Swirl Ice Cream

Carb Conquest Chocolate Ice Cream

Carb Conquest Vanilla Ice Cream

Chocolate Chip Ice Cream

Chocolate Ice Cream

Chocolate Peanut Butter Fudge Ice Cream

Chocolate Thunder Ice Cream

Combo Cream

Cotton Candy Ice Cream

Dulce De Leche Ice Cream

Fudge Swirl Ice Cream

Gold Caramel Toffee Swirli Ice Cream

Gold Double Nut Chocolate Ice Cream

Gold Georgian Bay Butter Pecan Ice Cream

Gold Peanut Butter Fudge Swirli Ice Cream

Gold Peanut Butter Fudge Tracks Ice Cream

Gold Thunder Bay Cherry Ice Cream

Gold Victorian Vanilla

Golden Vanilla Ice Cream

Heavenly Hash Ice Cream

Lite Neapolitan Ice Cream

Lite No Sugar Added Butter Pecan Ice Cream with Splenda

Lite No Sugar Added Vanilla with
Splenda
Mackinac Fudge Ice Cream
Mint Chocolate Ice Cream
Neapolitan Ice Cream
Peppermint Ice Cream
Praline Pecan Ice Cream
Scooperman Ice Cream
Tin Roof Ice Cream
Vanilla Ice Cream

Midwest Country Fare (Hy-Vee)

Chocolate Chip Ice Cream
Light Vanilla Ice Cream
Neapolitan Ice Cream
Peppermint Stick Ice Cream
Vanilla Ice Cream

Organic So Delicious Dairy Free ✓

Butter Pecan
Chocolate Peanut Butter
Chocolate Velvet
Creamy Lemon
Creamy Orange
Creamy Raspberry
Creamy Vanilla
Dulce De Leche
Mint Marble Fudge
Mocha Fudge
Neapolitan
Strawberry

Publix ◊

Banana Split Premium Ice Cream
Bear Claw Premium Ice Cream
Black Jack Cherry Premium Ice Cream
Buckeye's & Fudge Premium Limited
Edition Ice Cream
Butter Pecan Premium Homemade Ice
Cream
Butter Pecan Premium Ice Cream
Butter Pecan Premium Light Ice Cream
Caramel Mountain Tracks Premium
Limited Edition Ice Cream
Cherry Nut Premium Ice Cream
Chocolate Almond Premium Ice Cream
Chocolate Cherish Passion Premium Ice
Cream
Chocolate Chip Premium Homemade
Ice Cream

Chocolate Chip Premium Ice Cream
Chocolate Ice Cream
Chocolate Low Fat Ice Cream
Chocolate Marshmallow Swirl Ice
Cream
Chocolate Peanut Butter Swirl Ice
Cream
Chocolate Premium Ice Cream
Chocolate Premium Light Ice Cream
Coffee Almond Fudge Premium Light
Ice Cream
Coffee Premium Ice Cream
Double Chocolate Chunk Premium
Homemade Ice Cream
Dulce de Leche Premium Ice Cream
Egg Nog Premium Limited Edition Ice
Cream
French Silk Duo Premium Limited
Edition Ice Cream
French Vanilla Premium Ice Cream
Fudge Royal Ice Cream
Fudge Royal Low Fat Ice Cream
Heavenly Hash Premium Ice Cream
Maple Walnut Premium Limited Edition
Ice Cream
Mint Chocolate Chip Premium Ice
Cream
Monkey Business Premium Limited
Edition Ice Cream
Neapolitan Ice Cream
Neapolitan Low Fat Ice Cream
Neapolitan Premium Ice Cream
Neapolitan Premium Light Ice Cream
Otter Paws Premium Ice Cream
Peanut Butter Goo Goo Premium Ice
Cream
Peppermint Stick Premium Limited
Edition Ice Cream
Rum Raisin Premium Limited Edition
Ice Cream
Santa's White Christmas Premium Ice
Cream
Strawberry Premium Homemade Ice
Cream
Strawberry Premium Ice Cream
Strawberry Premium Light Ice Cream
Vanilla Ice Cream
Vanilla Low Fat Ice Cream

Vanilla Premium Homemade Ice Cream
Vanilla Premium Ice Cream
Vanilla Premium Light Ice Cream
Vanilla Strawberry Ice Cream

Purely Decadent Dairy Free ✓

Cherry Nirvana
Chocolate Obsession
Coconut Craze
Cookie Dough (Gluten-Free)
Mint Chocolate Chip
Mocha Almond Fudge
Peanut Butter Zig Zag
Pomegranate Chip
Praline Pecan
Purely Vanilla
Rocky Road
So Very Strawberry
Turtle Trails

Rice Dream ✓

Carob Almond
Organic Cocoa Marble Fudge
Organic Neapolitan
Organic Orange Vanilla
Organic Strawberry
Organic Vanilla

Safeway

Select - Caramel Cashew Ice Cream
Select - Chocolate Chunk Ice Cream
Select - Coffee Ice Cream
Select - Dutch Chocolate Ice Cream
Select - Fat Free Caramel Swirl Ice Cream
Select - Fat Free No Sugar Added Vanilla Ice Cream
Select - Light Peppermint Ice Cream
Select - Mocha Ice Cream
Select - Mother Load Ice Cream
Select - Ole' Vanilla Ice Cream
Select - Pecan Praline Ice Cream

Soy Dream ✓

French Vanilla
Green Tea
Mocha Fudge
Strawberry Swirl
Vanilla
Vanilla Fudge Swirl

Stop & Shop

Butterscotch Ripple Ice Cream
Chocolate Chip Ice Cream
Coffee Ice Cream
Country Club Ice Cream
Heavenly Hash Ice Cream
Natural Butter Pecan Ice Cream
Natural Chocolate Chip Ice Cream
Natural Chocolate Ice Cream
Natural Coffee Ice Cream
Natural French Vanilla Ice Cream
Natural Mint Chocolate Chip Ice Cream
Natural Mocha Almond Ice Cream
Natural Strawberry Ice Cream
Natural Vanilla Bean Ice Cream
Natural Vanilla Fudge Ripple Ice Cream
Neapolitan Ice Cream
Peppermint Stick Ice Cream
Strawberry Ice Cream
Vanilla Fudge Swirl Ice Cream
Vanilla Ice Cream

Straus Family Creamery ⑃

Ice Cream (All)

Tillamook

Ice Cream (All BUT Caramel Toffee
Crunch, Cookies and Cream, Cookie
Dough, German Chocolate Cake,
Marionberry Pie, Cows in Brownie
Batter and Lemon Blueberry Pie)

Turkey Hill ⓘ

All Natural Recipe - Chocolate
All Natural Recipe - Coffee
All Natural Recipe - Mint Chocolate Chip
All Natural Recipe - Neapolitan
All Natural Recipe - Nutty Neapolitan
All Natural Recipe - Vanilla Bean
Creamy Commotions - Moose Tracks
Duetto - Bananas Foster (Limited Edition)
Duetto - Cherry
Duetto - Chocolate and Coconut (Limited Edition)
Duetto - Lemon
Duetto - Mango
Duetto - Raspberry
Duetto - Root Beer

Duetto - Strawberry Banana
Dynamic Duos - Movie Night
Light Ice Cream - Banana Split
Light Ice Cream - Chocolate Chip
Light Ice Cream - Chocolate Nutty
   Moose Tracks
Light Ice Cream - Dulce de Chocolate
Light Ice Cream - Moose Tracks
Light Ice Cream - Raspberry Chocolate
   Chunk
Light Ice Cream - Vanilla Bean
No Sugar Added Ice Cream - Cherry
   Fudge Ripple
No Sugar Added Ice Cream - Dutch
   Chocolate
No Sugar Added Ice Cream - Peanut
   Brittle
No Sugar Added Ice Cream - Vanilla
   Bean
Premium Ice Cream - Banana Split
Premium Ice Cream - Black Cherry
Premium Ice Cream - Black Raspberry
Premium Ice Cream - Butter Pecan
Premium Ice Cream - Choco Mint Chip
Premium Ice Cream - Chocolate
   Marshmallow
Premium Ice Cream - Chocolate Peanut
   Butter Cup
Premium Ice Cream - Colombian Coffee
Premium Ice Cream - Dutch Chocolate
Premium Ice Cream - Eagles
   Touchdown Sundae
Premium Ice Cream - Egg Nog
   (Seasonal)
Premium Ice Cream - French Vanilla
Premium Ice Cream - Fudge Ripple
Premium Ice Cream - Gertrude Hawk
   Box of Chocolate (Limited Edition)
Premium Ice Cream - Neapolitan
Premium Ice Cream - Original Vanilla
Premium Ice Cream - Peaches 'n Cream
   (Seasonal)
Premium Ice Cream - Peanut Butter
   Ripple
Premium Ice Cream - Rocky Road
Premium Ice Cream - Rum Raisin
Premium Ice Cream - Strawberries &
   Cream

Premium Ice Cream - Vanilla &
   Chocolate
Premium Ice Cream - Vanilla Bean
Premium Ice Cream - Vanilla Swiss
   Almond (Limited Edition)
Stuff'd - Moose Tracks
Stuff'd - Nutty Chocolate Moose Tracks

Winn-Dixie ⓘ
Chocolate Chip Ice Cream
Classic Chocolate Ice Cream
Classic Neapolitan Ice Cream
Classic Vanilla Ice Cream

JUICE & JUICE DRINKS

Dole ⓘ
100% Juice Products

Giant
Frozen Concentrate 100% Grape Juice
Frozen Concentrate Cranberry Cocktail
Frozen Concentrate Grape Cocktail
Frozen Concentrate Lemonade
Frozen Concentrate Limeade
Frozen Concentrate Orange Juice
Frozen Concentrate Pink Lemonade
Frozen Concentrate White Grape
   Cocktail
Frozen Concentrate Wildberry Punch
Fruit Punch (Green, Red)

Great Value (Wal-Mart)
Frozen Concentrated 100% Grape Juice
Frozen Concentrated Apple Juice
Frozen Concentrated Country Style
   Orange Juice
Frozen Concentrated Florida Grapefruit
   Juice
Frozen Concentrated Fruit Punch
Frozen Concentrated Grape Juice Drink
Frozen Concentrated Lemonade
Frozen Concentrated Limeade
Frozen Concentrated Orange Juice
Frozen Concentrated Orange Juice w/
   Calcium
Frozen Concentrated Pink Lemonade

Hy-Vee
Apple Juice Frozen Concentrate
Fruit Punch Frozen Concentrate

Grape Juice Cocktail Frozen Concentrate
Lemonade Frozen Concentrate
Limeade Frozen Concentrate
Orange Juice Frozen Concentrate
Orange Juice with Added Calcium Frozen
Pineapple Juice From Concentrate
Pink Lemonade Frozen Concentrate

Laura Lynn (Ingle's)
Frozen Juice (All)

Meijer
Frozen Apple Juice Concentrate
Frozen Fruit Punch Concentrate
Frozen Grape Juice Concentrate
Frozen Grapefruit Juice Concentrate
Frozen Lemonade Concentrate
Frozen Limeade Concentrate
Frozen Orange Juice Concentrate
Frozen Orange Juice Concentrate High Pulp
Frozen Pink Lemonade Concentrate

Old Orchard
Old Orchard (All)

Publix ()
Frozen Concentrated Orange Juice

Stop & Shop
Frozen Concentrate 100% Grape Juice
Frozen Concentrate Apple Juice
Frozen Concentrate Cranberry Cocktail
Frozen Concentrate Fruit Punch
Frozen Concentrate Grape Cocktail
Frozen Concentrate Lemonade
Frozen Concentrate Limeade
Frozen Concentrate Orange Juice
Frozen Concentrate Pink Lemonade
Frozen Concentrate White Grape Cocktail
Frozen Concentrate Wildberry Punch

Welch's
Welch's (All)

Winn-Dixie ⓘ
Frozen Grape Juice Cocktail

MEAT

Applegate Farms ⓘ
Applegate Farms (All BUT Chicken Nuggets, Chicken Pot Pie, & Chicken Strips)

Bubba Burger ⚕
Bubba Burger (All)

Empire Kosher
Frozen Chicken
Frozen Ground Turkey
Frozen Whole Turkey & Turkey Breasts
Individually Quick Frozen Chicken Parts

Garrett County Farms
Frozen Chicken Apple Breakfast Links
Frozen Original Breakfast Links
Frozen Sunrise Maple Breakfast Links
Frozen Turkey Maple Breakfast Links

Jennie-O Turkey Store
Frozen Ground Seasoned Turkey
Frozen Ground Turkey
Frozen Turkey Breast (Gravy packet NOT GF)
Frozen Turkey Burgers
Prime Young Turkey - Frozen (Gravy packet NOT GF)

Kroger ⓘ
Frozen Plain Chicken Breast
Frozen Plain Chicken Thighs
Frozen Plain Chicken Wings
Frozen Plain Turkey Breast
Frozen Plain Turkey Thighs

Manor House (Safeway)
Frozen Enhanced Turkey

Meijer
Breast Split Frozen
Breast Tenders Frozen
Frozen Duckling
Frozen Turkey Breast
Frozen Turkey Breast Young

Perdue ⓘ
Individually Frozen - Chicken Breasts
Individually Frozen - Chicken Tenderloins
Individually Frozen - Chicken Wings

Philly-Gourmet
100% Pure Beef Homestyle Patties
All Beef Sandwich Steaks

Pilgrim's Pride
Marinated Individually Quick Frozen - Boneless/Skinless Breasts
Marinated Individually Quick Frozen - Boneless/Skinless Thighs
Marinated Individually Quick Frozen - Drum
Marinated Individually Quick Frozen - Drummettes
Marinated Individually Quick Frozen - Split Breast
Marinated Individually Quick Frozen - Tenderloins
Marinated Individually Quick Frozen - Thigh
Marinated Individually Quick Frozen - Wing Sections

Publix ()
Frozen Boneless Skinless Chicken Breasts
Frozen Boneless Skinless Chicken Cutlets
Frozen Chicken Breast Tenderloins
Frozen Chicken Wingettes

Quaker Maid Meats
100% Pure Beef Homestyle Patties
Philly Steak, The
Pure Beef Sandwich Steaks

Rosina ⓘ
Rosina Sausage Meatballs

Shelton's
Chicken Franks ♨
Smoked Chicken Franks ♨
Smoked Turkey Franks ♨
Turkey Bologna ♨
Turkey Breakfast Strips ♨
Turkey Burgers ♨
Turkey Franks ♨

NOVELTIES

Dibs
Chocolate
Mint

Vanilla

Dreyer's
Black Cherry/Strawberry/Kiwi/Mixed Berry No Sugar Added Fruit Bar
Cherry/Grape/Tropical Mini Snack Size Fruit Bars
Creamy Coconut Fruit Bar
Grape Fruit Bar
Lemonade Fruit Bar
Lime Fruit Bar
Lime/Strawberry/Wildberry Fruit Bar Pack
Orange & Cream Fruit Bar
Orange & Cream/Raps Cream/Lime Cream Mini Snack Size Fruit Bars
Raspberry/Strawberry/Tangerine No Sugar Added Fruit Bar
Strawberry Fruit Bar
Tangerine Fruit Bar

Edy's
see Dreyer's

Eskimo Pie ⓘ
Dark Chocolate Coated Vanilla Bar
Dark Chocolate Coated Vanilla Club
King Size Orginial Vanilla Bar
No Sugar Added Ice Cream Bar

Gaga's SherBetter ⓘ
SherBetter on a Stick - Chocolate
SherBetter on a Stick - Lemon
SherBetter on a Stick - Orange
SherBetter on a Stick - Raspberry

Giant
Chocolate Ice Cream Cups
Citrus Pops
Jr Pops
No Sugar Added Fudge Pops
Orange Cream Bars
Twin Pops
Vanilla Ice Cream Cup

Hood
Citrus Stix
Fudge Stix
Hoodsie Cups
Hoodsie Pops - 6 Flavor Assortment Twin Pops
Hoodsie Sundae Cups
Ice Cream Bar

Kids Karnival Stix
Kids Stix
Mix Stix
Orange Cream Bar
Pop Stix

Hy-Vee
Assorted Twin Pops
Chocolate & Strawberry Sundae Cups
Fat Free No Sugar Added Fudge Bars
Fudge Bars
Galaxy Bars
Pops - Cherry, Orange & Grape
Reduced Fat Galaxy Bars

Julie's Organic ()
Gluten-Free Ice Cream Sandwich

Kidz Dream ✓
Berry Blast
Orange Creamsicle

Lucerne (Safeway)
Fudge Ice Cream Bars
Orange Ice Cream Bars
Root Beer Float Ice Cream Bars
Toffee Brittle Ice Cream Bars
Vanilla Ice Cream Bars
Vanilla Sundae Ice Cream Bars
Vanilla Sundae Ice Cream Cups
Vanilla/Sherbet Ice Cream Bars

Meijer
Brr Bar
Dream Bars
Frozen Novelties - Gold Bar
Frozen Novelties - Toffee Bar
Fudge Bars
Ice Cream Bars
Juice Stix
No Sugar Added Fudge Bars
No Sugar Added Party Pops (Assorted)
Orange Glider
Red White and Blue Pops
Toffee Bars
Twin Pops

Minute Maid
Juice Bars - Orange, Cherry, and Grape

Nestlé Ice Cream
Frozen Lemonade Cup
Frozen Strawberry Lemonade Cup
Itzakadoozie Ice Pop

Laffy Taffy Push Up
Loaded Butterfinger Bar
Push-Up Orange
Push-Up Rainbow
Triple Blast Ice Pop

Organic So Delicious Dairy Free ✓
Creamy Fudge Bar
Creamy Vanilla Bar
Vanilla & Almonds Bar

Publix ()
Banana Pops
Cream Pops
Fudge Bar
Fudge Sundae Cups
Ice Cream Bar
Ice Cream Squares
No Sugar Added Fudge Pops
No Sugar Added Ice Cream Bars
No Sugar Added Ice Cream Squares
No Sugar Added Ice Pop
Orange, Cherry and Grape Junior Ice Pops
Red White and Blue Junior Ice Pops
Toffee Bar
Twin Pops
Vanilla Cups

Purely Decadent Dairy Free ✓
Purely Vanilla Bar
Vanilla Almond Bar

Rice Dream ✓
Vanilla Bites

Safeway
Assorted Ice Pops
Basic Red Vanilla Ice Cream
Kreme Koolers
Select - Caramel Caribou Ice Cream Bars
Select - Fruit Bars (All flavors)

Skinny Cow, The ⓘ
Chocolate Truffle Bars
French Vanilla Truffle Bars
Low Fat Fudge Bars
Skinny Mini Fudge Bars
Vanilla and Caramel Skinny Dippers
Vanilla and Mint Skinny Dippers

So Delicious Dairy Free ✓
Creamy Orange Bar

Creamy Raspberry Bar
Kidz - Assorted Fruit Pops
Kidz - Fudge Pops
Sweet Nothings ✓
Fudge Bar
Mango Raspberry Bar
Welch's
Welch's (All)

PIZZA & CRUSTS

Amy's Kitchen ⓘ ✓
Rice Crust Cheese Pizza
Rice Crust Spinach Pizza
Chebe 😋 ✓
Pizza Crust Mix
Conte's Pasta ✓
Margherita Pizza
Mushroom Florentine Pizza
Prebaked Pizza Shell
Ener-G 😋
Rice Pizza Shells
Yeast Free Rice Pizza Shells
Foods by George 😋
Pizza
Pizza Crusts
Gluten-Free & Fabulous 😋 ✓
Cheese Pizza
Pepperoni Pizza
Pizza Crust
Glutino 😋 ✓
Pizza - 3 Cheese with Brown Rice Crust
Pizza - Duo Cheese
Pizza - Spinach & Feta
Pizza - Spinach Soy Cheese with Brown
Rice Crust
Mariposa Baking Company 😋
Pizza Crust

POTATOES

Alexia Foods ⓘ 😋
Potato Products
Bob Evans ()
Seasoned Hashbrowns
Seasoned Home Fries

Diner's Choice
Diner's Choice (All)
Dr. Praeger's ✓
Potato Littles
Sweet Potato Littles
Sweet Potato Pancakes
Giant
Crinkle Cut French Fries
Crispy Fries
Extra Crispy Crinkle Cut Fries
Hash O' Brien
Puffs with Onions
Shoestring Fries
Shredded Hash Browns
Southwestern Style Hash Browns
Steak Fries
Straight Cut French Fries
Hy-Vee
Frozen Country Style Hash Brown
Potatoes
Frozen Crinkle Cut Fries
Frozen Criss Cut Potatoes
Frozen Steak Fries
Hash Browns Real Russet Potatoes
Ingles Markets
Broccoli & Cheese Potato
Kroger ⓘ
Plain Frozen Potatoes - Salted
Laura Lynn (Ingle's)
Frozen Potato Skins (All)
Meijer
Frozen French Fries
Frozen French Fries Crinkle Cut
Frozen French Fries Quickie Crinkles
Frozen French Fries Shoestring
Frozen French Fries Steak Cut
Frozen Hashbrowns
Frozen Hashbrowns - Shredded
Frozen Hashbrowns - Southern Style
Frozen Hashbrowns - Western Style
Frozen Potatoes - Tater Tots
Frozen Potatoes - Tater Treats
Ore-Ida ⓘ
ABC Tater Tots
Cottage Fries
Country Fries
Country Style Hashbrowns

Country Style Steak Fries
Crispers
Extra Crispy Crinkle Cut
Extra Crispy Fast Food Fries
Extra Crispy Seasoned Crinkle Cut
Fast Food Fries
French Fries
Golden Crinkles
Golden Fries
Golden Patties
Golden Twirls
Hash Browns
Pixie Crinkles
Potato Wedges with Skins
Potatoes O'Brien
Shoestrings
Southern Style Hash Browns
Steak Fries
Steam n' Mash Cut Russets
Steam n' Mash Cut Sweet Potatoes
Steam n' Mash Garlic Seasoned Potatoes
Steam n' Mash Three Cheese Potatoes
Tater Tots (All Varieties)
Waffle Fries
Zesties
Zesty Twirls

Publix ()

Crinkle Cut Fries
Golden Fries
Shoestring Fries
Southern Style Hash Browns
Steak Fries
Tater Bites
Tater Puffs

Safeway

Crinkle Cut Potatoes
Crispy Fries
French Fried Potatoes
Hash Browns - Country Style
Hash Browns - Shredded
Hash Browns - Southern Style
O'Brien Potatoes
Potato Sticks
Restaurant Style Crinkle Cut Potatoes
Shoestring Potatoes
Steak Cut Potatoes
Twice Baked Potatoes

Simply Potatoes

Simply Potatoes (All)

Smart Ones ⓘ

Broccoli & Cheddar Potatoes

Stop & Shop

Butter Twice Baked Potatoes
Cheddar Cheese Twice Baked Potatoes
Crinkle Cut French Fries
Crispy Fries
Extra Crispy Crinkle Cut Fries
Frozen Natural Wedges
Latkes
Puffs with Onions
Shoestring Fries
Shredded Hash Browns
Sour Cream & Chive Twice Baked
    Potatoes
Southwestern Style Hash Browns
Steak Fries
Straight Cut French Fries

PREPARED MEALS & SIDES

Amy's Kitchen ⓘ ✓

Asian Noodle Stir-Fry
Baked Ziti Bowl
Black Bean & Vegetable Enchilada
Black Bean & Vegetable Enchilada -
    Light in Sodium
Black Bean Enchilada Whole Meal
Brown Rice & Vegetable Bowl
Brown Rice & Vegetables Bowl - Light
    in Sodium
Brown Rice with Black-Eyed Peas &
    Veggies Bowl
Cheese Enchilada
Cheese Enchilada Whole Meal
Garden Vegetable Lasagna
Indian Mattar Paneer
Indian Mattar Paneer - Light in Sodium
Indian Mattar Tofu
Indian Palak Paneer
Indian Paneer Tikka
Indian Vegetable Korma
Mexican Casserole Bowl
Mexican Casserole Bowl - Light in
    Sodium

Mexican Tamale Pie
Rice Macaroni & Cheese
Santa Fe Enchilada Bowl
Shephard's Pie
Teriyaki Bowl
Thai Stir-Fry
Tofu Rancheros
Tofu Scramble

Bell & Evans ⓘ ✔
Chicken Burgers
Flavored Fully Cooked Breasts
Flavored Fully Cooked Wings
Gluten-Free Breaded Chicken Breasts
Gluten-Free Breaded Chicken Patties
Gluten-Free Chicken Nuggets
Gluten-Free Chicken Tenders
Gluten-Free Garlic Parmesan Breaded
   Chicken Breast
Gluten-Free Italian Style Breaded
   Chicken Patties
Grilled Chicken Breasts

Bob Evans ()
Bacon & Potato Brunch Bowl
Ham & Potato Brunch Bowl

Omelet Brunch Bowl with Potatoes
Omelet Brunch Bowl with Sausage
   Patties
Sausage & Potato Brunch Bowl

CedarLane Natural Foods
Five Layer Mexican Dip
Low Fat Black Bean Enchilada Meal
Low Fat Garden Veg Enchilada
Three Layer Enchilada Pie

Coleman Natural ✔
Gourmet Chicken Meatballs - Chipotle
   Cheddar
Gourmet Chicken Meatballs - Italian
   Parmesan
Gourmet Chicken Meatballs - Sun-
   Dried Tomato Basil Provolone

Coleman Organic ✔
Chicken Wings - Buffalo Style

Conte's Pasta ✔
Cheese Lasagna Microwave Meal
Cheese Ravioli
Cheese Ravioli Microwave Meal
Gnocchi
Manicotti w/Tomato Sauce Microwave
   Meal
Meat Lasagna Microwave Meal
Pierogi (Potato/Cheese/Onion)
Pierogi (Potato/Onion)
Spaghetti w/Meatballs And Tomato
   Sauce Microwave Meal
Spinach & Cheese Ravioli
Stuffed Shells
Stuffed Shells w/Tomato Sauce
   Microwave Meal
Vegetable Lasagna Microwave Meal

Contessa ⚕
Jambalaya
Paella
Roasted Chicken with Honey Sauce
Seafood Veracruz
Shrimp on the Bar-B
Shrimp Santa Fe
Shrimp Scampi
Whiskey Jack Shrimp

Delimex ⓘ
3-Cheese Taquitos
Beef Tamales

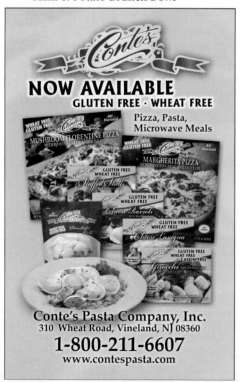

Beef Taquitos
Chicken & Cheese Tamales
Chicken Taquitos

Dr. Praeger's ✓
Broccoli Little
Potato Crusted Fillet Fish Sticks
Potato Crusted Fish Fillets
Potato Crusted Fishies
Spinach Littles

El Monterey
Beef Corn Taquitos
Cheese Enchilada Dinner
Chicken Corn Taquitos
Spicy Beef Enchilada Dinner
Steak Corn Taquitos

Empire Kosher
Fully Cooked Barbecue Chicken (Fresh Or Frozen)
Fully Cooked Barbecue Turkey (Fresh Or Frozen)

Farm Rich
Meatballs ⓘ

Garrett County Farms
Dino Shaped Chicken Bites
Uncured Beef Corn Dogs
Uncured Chicken Corn Dogs

Giant
Spinach, Artichoke & Cheese Dip
Wings - Buffalo
Wings - Honey BBQ

Gluten Free Café ✓
Asian Noodles
Fettuccini Alfredo
Homestyle Chicken & Vegetables
Lemon Basil Chicken
Pasta Primavera
Savory Chicken Pilaf

Glutenfreeda ⚋ ✓
Burritos (All)

Glutino ⚋ ✓
Chicken Pad Thai
Chicken Penne Alfredo
Chicken Pomodoro
Chicken Ranchero
Duo Penne Mushroom

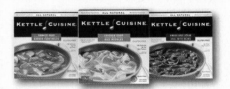

All natural. All gluten free.
All new packaging.

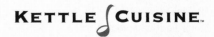

Look for our soups, chilis, and chowders
in your grocer's natural food freezer.
www.kettlecuisine.com

Macaroni & Cheese

Penne Alfredo

Goya

Classic Entrees - Ground Beef, Potatoes in Seasoned Sauce with Rice

Classic Entrees - Pigeon Peas & Rice

Classic Entrees - Rice with Chicken

Henry & Lisa's ✓

Gluten-Free Wild Alaskan Battered Fish Nuggets

Wild Alaskan Salmon Burgers

Ian's Natural Foods 🦴 ✓

Wheat and Gluten-Free Recipe Alphatots

Wheat and Gluten-Free Recipe Chicken Finger Kids Meal

Wheat and Gluten-Free Recipe Chicken Nuggets

Wheat and Gluten-Free Recipe Chicken Patties

Wheat and Gluten-Free Recipe Egg & Maple Cheddar Wafflewich

Wheat and Gluten-Free Recipe Fish Sticks

Wheat and Gluten-Free Recipe French Bread Pizza

Wheat and Gluten-Free Recipe French Toast Sticks

Wheat and Gluten-Free Recipe Lightly Battered Fish

Wheat and Gluten-Free Recipe Mac & Meat Sauce

Wheat and Gluten-Free Recipe Mac & No Cheese

Wheat and Gluten-Free Recipe Maple Sausage and Egg Wafflewich

Wheat and Gluten-Free Recipe Popcorn Turkey Corn Dogs

Ingles Markets

Chicken Santa Fe

Lemon Herb Chicken Piccata

Sante Fe Rice & Beans

Jennie-O Turkey Store

Frozen Italian Meatballs

Kettle Cuisine ✓

Angus Beef Steak Chili with Beans

Chicken Chili with White Beans

Chicken Soup with Rice Noodles

Grilled Chicken and Corn Chowder

New England Clam Chowder

Organic Carrot and Coriander Soup

Organic Mushroom and Potato Soup

Roasted Vegetable Soup

Three Bean Chili

Tomato Soup with Garden Vegetables

Mama Lucia

Sausage Meatballs Made with Beef

Margaritaville Shrimp 🦴 ✓

Island Lime Shrimp

Jammin Jerk Shrimp

Sunset Scampi

Moosewood

Chilaquile Casserole

Nate's

Bean, Rice & Cheese Taquito

Black Bean & Soy Cheese Taquito

Chunky Vegetable Taquito

Three Cheese Taquito

PJ's Organics

Bean & Cheese Tamale Meal

Beef Enchilada Meal

Chicken Enchilada Meal

Chicken Tamale Meal

Deluxe Chicken Taquito

Pork Tamale Meal

Traditional Chicken Taquito

Rice Expressions ⓘ

Rice Expressions (All)

Safeway

Select - Gourmet Club Eating Right Chicken Lettuce Wraps

Select - Gourmet Club Eating Right Ginger Chicken

Simply Enjoy (Giant)

Butter Chicken

Pad Thai with Chicken

Tikka Masala

Simply Enjoy (Stop & Shop)

Butter Chicken

Pad Thai with Chicken

Tikka Masala

Smart Ones ⓘ

Chicken Santa Fe

Creamy Tuscan Chicken

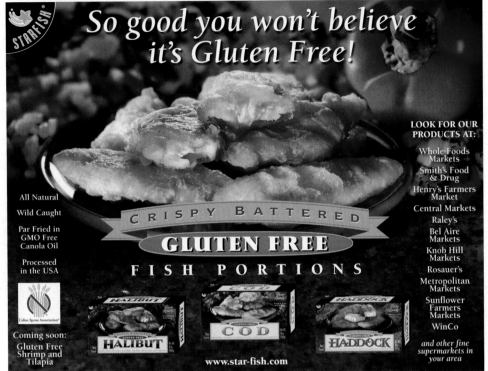
Fiesta Chicken
Grilled Chicken in Garlic Herb Sauce
Home-Style Chicken
Lemon Herb Chicken Piccata
Santa Fe Rice & Beans

South Beach Living 〰
Frozen Entrees - Caprese Style Chicken
Frozen Entrees - Savory Beef

Starfish
Gluten-Free Battered Cod ✓
Gluten-Free Battered Haddock ✓
Gluten-Free Battered Halibut ✓

Stop & Shop
Buffalo Style Wings
Honey BBQ Wings
Spinach, Artichoke & Cheese Dip

Tabatchnick Fine Foods
Balsamic Tomato & Rice
Black Bean Soup
Cabbage Soup
Corn Chowder
Cream of Broccoli
Cream of Spinach
Creamed Spinach

Lentil Soup
New England Potato
No Salt Spilt Pea Soup
Old Fashioned Potato
Southwest Bean
Split Pea Soup
Vegetarian Chili
Wilderness Wild Rice
Yankee Bean

Wellshire Farms ✓
Dino Shaped Chicken Bites
Uncured Beef Corn Dogs
Uncured Chicken Corn Dogs

SAUSAGE

Jones Dairy Farm ⑃
All Natural Golden Brown Fully Cooked
& Browned Sausage Patties
All Natural Golden Brown Light Fully
Cooked & Browned Sausage & Rice
Links

FAN GLUTENFREE TASTIC

Why are we calling attention to the fact that Jones All Natural Sausage contains no gluten and none of the ingredients hidden in other brands? Because we thought you'd like to know. It's just pork, salt and spices—has been for over 120 years. Plus our sausage is frozen so it's always fresh. Always fantastic.

Visit **jonesdairyfarm.com/gluten-free** for great recipes and special savings.

NO nitrites

NO MSG

NO artificial flavors

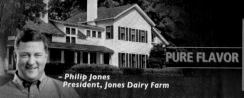

– *Philip Jones*
President, Jones Dairy Farm

PURE FLAVOR **SIMPLE PLEASURE**

SINCE 1889
JONES
DAIRY FARM®

ALL NATURAL SAUSAGE • HAM • BACON • CANADIAN BACON • BRAUNSCHWEIGER GF

All Natural Golden Brown Made From
  Beef Fully Cooked & Browned Sausage
  Links
All Natural Golden Brown Mild Fully
  Cooked & Browned Sausage Links
All Natural Golden Brown Spicy Fully
  Cooked & Browned Sausage Links
All Natural Hearty Pork Sausages
All Natural Light Pork Sausage & Rice
  Links
All Natural Little Pork Sausages
All Natural Original Pork Sausage Roll
All Natural Pork Sausage Patties

Shelton's
Turkey Breakfast Sausage Links
Turkey Italian Sausage Links
Turkey Sausage Patties

Wellshire Farms ✔
Frozen Chicken Apple Patties
Frozen Chicken Apple Sausage Links
Frozen Country Sage Sausage Links
Frozen Country Sage Sausage Patties
Frozen Original Breakfast Sausage Links
Frozen Original Breakfast Sausage
  Patties
Frozen Sunrise Maple Sausage Links
Frozen Sunrise Maple Sausage Patties
Frozen Turkey Maple Patties
Frozen Turkey Maple Sausage Links

SHERBET & SORBET

Dreyer's
Berry Rainbow Sherbet
Orange Cream Sherbet
Root Beer Float
Swiss Orange Sherbet
Tropical Rainbow Sherbet

Edy's
see Dreyer's

Gaga's SherBetter ⓘ
Chocolate
Lemon
Orange
Rainbow
Raspberry

Giant
Lemon Lime Sherbet
Orange Sherbet
Pineapple Sherbet
Rainbow Sherbet
Raspberry Sherbet

Guaranteed Value (Stop & Shop)
Rainbow Sherbet

Hood
New England Creamery - Black
  Raspberry Sherbet
New England Creamery - Orange
  Sherbet
New England Creamery - Rainbow
  Sherbet
New England Creamery - Wildberry
  Sherbet
Sherbet (All)

Hy-Vee
Lime Sherbet
Orange Sherbet
Pineapple Sherbet
Rainbow Sherbet
Raspberry Sherbet

Meijer
Cherry Sherbert
Lemonberry Twist Sherbet
Lime Sherbet
Orange Sherbet
Pineapple Sherbet
Rainbow Sherbet
Raspberry Sherbet

Publix ()
Cool Lime Sherbet
Exotic Fruit Medley Sherbet
No Sugar Added Sunny Orange Sherbet
Peach Mango Passion Sherbet
Rainbow Dream Sherbet
Raspberry Blush Sherbet
Sunny Orange Sherbet
Tropic Pineapple Sherbet
Tropical Swirl Sherbet

Safeway
Chocolate Sorbet
Key Lime Sherbet
Lemon Crunch Sherbet
Raspberry Sorbet

Sambazon
  Sambazon (All)
Turkey Hill ⓘ
  Sherbet - Fruit Rainbow
  Sherbet - Orange Grove
  Venice Premium Ice - Mango
  Venice Premium Ice -Cherry Lemon

VEGETABLES

Birds Eye Foods
  Baby Blends Baby Corn & Vegetable Blend
  Baby Blends Baby Corn, Bean & Pea Mix
  Baby Blends Baby Mixed Beans & Carrots
  Baby Blends Baby Pea & Vegetable Blend
  Baby Vegetables Baby Broccoli Florets
  Baby Vegetables Baby Gold & White Corn
  Baby Vegetables Baby Sweet Peas
  Baby Vegetables Baby White Corn Kernels
  Baby Vegetables Cauliflower Florets
  Baby Vegetables White Pearl Onions
  Box Sauce Creamed Spinach with Real Cream Sauce
  Box Sauce Green Beans & Lightly Toasted Almonds
  Box Sauce Pearl Onions In A Real Cream Sauce
  Box Sauce Peas & Pearl Onions In Lightly Season Sauce
  Box Sauce Roasted Potatoes & Broccoli
  Box Sauce Sweet Corn & Butter Sauce
  Box Sauce Tuscan Vegetables In Herbed Tomato Sauce
  Broccoli Stir-Fry
  Classic Vegetables Baby Lima Beans
  Classic Vegetables Broccoli Spears
  Classic Vegetables Classic Mixed Vegetables
  Classic Vegetables Cut Green Beans
  Classic Vegetables Cut Leaf Spinach
  Classic Vegetables French Cut Green Beans
  Classic Vegetables Sweet Garden Peas
  Classic Vegetables Sweet Kernel Corn
  Classic Vegetables Tender Broccoli Cuts
  Corn On The Cob Sweet Corn On The Cob
  Corn On The Cob Sweet Mini Corn On The Cob
  Deluxe Box Artichoke Hearts
  Deluxe Box Asparagus Spears
  Deluxe Box Baby Peas
  Deluxe Box Broccoli Florets
  Deluxe Box Brussels Sprouts
  Deluxe Box Fordhook Lima Beans
  Deluxe Box Sugar Snap Peas
  Farm Fresh Broccoli & Cauliflower
  Farm Fresh Broccoli, Carrots, & Water Chestnuts
  Farm Fresh Broccoli, Cauliflower & Carrots
  Farm Fresh Broccoli, Corn & Peppers
  Freshlike Baby Blends Blend, Baby Asparagus
  Freshlike Baby Blends Blend, Baby Corn
  Freshlike Baby Blends Blend, Baby, Beans/Carrot
  Freshlike Blends Blend, California
  Freshlike Blends Stir Fry Broccoli
  Freshlike Classic Vegetables Beans, Cut Green
  Freshlike Classic Vegetables Beans, French Cut Green
  Freshlike Classic Vegetables Broccoli, Cut
  Freshlike Classic Vegetables Carrots, Sliced
  Freshlike Classic Vegetables Corn, Cut
  Freshlike Classic Vegetables Mixed Vegetables
  Freshlike Classic Vegetables Peas, Garden
  Freshlike Classic Vegetables Veg For Soup
  Freshlike Classic Vegetables Veg For Stew
  Freshlike Deluxe Box Spinach, Chopped

Freshlike Select Vegetables Cauliflower Florets

Freshlike Select Vegetables Corn, Gold & White

Freshlike Select Vegetables Corn, White

Freshlike Select Vegetables Peas, Tiny

Freshlike Stir-Fry Blend, Broccoli Stir Fry

Pepper Stir-Fry

Premium Vegetables Broccoli Florets

Premium Vegetables California Blend

Premium Vegetables Normandy Blend

Premium Vegetables Whole Green Beans

Select Box - Cooked Winter Squash

Select Box Broccoli Spears

Select Box Chopped Broccoli

Select Box Chopped Spinach

Select Box Classic Mixed Vegetables

Select Box Cut Green Beans

Select Box French Cut Green Beans

Select Box Garden Peas

Select Box Leaf Spinach

Select Box Sweet Kernel Corn

Steam And Serve Balsamic Glazed Vegetables

Steam And Serve Beans with A Twist

Steam And Serve Italian Herb Harvest Vegetables

Steam And Serve Lemon Pepper Vegetables

Steam And Serve Savory Brussels Sprouts

Steam And Serve Spring Vegetables In Citrus Sauce

Steamfresh Lightly Sauced Corn with Butter Sauce

Steamfresh Lightly Sauced Roasted Red Potatoes with Chive Butter Sauce

Steamfresh Mixtures Asparagus, Corn & Baby Carrots

Steamfresh Mixtures Baby Broccoli Blend

Steamfresh Mixtures Baby Potato Blend

Steamfresh Mixtures Broccoli & Cauliflower

Steamfresh Mixtures Broccoli, Carrots, Sugar Snap Peas, Wtr Chs

Steamfresh Mixtures Broccoli, Cauliflower, & Carrots

Steamfresh Mixtures Italian Blend

Steamfresh Premium Broccoli Florets

Steamfresh Premium Brussels Sprouts

Steamfresh Premium Gold And White Corn

Steamfresh Premium Sugar Snap Peas

Steamfresh Premium Sweet Mini Corn On The Cob

Steamfresh Premium Whole Green Beans

Steamfresh Selects Broccoli Cuts

Steamfresh Selects Cut Green Beans

Steamfresh Selects Mixed Vegetables

Steamfresh Selects Super Sweet Corn

Steamfresh Selects Sweet Peas

Steamfresh Single Serve Baby Brussels Sprouts

Steamfresh Single Serve Super Sweet Corn

Steamfresh Single Serve Sweet Peas

Sugar Snap Stir-Fry

Grand Selections (Hy-Vee)

Frozen Caribbean Blend Vegetables

Frozen Normandy Blend Vegetables

Frozen Petite Green Peas

Frozen Petite Whole Carrots

Frozen Riviera Blend Vegetables

Frozen Sugar Snap Peas

Frozen Super Sweet Cut Corn

Frozen White Shoepeg Corn

Frozen Whole Green Beans

Great Value (Wal-Mart)

"Golden" Whole Kernel Corn Microwavable

Broccoli & Cauliflower

Broccoli Cuts

Broccoli Florets

Broccoli, Cauliflower, & Carrots

California Style Vegetable Mix

Cauliflower

Corn On The Cob

Cut Broccoli

Cut Corn On The Cob

Cut Green Beans

Cut Leaf Spinach

Extra Long, All Green Asparagus Spears
Microwavable Diced Carrots
Microwaveable Sweet Peas
Mixed Vegetables
Seasoned Mixed Garden Medley
Vegetable Medley

Hy-Vee
Corn On The Cob
Cream Style Golden Corn
Frozen Broccoli Cuts
Frozen Broccoli Florets
Frozen Brussels Sprouts
Frozen California Mix
Frozen Cauliflower Florets
Frozen Chopped Broccoli
Frozen Chopped Spinach
Frozen Crinkle Cut Carrots
Frozen Cut Golden Corn
Frozen Cut Green Beans
Frozen French Cut Green Beans
Frozen Italian Blend
Frozen Leaf Spinach
Frozen Mixed Vegetables
Frozen Oriental Vegetables
Frozen Sweet Peas
Frozen Winter Mix
Mini Corn On The Cob
Whole Kernel Golden Corn

Kroger ⓘ
Plain Frozen Vegetables

Laura Lynn (Ingle's)
Frozen Vegetables (All BUT Breaded Okra)

Meijer
Frozen Beans - Green Cut
Frozen Beans - Green French Cut
Frozen Beans - Green Italian Cut
Frozen Broccoli Chopped
Frozen Carrots Crinkle Cut
Frozen Carrots Whole Baby
Frozen Cauliflower Florets
Frozen Chinese Pea Pods
Frozen Collards Chopped
Frozen Corn - Whole Kernel
Frozen Corn - Whole Kernel Golden
Frozen Corn Cob Mini Ear
Frozen Corn on Cob

Frozen Edamame (Soybeans)
Frozen Mixed Vegetables
Frozen Okra - Chopped
Frozen Okra - Whole
Frozen Onions - Chopped
Frozen Organic Green Peas
Frozen Organic Mixed Vegetables
Frozen Peas - Green
Frozen Peas - Green Petite
Frozen Peas & Carrots
Frozen Peppers - Green, Chopped
Frozen Spinach - Chopped
Frozen Spinach - Leaf
Frozen Squash - Cooked
Frozen Vegetables - California Style
Frozen Vegetables - Fiesta
Frozen Vegetables - Florentine
Frozen Vegetables - Italian
Frozen Vegetables - Mexican
Frozen Vegetables - Oriental
Frozen Vegetables - Parisian Style
Frozen Vegetables - Stew Mix
Frozen Vegetables - Stir Fry

Safeway
Select - Organic Peas

Stahlbush Island Farms ⓘ
Stahlbush Island Farms (All)

VEGETARIAN MEAT

Quorn ()
Chicken-Style Tenders
Turkey-Style Roast

VEGGIE BURGERS

Dr. Praeger's ✔
Gluten-Free California Veggie Burger

Nature's Promise (Giant)
Garlic and Cheese Veggie Burger
Soy Vegetable Burger
Vegan Soy Vegetable Burger

Nature's Promise (Stop & Shop)
Garlic & Cheese Veggie Burger
Soy Vegetable Burger
Vegan Soy Vegetable Burger

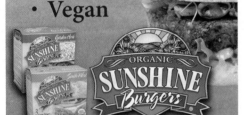

GLUTEN FREE
Veggie Burger

Made from sunflower kernels & brown rice. Available in five delicious flavors.

- **Organic**
- **Soy Free**
- **Vegan**

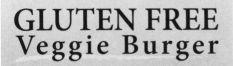

ORGANIC

www.sunshineburger.com

Sunshine Burger ⓘ ♨ ✔
- Barbecue
- Breakfast
- Falafel
- Garden Herb
- Original
- South West

WAFFLES & FRENCH TOAST

Glutino ♨ ✔
- Cinnamon French Toast

Nature's Path ⓘ ✔
- Buckwheat Wildberry Waffles
- Homestyle Waffles
- Mesa Sunrise Waffles

Van's All Natural
- Wheat-Free Apple Cinnamon Waffles
- Wheat-Free Blueberry Waffles
- Wheat-Free Buckwheat Waffles
- Wheat-Free Cinnamon French Toast
- Wheat-Free Flax Waffles
- Wheat-Free Homestyle Waffles
- Wheat-Free Mini Waffles

WHIPPED TOPPINGS

Cool Whip ✑
- Chocolate Whipped Topping
- Free Whipped Topping
- French Vanilla Whipped Topping
- Strawberry Whipped Topping
- Sugar Free Whipped Topping
- Whipped Topping

Giant
- Frozen Whipped Topping - Fat Free
- Frozen Whipped Topping - Lite
- Frozen Whipped Topping - Nondairy
- Frozen Whipped Topping - Regular
- Frozen Whipped Topping - Vanilla

Great Value (Wal-Mart)
- Fat Free Whipped Topping
- Light Whipped Topping
- Whipped Topping

Hy-Vee
- Frozen Extra Creamy Whipped Topping
- Frozen Fat Free Whipped Topping
- Frozen Lite Whipped Topping
- Frozen Whipped Topping

Lucerne (Safeway)
- Whipped Topping - Lactose Free
- Whipped Topping - Light
- Whipped Topping - Regular

Meijer
- Frozen Whipped Topping
- Frozen Whipped Topping Fat Free
- Frozen Whipped Topping Lite

Publix ◇
- Chocolate Whipped Topping (Bakery)

Stop & Shop
- Frozen Whipped Topping - Fat Free
- Frozen Whipped Topping - French Vanilla
- Frozen Whipped Topping - Lite
- Frozen Whipped Topping - Non Dairy
- Frozen Whipped Topping - Regular

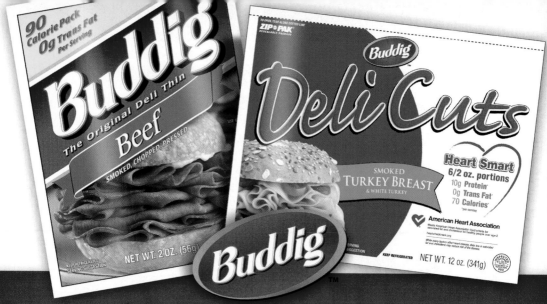

Free of Gluten. Full of Flavor.

Go gluten free with Buddig and Old Wisconsin.® Buddig Original and Deli Cuts are great-tasting, naturally high in protein and low in fat. Deli Cuts have recently been certified by the American Heart Association® to display their heart-check mark, making them an even better way to help you control your diet. Old Wisconsin products offer a wide range of hardwood-smoked beef and turkey meat snacks to fit your lifestyle. Enjoy naturally gluten free lunchmeat and snacks with the Buddig and Old Wisconsin family of products.*

Visit *buddig.com* and *oldwisconsin.com* to learn more or visit your local grocery retailer.

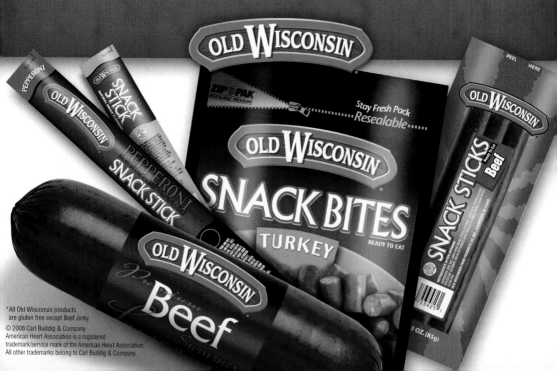

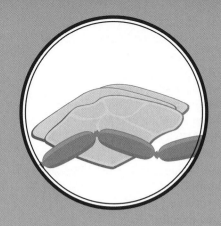

MEAT

BACON

Applegate Farms ⓘ
  Applegate Farms (All BUT Chicken Nuggets, Chicken Pot Pie, & Chicken Strips)

Boar's Head
  Meats (All)

Butcher's Cut (Safeway)
  Bacon (All Varieties, must have EST 13331)

Cloverdale Foods
  Meat Products (All)

Coleman Natural ✓
  Uncured Hickory Smoked Bacon

Garrett County Farms
  Classic Sliced Dry Rubbed Bacon
  Classic Sliced Turkey Bacon
  Sliced Applewood Bacon
  Sliced Canadian Style Bacon
  Thick Sliced Dry Rubbed Bacon
  Turkey Peppered Bacon

Giant
  Sliced Bacon - Regular
  Sliced Bacon - Thick Sliced

Global Gourmet
  Irish Bacon

Great Value (Wal-Mart)
  Hickory Fully Cooked Bacon
  Hickory Smoked Bacon
  Hickory Smoked Bacon Stack Pack
  Lower Sodium Bacon
  Peppered Bacon

Hormel
  Black Label - Bacon

  Canadian Style Bacon
  Fully Cooked Bacon
  Microwave Bacon
  Natural Choice - Canadian Bacon
  Natural Choice - Uncured Bacon
  Pillow Pack - Canadian Bacon

Hy-Vee
  Fully Cooked Turkey Bacon
  Hickory Smoked Fully Cooked Bacon

Jennie-O Turkey Store
  Extra Lean Turkey Bacon
  Turkey Bacon

Jones Dairy Farm ⛉
  Farm Fresh & Tender Sliced Canadian Bacon
  Slab Bacon
  Sliced Bacon - Regular
  Sliced Bacon - Thick

Kroger ⓘ
  Bacon - Plain

Meijer
  Bacon
  Bacon Lower Sodium

Oscar Mayer ⌒
  Bacon
  Center Cut Bacon
  Center Cut Naturally Smoked
  Lower Sodium Bacon
  Natural Hardwood Smoked Bacon
  Natural Smoked Uncured Bacon
  Naturally Hardwood Smoked Bacon
  Ready To Serve Bacon
  Ready To Serve Canadian Bacon
  Ready To Serve Hearty Thick Cut Bacon
  Smokehouse Thick Sliced Center Cut

Patrick Cudahy
Patrick Cudahy (All)

Plumrose ✓
Plumrose (All)

Publix ()
Bacon (All Varieties)

Range Brand
Bacon

Safeway
Pancetta Italian Bacon (Vacuum-
Packed)

Smith's
Smith's (All)

Stop & Shop
Center Cut Sliced Bacon
Lower Sodium Bacon
Maple Flavored Bacon
Regular Sliced Bacon

Wellshire Farms ✓
Bulk Maple Bacon
Canadian Style Bacon Nugget
Classic Sliced Dry Rubbed Bacon
Classic Sliced Turkey Bacon
Dry Rubbed Center Cut Bacon
Fully Cooked Hickory Smoked Bacon
Organic Dry Rubbed Bacon
Organic Turkey Bacon
PA Pork Applewood Smoked Bacon
Peppered Turkey Bacon
Sliced Canadian Brand Turkey Bacon
Sliced Canadian Style Bacon
Sliced Maple Bacon
Sliced Pancetta Bacon
Sliced Peppered Dry Rub Bacon
Sliced Traditional Dry Rubbed Bacon
Thick Sliced Dry Rubbed Bacon
Whole Pancetta Bacon

BEEF

Applegate Farms (i)
Applegate Farms (All BUT Chicken
Nuggets, Chicken Pot Pie, & Chicken
Strips)

Boar's Head
Meats (All)

Buddig ⸸
Original Buddig - Beef
Original Buddig - Corned Beef
Original Buddig - Pastrami

Butcher's Cut (Safeway)
Beef Burgers
Bulk Wrapped Corned Beef Brisket
Corned Beef
Corned Beef Brisket

Columbus Salame
Columbus Products (All)

Fast Classics (i)
Bacon Cheeseburger
Beef Burger

Fast Fixin' ()
Philly Beef
Restaurant Style - Black Angus Burger

Garrett County Farms
Corned Beef Brisket Half
Sliced Beef Bologna
Sliced Beef Salami
Sliced Corned Beef
Sliced Roast Beef
Whole Corned Beef Brisket
Whole Roast Beef

Great Value (Wal-Mart)
100% Pure Beef Patties (75/25)
100% Pure Beef Patties (80/20)
100% Pure Beef Patties (85/15)
Beef Philly Steak
Luncheon Meat
Thinly Sliced Seasoned Roast Beef

Homestyle Meals
Shredded Beef in BBQ Sauce

Hormel
Always Tender - Flavored Fresh Beef
Peppercorn
Deli Sliced Cooked Corned Beef
Deli Sliced Cooked Pastrami
Deli Sliced Seasoned Roast Beef
Natural Choice - Roast Beef
Pillow Pack - Dried Beef

Hy-Vee
Luncheon Meat
Quarter Pounders
Thin Sliced Beef
Thin Sliced Corned Beef

Thin Sliced Pastrami

Isaly's ◊
Deli Meats (All)

Land O' Frost
Lunchmeats (All BUT Taste Escapes Lemon Pepper Chicken)

Meijer
Beef Slice Chipped Meats
Corned Beef Sliced Chipped Meat
Pastrami Sliced Chipped Meat

Nature's Promise (Giant)
Deli Meats (All Varieties)

Nature's Promise (Stop & Shop)
Deli Meats (All Varieties)

Oscar Mayer 🖉
Deli Fresh Meats - Roast Beef Slow Roasted Shaved
Deli Fresh Meats - Shaved Cajun Seasoned Tray
Deli Fresh Meats - Shaved French Dip Tray

Papa Charlie's ⓘ
Thinly Sliced Seasoned Cooked Roast Beef

Plumrose ✓
Plumrose (All)

Primo Taglio (Safeway)
Cooked Corned Beef (Bulk Deli Meat)
Pastrami Coated with Spices (Bulk Deli Meat)
Seasoned Roast Beef (Coated with Seasonings) (Bulk Deli Meat)

Publix GreenWise Market ◊
Beef Back Ribs
Beef Cubed Steak
Beef for Stew

Publix ◊
Corned Beef (Pre-Packed Sliced Deli Lunch Meats)
Peppered Beef (Pre-Packed Sliced Deli Lunch Meats)

Redi•Serve ⓘ
Beef Burgers
Rib Quik

Saag's ⓘ ✓
Saag's Specialty Meats (All BUT Saag's British Bangers)

Sabrett
Hamburgers

Safeway
Cooked Corned Beef (Vacuum-Packed)
Corned Beef (Deli Counter)
Pastrami Coated with Seasonings (Vacuum-Packed)
Roast Beef - Coated with Garlic, Dextrose and Spices (Vacuum-Packed)

Smith's
Smith's (All)

Steak-Eze ◊
Angus Beef Philly Steak
Philly Beef

Thummann's
Meats (All BUT Franks for Deep Frying)

Wellshire Farms ✓
Corned Beef Brisket
Corned Beef Round
Pastrami Brisket
Pastrami Round
Sliced Beef Bacon
Sliced Beef Bologna
Sliced Beef Pastrami
Sliced Beef Salami
Sliced Corned Beef Round
Sliced Top Round Roast Beef
Whole Corned Beef Brisket
Whole Roast Beef

BOLOGNA

Applegate Farms ⓘ
Applegate Farms (All BUT Chicken Nuggets, Chicken Pot Pie, & Chicken Strips)

Boar's Head
Meats (All)

Cloverdale Foods
Meat Products (All)

Empire Kosher
Chicken Bologna - Slices
Turkey Bologna - Slices

Turkey Bologna Roll

Great Value (Wal-Mart)
Luncheon Meat

Hy-Vee
Beef Bologna
Bologna
Garlic Bologna
German Brand Bologna
Thick Bologna
Thin Bologna
Turkey Bologna

Midwest Country Fare (Hy-Vee)
Sliced Bologna
Thick Sliced Bologna

Nature's Promise (Giant)
Deli Meats (All Varieties)

Nature's Promise (Stop & Shop)
Deli Meats (All Varieties)

Old Wisconsin ⓘ
Old Wisconsin (All BUT Beef Jerky
Products)

Oscar Mayer ⌒
50% Less Fat Turkey Bologna
98% Fat Free Bologna
Beef Bologna
Beef Light Bologna
Bologna
Cheese Bologna
Light Bologna
Turkey Bologna

Perdue ⓘ
Deli Turkey Bologna

Plainville Farms
Plainville Farms (All BUT dressing,
turkey and cranberry relish)

Publix ()
Beef Bologna (Pre-Packed Sliced Deli
Lunch Meats)
German Bologna (Pre-Packed Sliced
Deli Lunch Meats)

Smith's
Smith's (All)

Wellshire Farms ✓
Sliced Turkey Bologna

CHICKEN

Applegate Farms ⓘ
Applegate Farms (All BUT Chicken
Nuggets, Chicken Pot Pie, & Chicken
Strips)

Bell & Evans ⓘ ✓
Fresh Chicken

Boar's Head
Meats (All)

Buddig
Buddig Fix Quix (All)
Deli Cuts - Rotisserie Chicken
Original Buddig - Chicken

Butcher's Cut (Safeway)
Boneless Skinless Chicken Breast
Young Chicken Thighs

Coleman Natural ✓
Bone-in Skin-on Chicken Thigh
Boneless Skinless Chicken Breast
Boneless Skinless Chicken Thigh
Chicken Breast Tenders
Drummettes
Drumsticks
Fresh for the Freezer Chicken
Split Breast
Whole Chicken
Wings

Coleman Organic ✓
Bone-in Skin-on Chicken Thigh
Boneless Skinless Chicken Breast
Boneless Skinless Chicken Thigh
Chicken Breast Tenders
Drummettes
Drumsticks
Fresh for the Freezer Chicken
Split Breast
Whole Chicken
Wings

Empire Kosher
Fresh Chill Pack Chicken & Turkey
Fresh Rotisserie Chicken
Fully Cooked Barbecue Chicken (Fresh
Or Frozen)

Fast Classics ⓘ
Buffalo Wings
Fire Roasted Chicken Breast

Honey BBQ Chicken Wings
Tomato Basil Chicken Breast

Fast Fixin' ()
Breakaway Chicken SteakEze
Grilled Chicken Breast
Grilled Chicken Breast - Fajita
Grilled Chicken Breast - Mesquite
Restaurant Style - Buffalo Wings
Restaurant Style - Italian Chicken Slices
Restaurant Style - Southwestern
  Chicken Slices

Great Value (Wal-Mart)
100% Natural Boneless Skinless Chicken
  Breasts
Boneless Skinless Chicken Breast Fillets
Chicken Drumsticks
Chicken Thighs
Chicken Wing Drumettes
Chicken Wing Sections
Luncheon Meat

Homestyle Meals
Shredded Chicken in BBQ Sauce

Hormel
Natural Choice - Grilled Chicken Strips
Natural Choice - Oven Roasted Chicken
  Strips

Hy-Vee
Boneless Skinless Chicken Thighs
  Flavored For Fajitas
Buffalo Style Flavored Chicken Wings
Herb Garlic Flavored Chicken Breasts
  with Rib Meat
Lemon Butter Flavored Chicken Breasts
  with Rib Meat
Thin Sliced Chicken

Jennie-O Turkey Store
Deli Chicken Breast - Buffalo Style
Deli Chicken Breast - Mesquite Smoked
Deli Chicken Breast - Oven Roasted

Land O' Frost
Lunchmeats (All BUT Taste Escapes
  Lemon Pepper Chicken)

Meijer
Chicken Slice Chipped Meat

Nature's Promise (Giant)
Deli Meats (All Varieties)

Oscar Mayer 〰
Chicken Strips & Cuts - Honey Roasted
  Chicken Breast Cuts
Chicken Strips & Cuts - Honey Roasted
  Chicken Breast Strips
Chicken Strips & Cuts - Oven Roasted
  Chicken Breast Cuts
Chicken Strips & Cuts - Oven Roasted
  Chicken Breast Strips
Deli Fresh Meats - Chicken Breast Oven
  Roasted
Deli Fresh Meats - Chicken Breast Oven
  Roasted Thin Sliced
Deli Fresh Meats - Chicken Breast
  Rotisserie Style Shaved
White Chicken Oven Roasted

Perdue ⓘ
Carving - Chicken Breast, Oven Roasted
Grilled Chicken Breast Strips - All
  Natural
Ground Breast of Chicken
Ground Chicken
Ground Chicken Burgers
Perfect Portions Boneless Skinless
  Chicken Breasts - All Natural
Perfect Portions Boneless Skinless
  Chicken Breasts - Herb & Pepper
Perfect Portions Boneless Skinless
  Chicken Breasts - Italian Style
Perfect Portions Boneless Skinless
  Chicken Breasts - Roasted Garlic with
  White Wine
Rotisserie Chicken - Barbecue
Rotisserie Chicken - Italian
Rotisserie Chicken - Lemon Pepper
Rotisserie Chicken - Oven Roasted
Rotisserie Chicken - Toasted Garlic
Rotisserie Chicken - Tuscany Herb
  Roasted
Rotisserie Oven Stuffer Roaster
Rotisserie Oven Stuffer Roaster Breast
Sauce N Toss Buffalo Style Chicken
  Wings
Sauce N Toss Honey BBQ Chicken
  Wings
Seasoned Oven Ready Roaster

Short Cuts Carved Chicken Breast - Grilled Southwestern Style

Short Cuts Carved Chicken Breast - Honey Roasted

Short Cuts Carved Chicken Breast - Original Roasted

Tender & Tasty Products

Pilgrim's Pride

Buffalo Wings - Fully Cooked

Chicken - Marinated (Chill Pack in A Tray)

Marinated Italian Chicken Breasts (Chill Pack in Tray)

Marinated Lemon-Pepper Chicken Breasts (Chill Pack in Tray)

Primo Taglio (Safeway)

Chicken Breast (Oven Roasted) Browned in Hot Cottonseed Oil (Bulk Deli Meat)

Publix ()

Apple Wood Smoked Rotisserie Chicken (Deli)

Barbecue Flavored with Barbecue Seasoning and Sauce Rotisserie Chicken (Deli)

Barbecue Flavored with Barbecue Seasoning Rotisserie Chicken (Deli)

Lemon Pepper Flavored with Lemon & Herb Seasoning Rotisserie Chicken (Deli)

Original Roasted Rotisserie Chicken (Deli)

Safeway

Deli Roasted Chicken (Deli Counter)

Steak-Eze ()

Fastcut Chicken

Thummann's

Meats (All BUT Franks for Deep Frying)

Ukrop's

Kitchen Entrees - Grilled Chicken Breast (Deli)

Kitchen Entrees - Grilled Chicken Breast with Honey BBQ Sauce (Deli)

Kitchen Entrees - Grilled Chicken Breast with Lemon Sauce (Deli)

Kitchen Entrees - Italian Chicken Breast (Deli)

Kitchen Entrees - Jamaican Jerk Chicken Breast (Deli)

Kitchen Entrees - Jamaican Jerk Chicken Breast with Caribbean Rice (Deli)

Kitchen Entrees - Parmesan Chicken Tenders (Deli)

Kitchen Entrees - Rotisserie Chicken (Deli)

Wellshire Farms ✓

Organic Chicken Franks

Sliced Oven Roasted Chicken Breast

HAM & PROSCIUTTO

Applegate Farms ⓘ

Applegate Farms (All BUT Chicken Nuggets, Chicken Pot Pie, & Chicken Strips)

Boar's Head

Meats (All)

Buddig ♺

Deli Cuts - Brown Sugar Ham

Deli Cuts - Honey Ham

Deli Cuts - Smoked Ham

Original Buddig - Ham with Natural Juices

Original Buddig - Honey Ham with Natural Juices

Butcher's Cut (Safeway)

Cooked Ham - 95% Fat Free

Shank Cut Ham

Spiral Sliced Ham (Glaze packet is NOT GF)

Cloverdale Foods

Meat Products (All)

Columbus Salame

Columbus Products (All)

Garrett County Farms

Black Forest Boneless Ham Nugget

Black Forest Deli Ham

Sliced Black Forest Ham

Sliced Breakfast Ham

Sliced Turkey Ham

Sliced Turkey Ham Steak

Sliced Virginia Brand Boneless Ham Steak

Sliced Virginia Brand Deli Ham

Virginia Deli Ham

Giant
Cooked Ham - 97% Fat Free

Great Value (Wal-Mart)
97% Fat Free Baked Ham
97% Fat Free Cooked Ham
97% Fat Free Honey Ham
Luncheon Meat
Sliced Chopped Ham
Sliced Turkey Ham
Thinly Sliced Smoked Ham
Thinly Sliced Smoked Honey Ham

Hormel
Black Label - Chopped Ham
Cure 81 - Bone-In Ham
Cure 81 - Boneless Ham
Cure 81 - Old Fashioned Spiral Ham
Deli Sliced Black Forest Ham
Deli Sliced Cooked Ham
Deli Sliced Double Smoked Ham
Deli Sliced Honey Ham
Deli Sliced Prosciutto Ham
Diced Ham
Ham Patties
Julienne Ham
Luncheon Meat
Natural Choice - Cooked Deli Ham
Natural Choice - Honey Deli Ham
Natural Choice - Smoked Deli Ham

Hy-Vee
96% Sliced Cooked Ham
Brown Sugar Spiral Sliced Ham
Chopped Ham
Cooked Ham
Deli Thin Slices - Honey Ham
Deli Thin Slices - Smoked Ham
Honey & Spice Spiral Sliced Ham
Thin Sliced Ham with Natural Juices
Thin Sliced Honey Ham with Natural
    Juices

Isaly's ()
Deli Meats (All)

Jennie-O Turkey Store
Refrigerated Honey Cured Turkey Ham
Refrigerated Turkey Ham

Jones Dairy Farm ⚱
Country Carved Honey & Brown Sugar
    Cured Ham Slices
Farm Fresh & Tender Ham Slices
Farm Fresh & Tender Ham Steak
Farm Fresh & Tender Hams

Krakus
Ham (All)

Land O' Frost
Lunchmeats (All BUT Taste Escapes
    Lemon Pepper Chicken)

Meijer
Double Smoked Ham
Ham Sliced Chipped Meats
Honey Ham - 97% Fat Free
Honey Roasted Ham
Sliced Cooked Ham - 97% Fat Free

Nature's Promise (Giant)
Deli Meats (All Varieties)

Nature's Promise (Stop & Shop)
Deli Meats (All Varieties)

Oscar Mayer ᕬ
Baked Ham
Boiled Ham
Chopped Ham
Chopped Honey Ham
Chopped with Smoke Flavor Ham
Deli Fresh Meats - Black Forest Shaved
    Tray
Deli Fresh Meats - Cracked Black
    Peppered Shaved Tray
Deli Fresh Meats - Ham Brown Sugar
    Shaved
Deli Fresh Meats - Ham Brown Sugar
    Thin Sliced
Deli Fresh Meats - Ham Cooked
Deli Fresh Meats - Ham Cooked 96%
    Fat Free
Deli Fresh Meats - Ham Honey Shaved
Deli Fresh Meats - Ham Smoked 97%
    Fat Free Thin Sliced
Deli Fresh Meats - Ham Smoked Shaved
Deli Fresh Meats - Ham Virginia Brand
    Shaved
Deli Thin Honey Ham
Honey 96% Fat Free Ham
Honey Ham

Natural Smoked Ham
Smoked 96% Fat Free Ham

Patrick Cudahy
Patrick Cudahy (All)

Perdue ⓘ
Carving - Turkey Ham, Honey Smoked
Deli Turkey Ham - Hickory Smoked
Slicing - Turkey Ham

Plainville Farms
Plainville Farms (All BUT dressing,
turkey and cranberry relish)

Plumrose ✓
Plumrose (All)

Primo Taglio (Safeway)
Black Forest Ham with Natural Juices
(Bulk Deli Meat)
Maple Ham (Old Fashioned) with
Natural Juices (Bulk Deli Meat)
Prosciutto Dry Cured Ham (Bulk Deli
Meat)

Publix ⟨⟩
Cooked Ham (Pre-Packed Sliced Deli
Lunch Meats)
Extra Thin Sliced Honey Ham (Pre-
Packed Sliced Deli Lunch Meats)
Hickory Smoked Ham - Semi-Boneless,
Fully Cooked
Honey Cured Bone-In Ham - Brown
Sugar Glazed
Honey Cured Bone-In Ham with Brown
Sugar Glaze Mix Packet
Honey Kut Ham (Pre-Packed Sliced Deli
Lunch Meats)
Low Salt Ham (Pre-Packed Sliced Deli
Lunch Meats)
Sweet Ham (Pre-Packed Sliced Deli
Lunch Meats)
Tavern Ham (Pre-Packed Sliced Deli
Lunch Meats)
Virginia Brand Ham (Pre-Packed Sliced
Deli Lunch Meats)

Saag's ⓘ ✓
Saag's Specialty Meats (All BUT Saag's
British Bangers)

Safeway
Black Forest Ham with Natural Juices
(Vacuum-Packed)

Old Fashioned Maple Ham with Natural
Juices (Vacuum-Packed)
Prosciutto Dry Cured Ham (Vacuum-
Packed)

Smith's
Smith's (All)

Stop & Shop
Cooked Ham - 97% Fat Free
Cooked Ham with Natural Juices - 98%
Fat Free
Danish Brand Ham with Natural Juices -
97% Fat Free

Thummann's
Meats (All BUT Franks for Deep Frying)

Ukrop's
Kitchen Entrees - Spiral Sliced Ham
(Deli)

Wellshire Farms ✓
Black Forest Boneless Half Ham
Black Forest Boneless Ham Nugget
Black Forest Deli Ham
Black Forest Quarter Ham
Glazed Boneless Half Ham
Old Fashioned Traditional Boneless Half
Ham
Old Fashioned Traditional Boneless
Whole Ham
Semi Boneless Half Ham
Sliced Breakfast Ham
Sliced Tavern Ham
Sliced Turkey Ham
Sliced Virginia Brand Ham
Smoked Ham Hocks
Smoked Ham Shanks
Spiral Sliced Glazed Boneless Half Ham
Spiral Sliced Glazed Boneless Whole
Ham
Turkey Ham Nuggets
Turkey Ham Steak
Virginia Brand Boneless Ham Steak
Virginia Brand Buffet Ham
Virginia Brand Deli Ham
Virginia Brand Honey Ham Nugget

Winn-Dixie ⓘ
Premium Ham

Hot Dogs & Franks

Applegate Farms ⓘ
  Applegate Farms (All BUT Chicken Nuggets, Chicken Pot Pie, & Chicken Strips)

Butcher's Cut (Safeway)
  Jumbo Franks (includes Chicken & Pork)
  Jumbo Turkey Franks

Cloverdale Foods
  Meat Products (All)

Coleman Natural ✓
  Beef Hot Dog
  Beef-Pork Frank

Empire Kosher
  Turkey Franks

Garrett County Farms
  4XL Big Beef Franks
  Chicken Franks
  Old Fashioned Beef Franks
  Original Deli Frank
  Premium Beef Frank
  Turkey Franks

Jennie-O Turkey Store
  Turkey Franks

Midwest Country Fare (Hy-Vee)
  Bun Length Hot Dogs
  Cheezy Jumbo Hot Dogs
  Hot Dogs
  Jumbo Hot Dogs

Oscar Mayer ⌇
  98% Fat Free Wieners
  Beef & Cheddar Premium Franks
  Beef Smokies Sausage
  Bun Length Turkey Hot Dogs
  Bun-Length Beef Franks
  Bun-Length Wieners
  Hot And Spicy XXL Hot Dogs
  Jalapeno & Cheddar Premium Franks
  Jumbo Beef Franks
  Jumbo Wieners
  Light Beef Franks
  Light Wieners
  Mini Beef Hot Dogs
  Premium Beef XXL Hot Dogs
  Regular Beef Franks
  Regular Wieners
  Smoked XXL Hot Dogs
  The Cheesiest Cheese Dogs
  Turkey Cheese Dogs
  Turkey Franks
  Turkey Hot Dogs
  Wieners

Publix ◇
  Beef Franks
  Beef Hot Dogs
  Meat Franks
  Meat Hot Dogs

Rocky Dogs ✓
  Chicken Hot Dogs

Saag's ⓘ ✓
  Saag's Specialty Meats (All BUT Saag's British Bangers)

Sabrett
  All Beef Frankfurters
  Pork & Beef Frankfurters

Safeway
  Jumbo Beef Franks
  Select - Beef Franks

Smith's
  Smith's (All)

Thummann's
  Meats (All BUT Franks for Deep Frying)

Wellshire Farms ✓
  4XL Big Beef Franks
  Cheese Frank
  Cocktail Franks
  Old Fashioned Beef Franks
  Organic Chicken Franks
  Organic Turkey Franks
  Original Deli Frank
  Premium Beef Franks
  Turkey Franks

Winn-Dixie ⓘ
  Jumbo Meat Franks

Meat Alternatives

El Burrito
  Soy Breakfast Sausage
  Soy Pepperoni Crumbles
  Soyground
  Soyrizo

Soytaco

Lightlife ()
Tofu Pups

Pepperoni

Boar's Head
Meats (All)

Garrett County Farms
Sliced Uncured Pepperoni

Hormel
Pepperoni
Pillow Pack - Pepperoni
Pillow Pack - Turkey Pepperoni

Hy-Vee
Pepperoni

Patrick Cudahy
Patrick Cudahy (All)

Primo Naturale
Pepperoni Stick
Whole Large Diameter Pepperoni

Pork

Cloverdale Foods
Meat Products (All)

Coleman Natural ✓
Hampshire Pork Baby Back Ribs
Hampshire Pork Chops
Hampshire Pork Loin
Hampshire Pork St. Louis Ribs
Hampshire Pork Tenderloins

Columbus Salame
Columbus Products (All)

Ejay's
All Natural Salt Port

Fast Fixin' ()
Ribz For Sandwiches

Great Value (Wal-Mart)
Luncheon Meat

Homestyle Meals
Pork Baby Back Ribs with BBQ Sauce
Shredded Pork in BBQ Sauce
Whole Bulk St. Louis Ribs with BBQ Sauce

Hormel
Always Tender - Adobo Pork Cubes Flavored Fresh Pork
Always Tender - Citrus Flavored Fresh Pork
Always Tender - Fajita Pork Strips Flavored Fresh Pork
Always Tender - Lemon-Garlic Flavored Fresh Pork
Always Tender - Mesquite Flavored Fresh Pork
Always Tender - Mojo Criollo Flavored Fresh Pork
Always Tender - Onion-Garlic Flavored Fresh Pork
Always Tender - Original Flavored Fresh Pork
Always Tender - Portabella Mushroom Flavored Fresh Pork
Always Tender - Roast Flavored Fresh Pork
Always Tender - Sun-Dried Tomato Flavored Fresh Pork

Plumrose ✓
Plumrose (All)

Primo Naturale
Sliced Sopressata
Sopressata
Whole Sopressata

Primo Taglio (Safeway)
Mortadella - Black Pepper Added (Bulk Deli Meat)
Sopressata (Bulk Deli Meat)

Publix GreenWise Market ()
Cajun Pork Sausage

Publix ()
Spanish Style Pork (Pre-Packed Sliced Deli Lunch Meats)

Safeway
Mortadella - Pistachio Nuts and Black Pepper Added (Vacuum-Packed)
Select - Signature Ribs St. Louis Style Smoke House
Sopressata (Vacuum-Packed)

Smith's
Smith's (All)

Ukrop's
    Kitchen Entrees - Roasted Pork Loin
    (Deli)
    Kitchen Entrees - Southern Style Pork
    BBQ (Deli)
    Kitchen Entrees - Virginia Pork BBQ
    (Deli)
Wellshire Farms ✓
    Organic Pork Andouille

Salami

Boar's Head
    Meats (All)
Columbus Salame
    Columbus Products (All)
Empire Kosher
    Turkey Salami - Slices
    Turkey Salami Roll
Hormel
    Homeland - Hard Salami
    Pillow Pack - Hard Salami
Hy-Vee
    Cooked Salami
Midwest Country Fare (Hy-Vee)
    Sliced Cooked Salami
Old Wisconsin ⓘ
    Old Wisconsin (All BUT Beef Jerky
    Products)
Oscar Mayer ✐
    50% Less Fat Turkey Cotto Salami
    Cotto Salami
    Hard Salami
    Salami Beef Deli Thin
    Turkey Cotto Salami
Perdue ⓘ
    Deli Turkey Salami
Primo Naturale
    Chubb Genoa Salami
    Chubb Salami Original
    Chubb Salami with Black Pepper
    Chubb Salami with Herbs
    Sliced Hard Salami
    Sliced Original Salami
    Sliced Premium Genoa Salami
    Sliced Salami with Herbs

    Whole Black Pepper Salami
    Whole Genoa Salami
    Whole Hard Salami
    Whole Herb and Wine Salami
    Whole Original Salami
Primo Taglio (Safeway)
    Cervelat Salami (Bulk Deli Meat)
    Genoa Salami (Bulk Deli Meat)
    Salami (Peppered) Coated with Gelatin
    & Black Pepper (Bulk Deli Meat)
Publix ◊
    Hard Salami - Reduced Fat (Pre-Packed
    Sliced Deli Lunch Meats)
Saag's ⓘ ✓
    Saag's Specialty Meats (All BUT Saag's
    British Bangers)
Safeway
    Genoa Salami (Deli Counter)
    Genoa Salami (Vacuum-Packed)
    Hard Salami (Deli Counter)
    Peppered Salami - Coated with Black
    Pepper and Gelatin (Vacuum-Packed)
Smith's
    Smith's (All)
Thummann's
    Meats (All BUT Franks for Deep Frying)

Sausage

Applegate Farms ⓘ
    Applegate Farms (All BUT Chicken
    Nuggets, Chicken Pot Pie, & Chicken
    Strips)
Boar's Head
    Meats (All)
Bob Evans ◊
    Bratwurst (All BUT Beer Brats)
    Kielbasa
    Sausage (All)
    Smoked Sausage
Butcher's Cut (Safeway)
    Bratwurst
    Italian Sausage - Mild
    Italian Sausage - Regular
    Polska Kielbasa
    Smoked Sausage

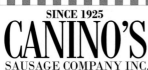

SINCE 1925

CANINO'S
SAUSAGE COMPANY INC.

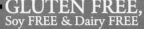

— QUICK FACTS —

- **GLUTEN FREE,** Soy FREE & Dairy FREE
- Contains NO MSG, Nitrates, Preservatives, or Artificial Colors
- Contains ALL NATURAL ingredients
- ALL PRODUCTS made with ONLY the finest ground pork
- LESS FAT than the USDA recommended amount
- Colorado Company since 1925

Canino's Sausage Company
Bratwurst
Breakfast Sausage
German Brand Sausage
Hot Italian
Hot! Chorizo
Mild Italian
Polish Sausage
Spicy Cajun Style Sausage
Sweet Italian Sausage

Cloverdale Foods
Meat Products (All)

Coleman Natural
Bratwurst
Polish Kielbasa

Coleman Organic
Apple Chicken Sausage
Mild Italian Chicken Sausage
Spinach & Feta Chicken Sausage
Sun-Dried Tomato & Basil Chicken Sausage

Garrett County Farms
Andouille Sausage

Chorizo Sausage
Polska Kielbasa
Turkey Andouille
Turkey Kielbasa

Great Value (Wal-Mart)
Fully Cooked Beef Breakfast Patties
Fully Cooked Maple Pork Sausage Patties
Fully Cooked Original Pork Sausage Patties
Fully Cooked Sausage Links
Fully Cooked Spicy Pork Sausage Patties
Hot Pork Sausage
Mild Pork Sausage
Sage Pork Sausage

Hans All Natural
Chipotle Pepper Chicken Sausage
Mild Italian Chicken Sausage
Organic Breakfast Links Chicken Sausage
Skinless Chicken Breakfast Links
Spicy Andouille Chicken Sausage
Spicy Chorizo Chicken Sausage
Spinach & Feta Cheese Chicken Sausage
Spinach, Fontina & Garlic Chicken Sausage
Sun-Dried Tomato & Basil Chicken Sausage
Sun-Dried Tomato Provolone Chicken Sausage
Sweet Apple Chicken Sausage

Hormel
Crumbled Sausage
Little Sizzlers - Sausage Links & Patties
Smokies

Hy-Vee
Beef Sausage
Beef Summer Sausage
Bratwurst
Bratwurst - Grill Pack
Little Smokies
Polish Sausage Link
Polish Sausage Rope
Sausage Links
Sausage Patties
Smoked Bratwurst
Smoked Sausage

Smoked Sausage with Cheddar Cheese

Jennie-O Turkey Store
Breakfast Lover's Turkey Sausage
Extra Lean Smoked Kielbasa Turkey Sausage
Extra Lean Smoked Turkey Sausage
Fresh Breakfast Sausage - Maple Links
Fresh Breakfast Sausage - Mild Links
Fresh Breakfast Sausage - Mild Patties
Fresh Dinner Sausage - Cheddar Turkey Bratwurst
Fresh Dinner Sausage - Hot Italian
Fresh Dinner Sausage - Lean Turkey Bratwurst
Fresh Dinner Sausage - Sweet Italian
Fully Cooked Frozen Sausage Links & Patties

Johnsonville
Johnsonville (All BUT Beer Brats)

Jones Dairy Farm
Chub Braunschweiger Liverwurst - 20% Bacon
Chub Braunschweiger Liverwurst - Light
Chub Braunschweiger Liverwurst - Original
Chub Braunschweiger Liverwurst with Onion
Chunk Braunschweiger - Light
Chunk Braunschweiger - Original
Sliced Braunschweiger

Krakus
Polish Kielbasa (All)

Nature's Promise (Giant)
Italian Spicy Pork Sausage
Mild Italian Chicken Sausage
Red Pepper and Provolone Pork Sausage
Spiced Apple Chicken Sausage
Spinach and Feta Chicken Sausage
Sun Dried Tomato and Basil Chicken Sausage

Nature's Promise (Stop & Shop)
Italian Spicy Pork Sausage
Mild Italian Chicken Sausage
Red Pepper & Provolone Pork Sausage
Spiced Apple Chicken Sausage
Spinach & Feta Chicken Sausage

Sun Dried Tomato & Basil Chicken Sausage

Old Wisconsin ⓘ
Old Wisconsin (All BUT Beef Jerky Products)

Oscar Mayer ⌇
Beef Summer Sausage
Little Smokies
Sausage Smokies Sausage
Summer Sausage

Patrick Cudahy
Patrick Cudahy (All)

Perdue ⓘ
Seasoned Fresh Lean Turkey Sausage - Sweet Italian
Turkey Breakfast Sausage

Primo Naturale
Sliced Dried Chorizo
Stick Dried Chorizo
Whole Chorizo

Publix GreenWise Market ⟨⟩
Chicken Sausage - Herb & Tomato
Chicken Sausage - Hot Italian
Chicken Sausage - Mild Italian
Pork Sage Sausage
Romano Pork Sausage

Publix ⟨⟩
Fresh Bratwurst
Fresh Chorizo
Fresh Italian - Hot
Fresh Italian - Mild
Fresh Turkey Italian - Hot
Fresh Turkey Italian - Mild

Saag's ⓘ ✔
Saag's Specialty Meats (All BUT Saag's British Bangers)

Sabrett
Hot Sausage
Italian Sausage

Safeway
Select - Sausage, Beef Hot Link
Select - Sausage, Beef Smoked
Select - Sausage, Cajun Style Link
Select - Sausage, Chicken Andouille
Select - Sausage, Chicken Apple
Select - Sausage, Italian
Select - Sausage, Italian Pork

Select - Sausage, Polish
Select - Sausage, Turkey Chicken
  Parmesan Basil
Select - Sausage, Turkey Chicken Sun
  Dried Tomato

Smith's
Smith's (All)

Thummann's
Meats (All BUT Franks for Deep Frying)

Villa Roma
Villa Roma (All)

Wellshire Farms ✓
Mild Italian Style Turkey Dinner Link
  Sausage
Morning Maple Turkey Breakfast Link
  Sausage
Organic Polska Kielbasa
Organic Turkey Andouille
Organic Turkey Kielbasa
Polska Kielbasa
Pork Andouille Sausage
Pork Chorizo Sausage
Pork Linguica Sausage
Pork Liverwurst
Smoked Bratwurst
Turkey Andouille Sausage
Turkey Kielbasa
Turkey Liverwurst

Winn-Dixie ⓘ
Turkey Smoke Sausage

SEAFOOD

Aqua Star
Cooked Seasoned Shrimp
Crab (All Natural & Plain)
Fish (All Natural & Plain)
Marinated Fish (All BUT Teriyaki
  Salmon)
Marinated Shrimp
Parmesan Shrimp Scampi
Shrimp (All Natural & Plain)
Shrimp Rings with Cocktail Sauce

Captains Choice (Safeway)
Cod Fillets
Cooked Tail On Shrimp

Great Value (Wal-Mart)
Alaskan Pink Salmon

Wild Planet ⚥
Albacore (All)
Salmon (All)
Shrimp (All)

TOFU & TEMPEH

Azumaya
Tofu (All)

Giant
Tofu - Extra Firm
Tofu - Firm

House Foods
Tofu (All BUT Agedashi Tofu)

Lightlife ()
Organic Flax Tempeh
Organic Soy Tempeh
Organic Veggie Tempeh
Organic Wild Rice Tempeh

Mori-Nu
Organic Silken Tofu
Silken Extra Firm Tofu
Silken Firm Tofu
Silken Lite Firm Tofu
Silken Soft Tofu

Nasoya
Extra Firm Tofu
Firm Tofu
Lite Firm Tofu
Lite Silken Tofu
Silken Tofu
Soft Tofu
Super Firm Cubed

Stop & Shop
Tofu - Extra Firm
Tofu - Firm

Sunergia ()
More Than Tofu Line (All)
Nufu Line (All)

Turtle Island Foods
Organic Five-Grain Tempeh
Original Soy Tempeh
Spicy Veggie Tempeh

Vitasoy
- Firm Tofu
- Regular Tofu
- Silken Tofu

WestSoy ✔
- Vacuum Packed Extra Firm
- Vacuum Packed Firm Reduced Fat
- Water Packed Firm Organic
- Water Packed Soft Organic

TURKEY

Applegate Farms ⓘ
- Applegate Farms (All BUT Chicken Nuggets, Chicken Pot Pie, & Chicken Strips)

Boar's Head
- Meats (All)

Buddig ⚇
- Deli Cuts - Honey-Roasted Turkey
- Deli Cuts - Oven-Roasted Turkey
- Deli Cuts - Smoked Turkey
- Original Buddig - Honey-Roasted Turkey
- Original Buddig - Oven-Roasted Turkey
- Original Buddig - Turkey

Butcher's Cut (Safeway)
- Ground Turkey
- Oven Roasted Turkey Breast - 98% Fat Free & Regular

Columbus Salame
- Columbus Products (All)

Empire Kosher
- Fresh Ground Turkey
- Fully Cooked Barbecue Turkey (Fresh Or Frozen)
- Honey Smoked Turkey Breast-Skinless
- Preferred - Signature Edition Smoked Turkey Breast, Skinless
- Preferred - Signature Edition Turkey Breast Pastrami, Skinless
- Preferred - Signature Edition Turkey Pastrami, Skinless
- Premier - Signature Edition All Natural Turkey Breast Skinless
- Premier - Signature Edition All Natural Turkey Breast with Skin

- Signature Edition - Oven Prepared Turkey Breast
- Signature Edition - Smoked Turkey Breast
- Smoked Turkey Breast - Slices
- Turkey Breast - Slices
- Turkey Pastrami - Slices
- White Turkey Roll

Garrett County Farms
- Pan Roasted Turkey Breast
- Sliced Roasted Turkey Breast
- Sliced Smoked Turkey Breast
- Smoked Turkey Breast

Giant
- Honey Turkey Breast - 97% Fat Free
- Oven Roasted Turkey Breast - 97% Fat Free
- Smoked Turkey Breast

Great Value (Wal-Mart)
- Fat Free Turkey Breast
- Luncheon Meat
- Sliced Fat Free Smoked Turkey Breast
- Sliced Fat Free Turkey Breast
- Sliced Honey Turkey Breast
- Thinly Sliced Oven Roasted Turkey Breast
- Thinly Sliced Smoked Turkey Breast

Hormel
- Deli Sliced Oven Roasted Turkey Breast
- Deli Sliced Smoked Turkey Breast
- Julienne Turkey
- Natural Choice - Honey Deli Turkey
- Natural Choice - Oven Roasted Deli Turkey
- Natural Choice - Smoked Deli Turkey

Hy-Vee
- All Natural Fresh Turkey
- All Natural Frozen Turkey
- Butter Basted Turkey
- Deli Thin Slices - Honey Roasted Turkey Breast
- Deli Thin Slices - Oven Roasted Turkey Breast
- Moisture Enhanced Fresh Turkey
- Moisture Enhanced Frozen Turkey
- Thin Sliced Honey Turkey
- Thin Sliced Turkey

Ingles Markets
Best Turkey Deli Meat
Honey Roasted Breast
Mesquite Smoked Breast
Roasted Breast

Isaly's ()
Deli Meats (All)

Jennie-O Turkey Store
Festive Tender Cured Turkey
Flavored Tenderloins - Applewood Smoked
Flavored Tenderloins - Lemon-Garlic
Flavored Tenderloins - Roast Flavor
Flavored Tenderloins - Seasoned Pepper
Flavored Tenderloins - Tequila Lime
Flavored Tenderloins - Tomato Basil
Fresh Ground Turkey - Extra Lean
Fresh Ground Turkey - Italian
Fresh Ground Turkey - Lean
Fresh Ground Turkey - Taco Seasoned
Fresh Lean Turkey Patties
Fresh Tray - Breast Slices
Fresh Tray - Breast Strips
Fresh Tray - Tenderloins
Grand Champion - Hickory Smoked Turkey Breast (Deli)
Grand Champion - Homestyle Pan Roasted Turkey Breast (Deli)
Grand Champion - Honey Cured Turkey Breast (Deli)
Grand Champion - Mesquite Smoked Turkey Breast (Deli)
Grand Champion - Oven Roasted Turkey Breast (Deli)
Grand Champion - Tender Browned Turkey Breast (Deli)
Hickory Smoked Turkey Breast - Garlic Pesto (Deli)
Hickory Smoked Turkey Breast - Honey Cured (Deli)
Hickory Smoked Turkey Breast - Sun Dried Tomato (Deli)
Hickory Smoked Turkey Breast- Cracked Pepper (Deli)
Natural Choice - Oven Roasted Turkey Breast (Deli)
Natural Choice - Peppered Turkey Breast (Deli)
Natural Choice - Tender Browned Turkey Breast (Deli)
Oven Ready Turkey - Garlic & Herb
Oven Ready Turkey - Homestyle
Oven Ready Turkey Breast (Gravy packet NOT GF)
Oven Roasted Turkey Breast (Deli)
Pan Roasts with Gravy - White & White/Dark Combo
Prime Young Turkey - Fresh (Gravy packet NOT GF)
Refrigerated Dark Turkey Pastrami
Refrigerated Qtr Turkey Breasts - Cajun-Style
Refrigerated Qtr Turkey Breasts - Cracked Pepper
Refrigerated Qtr Turkey Breasts - Hickory Smoked
Refrigerated Qtr Turkey Breasts - Honey Cured
Refrigerated Qtr Turkey Breasts - Oven Roasted
Refrigerated Qtr Turkey Breasts - Sun-Dried Tomato
Smoked Turkey Breast - Hickory (Deli)
Smoked Turkey Breast - Honey Cured (Deli)
Smoked Turkey Breast - Mesquite (Deli)
Smoked Turkey Wings & Drumsticks
So Easy - Slow Roasted Turkey Breast
Turkey Breast - Apple Cinnamon (Deli)
Turkey Breast - Garlic Peppered (Deli)
Turkey Breast - Honey Maple (Deli)
Turkey Breast - Honey Mesquite (Deli)
Turkey Breast - Hot Red Peppered (Deli)
Turkey Breast - Italian Style (Deli)
Turkey Breast - Maple Spiced (Deli)
Turkey Breast - Mesquite Smoked (Deli)
Turkey Breast - Peppered (Deli)
Turkey Breast - Smoked (Deli)
Turkey Breast - Smoked Peppered (Deli)
Turkey Breast - Tender Browned (Deli)
Turkey Breast - Tomato Basil (Deli)

Land O' Frost
Lunchmeats (All BUT Taste Escapes Lemon Pepper Chicken)

Meijer
Fresh Hen Turkey
Fresh Tom Turkey
Fresh Turkey Breast
Gold - Hen Turkey
Gold - Tom Turkey
Hen Turkey
Hickory Smoked Turkey Breast
Honey Roasted Turkey Breast
Tom Turkey
Turkey Basted with Timer
Turkey Breast Fresh
Turkey Breast Zipper 97% Fat Free
Turkey Fresh Natural
Turkey Sliced Chipped Meat

Nature's Promise (Giant)
Deli Meats (All Varieties)

Nature's Promise (Stop & Shop)
Deli Meats (All Varieties)

Norwestern
Deli Turkey - Hickory Smoked
Deli Turkey - Oven Roasted
Deli Turkey - Turkey Pastrami

Oscar Mayer ↶
Deli Fresh - Turkey Breast Oven Roasted 98% Fat Free
Deli Fresh Meats - Turkey Breast Honey Smoked Shaved
Deli Fresh Meats - Turkey Breast Honey Smoked Thin Sliced
Deli Fresh Meats - Turkey Breast Mesquite Shaved
Deli Fresh Meats - Turkey Breast Mesquite Thin Sliced
Deli Fresh Meats - Turkey Breast Oven Roasted
Deli Fresh Meats - Turkey Breast Oven Roasted Shaved
Deli Fresh Meats - Turkey Breast Oven Roasted Thin Sliced
Deli Fresh Meats Turkey Breast Smoked
Deli Fresh Meats Turkey Breast Smoked Shaved
Deli Fresh Meats Turkey Breast Smoked Thin Sliced
Deli Fresh Meats Turkey Smoked 97% Fat Free
Deli Fresh Singles - Smoked Shaved Turkey Breast
Honey Smoked Lean White Turkey
Oven Roasted White Turkey
Smoked White Turkey
Turkey Breast Hickory Smoked 98% Fat Free
Turkey Breast Honey Roasted/Oven Roasted/Hickory Smoked Variety Pack
Turkey Breast Oven Roasted
Turkey Ham
Turkey Ham - Smoked Chopped 50% Less Fat
Turkey Smoked White 95% Fat Free
Turkey White Smoked

Patrick Cudahy
Patrick Cudahy (All)

Perdue ⓘ
Carving - Turkey Breast, Hickory Smoked
Carving - Turkey Breast, Honey Smoked
Carving - Turkey Breast, Mesquite Smoked
Carving - Turkey Breast, Oven Roasted
Carving - Whole Turkey
Carving Classics - Pan Roasted Turkey Breast, Cracked Pepper
Carving Classics - Turkey Breast Pan Roasted
Carving Classics - Turkey Breast Pan Roasted, Honey Smoked
Deli Dark Turkey Pastrami - Hickory Smoked
Deli Pick Ups - Sliced Turkey Breast, Golden Browned
Deli Pick Ups - Sliced Turkey Breast, Honey Smoked
Deli Pick Ups - Sliced Turkey Breast, Mesquite Smoked
Deli Pick Ups - Sliced Turkey Breast, Oven Roasted
Deli Pick Ups - Sliced Turkey Breast, Smoked

Deli Pick Ups - Sliced Turkey Ham, Honey Smoked

Deli Turkey Breast - Oil Browned

Fresh Ground Breast of Turkey

Fresh Lean Ground Turkey

Ground Turkey Burgers

Healthsense - Turkey Breast, Oven Roasted (Fat Free, Reduced Sodium)

Rotisserie Turkey Breast

Short Cuts Carved Turkey Breast - Oven Roasted

Whole Turkeys Seasoned with Broth

Plainville Farms

Plainville Farms (All BUT dressing, turkey and cranberry relish)

Plumrose ✔

Plumrose (All)

Primo Taglio (Safeway)

Dinner Roast Turkey Breast (Bulk Deli Meat)

Honey Maple Turkey Breast (Bulk Deli Meat)

Mesquite Smoked Turkey Breast with Natural Mesquite Smoke Flavoring Added (Bulk Deli Meat)

Natural Hickory Smoked Peppered Turkey Breast with Natural Smoke Flavoring (Bulk Deli Meat)

Natural Hickory Smoked Turkey Breast with Natural Smoke Flavoring (Bulk Deli Meat)

Pan Roasted Turkey Breast Browned in Hot Cottonseed Oil (Bulk Deli Meat)

Salsa Seasoned Cooked and Cured Turkey Breast (Bulk Deli Meat)

Publix ()

Extra Thin Sliced Oven Roasted Turkey Breast (Pre-Packed Sliced Deli Lunch Meats)

Extra Thin Sliced Smoked Turkey Breast (Pre-Packed Sliced Deli Lunch Meats)

Fresh Young Turkey - Whole

Fresh Young Turkey Breast

Fully Cooked Smoked Turkey (Whole)

Fully Cooked Smoked Turkey Breast

Fully Cooked Turkey Breast (Deli)

Fully Cooked Turkey, Whole (Deli)

Ground Turkey

Ground Turkey Breast

Smoked Turkey (Pre-Packed Sliced Deli Lunch Meats)

Turkey Breast (Pre-Packed Sliced Deli Lunch Meats)

Saag's ⓘ ✔

Saag's Specialty Meats (All BUT Saag's British Bangers)

Safeway

Cracked Pepper Turkey Breast with Natural Smoke Flavoring (Vacuum-Packed)

Hickory Smoked Turkey Breast with Natural Smoke Flavoring (Vacuum-Packed)

Oven Roasted Turkey Breast (Vacuum-Packed)

Roasted Turkey Breast (Deli Counter)

Stop & Shop

Oven Roasted Turkey Breast - Fat Free

Smoked Turkey Breast

Thummann's

Meats (All BUT Franks for Deep Frying)

Wellshire Farms ✔

Pan Roasted Turkey Breast

Sliced Oven Roasted Turkey Breast

Sliced Smoked Turkey Breast

Smoked Turkey Breast

Whole Turkey Ham

MISCELLANEOUS

Hy-Vee

Ham & Cheese Loaf

Old Fashioned Loaf

Pickle Loaf

Spiced Luncheon Loaf

Midwest Country Fare (Hy-Vee)

Sliced Dutch Brand Loaf

Sliced Pickle Loaf

Oscar Mayer ᏻ

Salami/Bologna/Ham Variety Pack

Publix ()

Olive Loaf (Pre-Packed Sliced Deli Lunch Meats)

Pickle & Pimento Loaf (Pre-Packed
   Sliced Deli Lunch Meats)
Winn-Dixie ⓘ
   Luncheon Meat

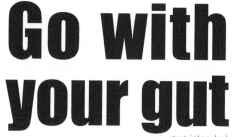

Go with your gut

pun intended

Is your gut telling you something may be wrong with your diet?

When your immune system is activated by incompatible foods it can cause a wide range of symptoms: IBS, migraine headaches, weight issues, joint pain, skin and respiratory problems, ADD/Hyperactivity, fatigue and many more.

Almost 70% of the immune system is in the gut.

There's one simple blood test, scientifically proven, that tells you which foods may be a problem for you.

*According to a study conducted at Baylor University, **98%** of people following The ALCAT Rotation Diet either lost weight or improved body mass.*

Call today or visit us on the web at www.ALCAT.com to request information about getting tested in your area.